Infection, Resistance, and Immunity

Infection, Resistance, and Immunity

Julius P. Kreier
Richard F. Mortensen

The Ohio State University

1817

HARPER & ROW, PUBLISHERS, New York
Grand Rapids, Philadelphia, St. Louis, San Francisco,
London, Singapore, Sydney, Tokyo

Sponsoring Editor: Glyn Davies
Project Editor: Thomas R. Farrell
Art Direction/Cover Coordinator: Heather A. Ziegler
Cover Design: Catherine Cannizzaro
Production: Kewal K. Sharma

INFECTION, RESISTANCE, AND IMMUNITY

Library of Congress Cataloging-in-Publication Data

Kreier, Julius P.
   Infection, resistance, and immunity / Julius P. Kreier, Richard F. Mortensen.
      p.   cm.
   ISBN 0-06-043791-X
   1. Host-parasite relationships.   2. Immunity.   3. Infection.
I. Mortensen, Richard F.   II. Title.
QR99.K74   1990
616.07'9—dc20   89-20001
                                                                      CIP

90 91 92   9 8 7 6 5 4 3 2 1

Contents

7. The Inducible Defense System: Antibody Molecules and Antigen–Antibody Reactions   82

Melanie S. Kennedy and Janice Blazina

8. The Inducible Defense System: The Induction and Development of the Inducible Defense   103

Diane W. Taylor

9. Specific Host Resistance: The Effector Mechanisms   129

13. The Bacteria   204

14. The Viruses   228

Paul J. Cote

18. Disease Transmission, Epidemiology, and Epizootiology 305

William Collins

19. The Immunological System and Neoplasia 318

James R. Blakeslee, Jr.

Contributors

James R. Blakeslee, Jr.
Department of Veterinary Pathobiology
College of Veterinary Medicine
The Ohio State University

Janice Blazina
Department of Pathology
College of Medicine
The Ohio State University

William Collins
Malaria Branch
Division of Parasitic Diseases
Centers for Disease Control

Paul J. Cote
Division of Molecular Virology
    and Immunology
School of Medicine
Georgetown University

Frank Kapral
Department of Medical Microbiology
    and Immunology
College of Medicine
The Ohio State University

Melanie S. Kennedy
Department of Pathology
College of Medicine
The Ohio State University

Susan L. Koletar
Department of Medicine
College of Medicine
The Ohio State University

Charles G. Orosz
Department of Surgery
College of Medicine
The Ohio State University

Michael F. Para
Department of Medicine
College of Medicine
The Ohio State University

John A. Schmitt, Jr.
Department of Botany
The Ohio State University

Diane W. Taylor
Department of Biology
Georgetown University

Caroline C. Whitacre
Department of Medical Microbiology
    and Immunology
College of Medicine
The Ohio State University

Lola Winter
Department of Microbiology,
    Immunology and Parasitology
New York State College of Veterinary
    Medicine
Cornell University

Preface

This text, designed to introduce students to the principles of infection and resistance, was developed as a result of experiences gained through teaching an undergraduate course in introductory immunology and pathogenic microbiology at The Ohio State University. The course was developed over 30 years ago by Dr. Matthew Dodd, late professor of microbiology at The Ohio State University, and has been taught over the years by various professors, we being the most recent. The course attracts large numbers of students, including those majoring in microbiology, nursing, medical and dental technology, and premedical, preveterinary, and predental fields.

The text presents a holistic view of host–parasite interaction and covers parasite invasive strategies, host defense mechanisms (both constitutive and inducible), and host defense evading strategies used by parasites.

The text begins with an introduction to principles of infection and resistance, providing a brief history of the development of microbiology and immunology to acquaint the reader with the origins of the disciplines. It then presents constitutive defense mechanisms, inflammation, and the inducible defenses. The inducible defenses are covered in a series of chapters that deal with antigens, antibodies, antigen antibody reactions, induction and development of the inducible defenses, and the effector mechanisms of the inducible defenses. The section on inducible defenses concludes with chapters on the untoward consequences of the defensive responses, and on graft and transplantation immunology.

The next section of the book deals primarily with the parasite component of the host–parasite system. In particular, it discusses mechanisms of pathogenicity and virulence. In this section selected examples of infectious processes caused by bacteria, viruses, worms, protozoa, and fungi are presented. The role of host responses in pathogenesis of disease is also treated in this section. The book concludes with chapters on immunization, disease transmission, and the immunological system and neoplasia.

In our attempt to provide the student with a holistic view of the interaction of parasites and their hosts and to help students better understand the role of immunity in the broader relationship between parasite and host, we have chosen to present the host component of the host–parasite system before the parasite component.

In the past, we have usually assigned two texts for our course, one on pathogenesis of infectious disease and another on immunology. The result has never been completely satisfactory. Immunology texts, in particular, have been a problem for the beginning student, as they contain too much information and too much detail. We hope that this text, which is written for a one-semester introductory course in infectious disease and immunology, will open up to students the fascinating fields of immunology, infectious disease, human medicine, and veterinary medicine.

Grateful acknowledgment is made to the following reviewers: Carl Henrikson, Towson State University; Edward Hoffman, University of Florida; Robert Kearns, University of Dayton; Lida Mattman, Wayne State University; David Prescott, University of Colorado; Margaret Sullivan, University of Arkansas; and William Wellnitz, Augusta College.

JULIUS P. KREIER
RICHARD F. MORTENSEN

Infection, Resistance, and Immunity

Chapter

1

Principles of Infection and Resistance

THE NATURE OF PARASITES

Parasitism is a life-style that has been adopted by many types of living things. There are parasitic forms among most groups of multicellular plants and animals, among the fungi, and in most groups of unicellular organisms. All viruses are parasites. There are many species of parasites that inhabit the bodies of either plants or animals. Examples of parasitic flowering plants are dodder, indian pipe, and mistletoe. Various species of hookworms, ascarids, and trichinella are common in humans and other animals, and many species of nematode infest the roots of plants. The

1

organism that causes athletes foot is a parasitic fungus. Unicellular protozoa cause malaria and dysentery. A large variety of species of bacteria are parasitic; anthrax, diphtheria, tuberculosis, and brucellosis, for example, are diseases caused by parasitic bacteria (Figure 1.1).

Some of the parasitic organisms cause severe disease, others draw nourishment from their hosts but do little harm, and some benefit the host while benefiting themselves. The obligatorily parasitic viruses may cause severe disease or may be harmless commensals.

The term *parasite* is used with several meanings. In common medical and veterinary terminology it may be used to describe a blood-sucking arthropod, such as a flea or louse; a worm inhabiting the digestive tract, such as a hookworm or tapeworm; or a protozoan such as the amoeba that causes amoebic dysentery. In this usage bacteria and viruses are not included among the parasites, and they are not studied in conventional courses on parasitology. In the usage followed in this book, all organisms living in or on the bodies of other organisms and drawing their sustenance from them are considered to be parasites; thus the group includes bacteria and viruses as well as arthropods, worms, and protozoa.

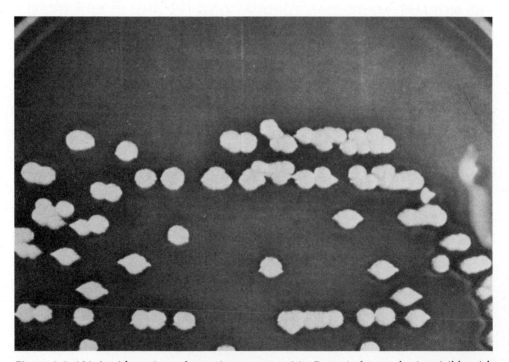

Figure 1.1 (A) A wide variety of organisms are parasitic. Bacteria form colonies visible with the naked eye when streaked on nutrient agar.

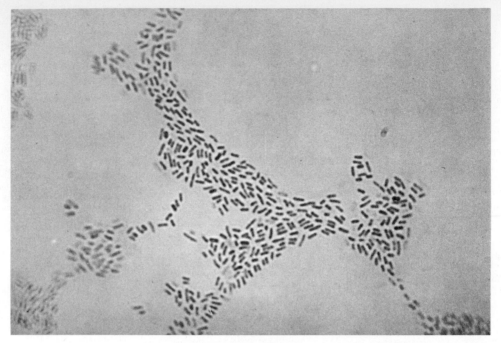

Figure 1.1 (*Continued*) (B) Microscopic examination of bacteria streaked out on a micro-scope slide and stained reveals the individual organisms, in this case bacilli.

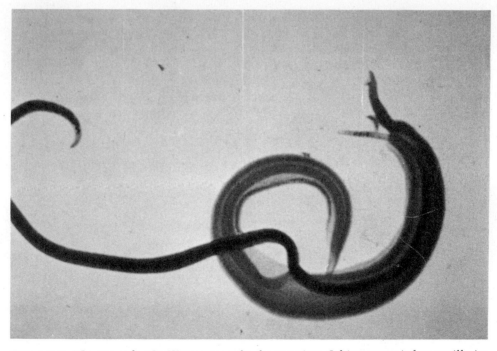

Figure 1.1 (*Continued*) (C) Worms may also be parasites. Schistosomes infect capillaries in the liver and bladder of humans.

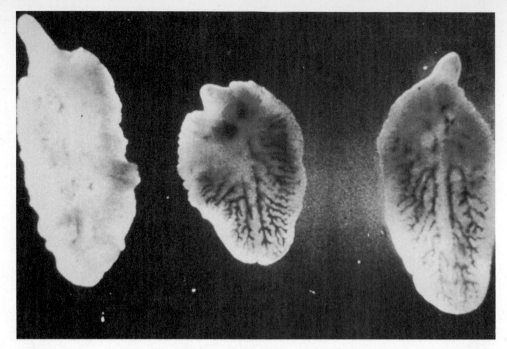

Figure 1.1 (*Continued*) (D) Liver flukes of various species infect man and other animals, causing severe diseases.

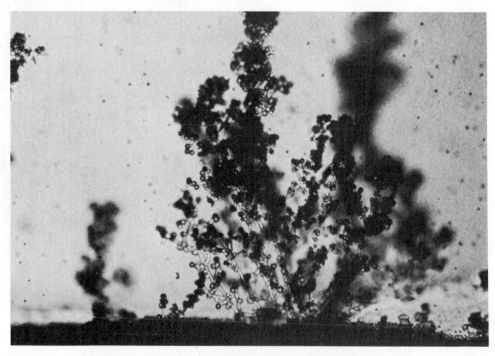

Figure 1.1 (*Continued*) (E) Many fungi grow on and in the bodies of plants and animals, sometimes as harmless commensals and sometimes as pathogens. *Candida albacans*, shown above, is a common parasite of humans.

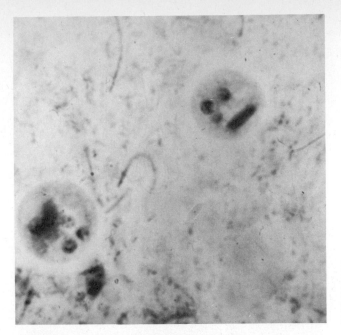

Figure 1.1 (*Continued*) (F) Protozoa inhabit blood and body cavities. *Entamoeba histolytica* is a common inhabitant of the colons of humans. The cyst form shown here is passed in the feces.

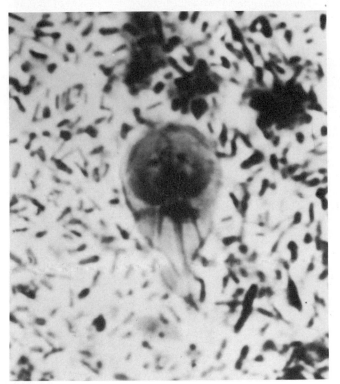

Figure 1.1 (*Continued*) (G) *Giardia intestinalis* inhabits the intestines of humans and possibly other animals. It causes diarrhea. It and *E. histolytica* are both spread by ingestion of cysts (spores) in food and water.

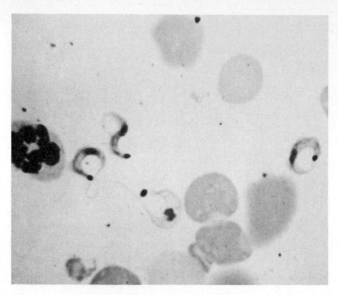

Figure 1.1 (*Continued*) (H) *Trypanosoma cruzi* grows in the blood and tissues of humans and other animals, causing Chagas' disease.

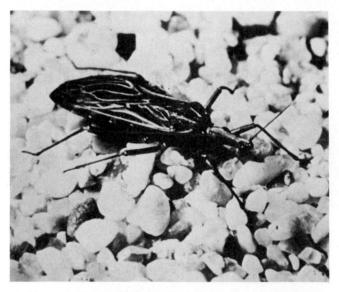

Figure 1.1 (*Continued*) (I) The reduviid bug, a bloodsucking insect, spreads *T. cruzi.* The trypanosome is a parasitic insect that serves as its vector.

TYPES OF HOST–PARASITE RELATIONSHIPS

As noted in the previous section, parasites are organisms that live in or on the bodies of another organism, the host, and derive their sustenance from it. It is not generally in the interest of a parasite to seriously harm its host because then the parasite would be in danger of losing its support. In fact, many parasites cause little harm to their hosts. Serious harm usually indicates a poor adaptation of the host and parasite. Some damage to the host may be a necessary part of the parasite's life cycle, however, and thus be unavoidable.

Damage associated with parasite entry into the host and migration to its site of development is often associated with a parasitic relationship. Some parasitic worms—the hookworm, for example—penetrate the skin to initiate infection and cause local injury characterized by development of a rash; they may also pass through the lungs during their migration to the digestive tract, thus causing pneumonia.

A variety of parasites cause injury as part of their mechanism of dispersal from one host to another. Most viruses of the respiratory tract, such as the influenza virus, and some bacteria, such as the organisms causing tuberculosis and diphtheria, cause considerable irritation to the mucosa of the respiratory tract. This irritation causes increased fluid release, with coughing and sneezing that facilitate the exit of the parasite from the host. The diarrhea caused by bacteria and viruses infecting the intestines also serves to spread these parasites.

One of the more unusual mechanisms for spread of a parasite, and one that is damaging to the host, was developed by the neurotrophic rabies virus. The virus, which grows in the host's brain and its salivary glands, causes changes in the host's behavior so that it attacks other potential hosts, inoculating infected saliva during the attack. In most of the host species of the rabies virus, the damage to the nervous system that causes these changes is finally fatal to the host. However, in bats and skunks, which are probably the hosts in which the rabies virus maintains itself between epidemics, damage is limited and spread is not dependent on changes in the host's behavior. The occurrence of some damage as a result of parasitization does not change the fact that it is usually not in the interest of a parasite to severely damage its host.

Our understanding of host–parasite relationships has developed and changed with the passage of time, as have the terms used to describe them. Originally the term *parasitic* was used for any relationship in which two organisms live together in an intimate association. The term *symbiotic* has now come to be used as the general term to describe any relationship in which two organisms live together in an intimate association (Figure 1.2). In this usage symbiotic relationships are considered to be *mutualistic* if both members of the pair benefit, *commensal* if the symbiont benefits and the host is not harmed, or *parasitic* if the symbiont benefits and the host is harmed to a greater or lesser degree. The term *parasitosis* is sometimes used to designate a parasitic relationship that is particularly harmful to the host.

In practice the categories into which host–parasite relationships have been divided are somewhat arbitrary and grade one into the other. This is as one should

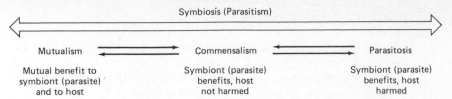

Figure 1.2 Symbiotic relationships may vary over time. Depending on environmental factors such as host resistance, the relationship of a given host–parasite pair may shift between mutually beneficial (mutualism) and harmful to the host (parasitosis). Intermediate stages of toleration (commensalism) may occur.

expect, as host–parasite relationships are subject to and are the results of evolution, and at any given time transformation from one relationship to another may not be complete. Evolution toward mutual interdependence between host and parasite has been realized to a remarkable degree in some instances. As a result of evolutionary change, for example, some mutualistic relationships have become so intimate that the members of the pair are no longer considered separate individuals. This is the case with chloroplasts and the plant cells in which they occur, and with the mitochondria inhabiting plant and animal cells.

Parasites may be distinguished from predators and from saprophytes. Predators are organisms that hunt, catch, and kill other organisms before eating them. Usually prey and predator are similar in size. The prey may be somewhat smaller than the predator, as is a mouse preyed on by a cat; or larger, as is a deer preyed on by wolves. Parasites, on the other hand, are almost always much smaller than their hosts. Fleas, for example, are much smaller than dogs, and the pneumococcus is much smaller than the human in which it causes pneumonia. The major difference between parasites and predators is not size, however, but behavior. Parasites such as fleas and bacteria do not hunt, catch, and kill their prey before eating it; rather, they eat it while it continues to live.

Saprophytes, unlike parasites and predators, neither feed on the still-living nor kill before eating; they eat dead organisms that they did not kill. Animals such as buzzards, which scavenge for their living, eating dead animals, are in a sense saprophytes, but in conventional usage the term *saprophytes* is reserved for microorganisms such as bacteria, protozoa, and fungi that digest and thus degrade the bodies of dead plants and animals.

As noted earlier, parasites live in or on another organism and gain their sustenance from it. They draw their nourishment from the living bodies of their hosts. The parasitic worms and arthropods that live on the surface of the body or in the lumens of the hollow organs such as the intestines are usually described as *infesting* their hosts. The bacteria, fungi, protozoa, and viruses that are parasitic are usually described as *infecting* their hosts.

The implication of the word *infection* is a generalized invasion of the host's tissues, whereas an *infestation* is more superficial. Parasites that are described as causing infestations are also usually larger than those described as causing infections. The distinction between the terms, however, is not sharp. Dermatomycoses caused by fungi are usually referred to as infections, for example, and parasitization by relatively large worms such as trichinella, which invade the tissues of the body, is usually considered an infection.

Some of the difficulty in the terminology used to describe host–parasite relationships is the result of historical accident. Classical parasitology (the science that deals with the parasitic protozoa, worms, and arthropods) developed as a part of zoology. The study of parasitic bacteria and viruses was a province of microbiology. As a result of this separate development, separate terminologies developed to describe essentially similar processes.

People studying microbes became aware quite early that infection with some microbes would result in disease, whereas with others infection either did not result in disease or did not occur at all. Failure by a given microorganism to induce disease in a particular organism may be a result of host specificity. Because of host specificity, a microorganism that produces disease in one animal may be totally harmless to another. It may fail to infect or it may infect but produce no disease. The virus that causes canine distemper, for example, is totally incapable of infecting humans, and the bacteria that cause tuberculosis in chickens do not generally infect cattle or humans.

Some degree of host specificity is the rule for most host–parasite interactions. When parasites do succeed in infecting new hosts, the results can be devastating. *Trypanosoma brucei,* a protozoan, exists in many species of antelope in Africa, where it causes little or no harm. In domestic cattle, however, the same organism usually produces a rapidly fatal disease. Some variants of *T. brucei* that normally occur in antelope can produce severe disease when they infect humans.

Microbes capable of causing infections that result in disease are called *pathogens.* Infection even with a potentially pathogenic microorganism, however, does not always result in disease. If we wish to describe the degree of pathogenicity of a microbe, we refer to its virulence. *Virulence* is a quantitative term. Infection of a susceptible animal with a highly virulent pathogen will almost always result in disease, whereas infection with a pathogen of low virulence will often fail to produce disease or only produce a mild disease. One must in any case distinguish between infection and disease. Infection is the successful colonization of a host by a parasite; disease is the disorder that may result from the infection.

There are, of course, many microbes that cannot produce even infection, let alone disease. The great bulk of free-living microbes are of this type. There are many free-living microbes that dwell in soil and water. They may prey on other microbes, as do the free-living amoeba, or they may live as saprophytes. Some free-living microbes can, under some circumstances, cause infection and disease. Normally free-living microbes that can opportunistically cause infection are called *facultative parasites. Legionella pneumonia* is a free-living aquatic bacterium. If it is inhaled in an aerosol such as is produced by the cooling towers of some water-cooled air conditioners, it is capable of causing infection in the lungs and severe pneumonia. Another example of a facultative parasite is the aquatic amoeba *Naegleria fowleri* which, if sucked into the nose with the water in which it is growing, may invade the brain through the nasal passages and cause meningitis.

One may contrast the life-style of a free-living organism that may accidentally or only occasionly colonize a host with the life-style of an organism that can only live as a parasite. These latter are called *obligate parasites.* All viruses are obligate parasites, but obligate parasitism occurs among all classes of parasites. Plasmodia that cause malaria are obligately parasitic protozoa, trichinella are obligately parasitic worms, and dodder is an obligately parasitic plant. There are some parasites that are obligate parasites during some stages of their life cycles and free-living in others. The common flea, for example, is free-living in its larval stage but is parasitic as an adult.

THE NORMAL MICROBIAL POPULATIONS ON AND IN MULTICELLULAR ORGANISMS

If one is to understand host–parasite relationships and the relationship of microbes to disease, one must be aware that microbes normally live on the outer surfaces of plants and animals. In animals they also live throughout the digestive tract, in the upper portions of the respiratory tract, and the lower portions of the reproductive tract. In healthy plants and animals few microbes live within the tissues of the body, and in healthy animals the lungs, bladder, and uterus are normally free of microbes.

The microbes that live on the body's surfaces and in the hollow organs are usually considered to be commensals benefiting from the association. Commensals gain food and shelter for themselves and do little or no harm to their hosts. In some cases these microbes can be shown to benefit their hosts, and the relationship is thus mutualistic. The microbial inhabitants of the lower bowel of humans, for example, benefit their hosts. If they are eliminated by antibiotic treatment, the microbes that then may colonize the region may cause severe diarrhea. The microbes living in the rumen of cattle are clearly mutualistic since they digest cellulose for the host animals.

Many of the microbes normally colonizing the skin and digestive tracts of animals, including those that may be considered commensals or mutualists, may, if circumstances are appropriate, become pathogens. Any break in the skin is usually followed by at least a local infection. The infecting organisms are most commonly ones living on the skin. In a similar way, injury to the bowel is followed by infection in the body cavity by the organisms usually growing in the bowel. In this case organisms that in one situation have a mutualistic relationship to their hosts become disease-causing microorganisms under changed circumstances.

These examples illustrate the role of host resistance in host–parasite relationships. Diseases such as acquired immunodeficiency syndrome (AIDS), which weakens or destroys host resistance mechanisms, and medical treatments that permit graft acceptance or destroy tumors but also weaken the host defense mechanisms have shown clearly the degree to which host–parasite interaction is a dynamic equilibrium. When host resistance is impaired, organisms that are normally present may cause disease (Figure 1.3).

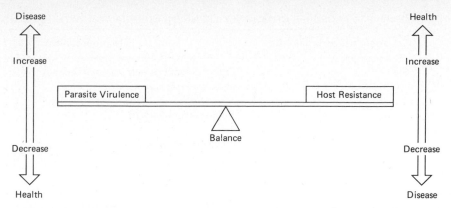

Figure 1.3 The host and parasite exist in a balance. Any decrease in host resistance or increase in parasite virulence can result in development of disease in host–parasite relationships that had previously been innocuous.

MICROBIAL POPULATIONS NORMALLY ASSOCIATED WITH HUMANS

The symbiotic association of microorganisms with humans (as with other animals and plants) is a normal occurrence. Microorganisms are established on the skin, and in the mouth, digestive tract, and genitourinary tract of humans. Many microorganisms of the normal population inhabit their hosts only sporadically and are therefore referred to as *transient normal flora* or *transient microbial populations*. Those that stay permanently are called *resident microbes.* Not all of the microorganisms normally occurring in association with humans have been described. This is in part because many of them are difficult to grow in culture and thus are difficult to study.

Only a small fraction of the many microorganisms in the environment are able to establish themselves and grow in association with the microbes that normally exist in a relationship with humans. The prevention of colonization by microbes not part of the normal population by the ones normally present is called *competitive exclusion.* Often the benefit derived by the host from the resident microbial population is a result of the competitive exclusion of pathogenic microorganisms. Because of competitive exclusion, the most abundant microorganisms among the normal microbial populations colonizing humans play a role in maintaining health. Some microorganisms, however, may directly benefit the host by producing substances useful to the host.

Some of the most common microbes normally inhabiting the bodies of humans and their locations in tissues and organs are listed in Table 1.1.

Skin

A wide range of organisms normally live on the skin of humans. The populations include animals such as mites and bacteria such as staphylococci. The microbial

Table 1.1 MICROBES COMMONLY LIVING IN ASSOCIATION WITH HUMANS

Location: tissue/organ/site	Microorganism
Skin	Diphtheroids (resemble *C. diphtheriae*)
	Propionibacterium acnes
	Staphylococcus epidermidis
	Pityrosporum (yeast)
Mouth	
Tongue	*Streptococcus salivarius*
Teeth	*S. sanguis*
Mucosa	*S. mitis*
Dental plaque	*Strep. sp., Actinomyces, Nocardia, Bacterionema, Veillonella*
Gingival surfaces	*Bacteriodes sp., Fusobacterium sp.*
Digestive tract	
Small intestine	*Streptococci, Lactobacilli, Candida albicans*
Large intestine	Anaerobes
	Bacteroides
	Facultative anaerobes
	Lactobacillus, Streptococcus faecalis, Klebsiella, Proteus, Escherichia coli
Urinary tract	*Streptococcus sp.*
	Mycobacterium
	Bacteriodes
Vaginal tract	Low pH (in sexually mature females)
	Lactobacilli
	Neutral pH (in immature and postmenopausal females)
	Streptococci mixed with other microbes

populations are large. Estimates based on colony counts usually exceed 200,000 per cm^2. The organisms are often found in clusters. Their precise location on and in the skin is determined by many factors. Moist and hairy areas, for example, have more organisms on them than do smooth and dry areas. There are three main types of microbes on the skin. These are diphtheroids, Gram-positive cocci, and yeasts.

Diphtheroids are Gram-positive pleomorphic rods of low virulence. The diphtheroids resident on the skin are similar to but clearly different from *Corynebacterium diphtheriae,* the related organism that is the causative agent of diphtheria. The diphtheroid found in the largest numbers on human skin is *Propionibacterium acnes,* which is anaerobic and grows in the hair follicles. Its growth is enhanced by the oily secretions of the sebaceous glands. *Propionibacterium acnes* has been implicated as a cause of acne. *Propionibacterium acnes* alone does not cause acne, however. Host factors are important contributors. It is well known that acne is most common during adolescence, and thus hormonal factors may be important. Other microbes such as staphylococci, as well as diet, may also be factors in the development of acne.

In addition to the anaerobic *P. acnes,* aerobic diphtheroids are always present in cultures obtained from the skin. The diphtheroids release fatty acids from sebum and thus contribute to the maintenance of the normal level of free fatty acids on the skin. Free fatty acids inhibit the growth of many potentially pathogenic microbes.

The second most abundant group of bacteria on the skin are Gram-positive cocci. Many of these cocci resemble the pathogenic *Staphylococcus aureus,* but differ in that they do not produce coagulase. Coagulase production is a distinguishing feature used to differentiate pathogenic from nonpathogenic staphylococci (see Chapter 12). The various commensal micrococci and staphylococci that are present probably prevent colonization of the skin by other potentially pathogenic Gram-positive bacteria. The nonpathogenic Gram-positive cocci normally present on the skin are often collectively called *Staphylococcus epidermidis.* The Gram stain and other attributes of bacteria are described in Chapter 13. The pathogenic *S. aureus* frequently colonizes the nose and the perianal region of a healthy person. When this occurs in doctors, nurses, and other health personnel, they may infect patients with whom they have contact.

Yeasts of the genus *Pityrosporum* make up the third-most numerous group of microorganisms on the skin. Extensive growth of these yeasts may result in minor skin diseases that range from scaliness to dandruff.

Mouth

Normally there are 10^9 bacteria in each milliliter of saliva and 10^{11} in each gram of deposit on the teeth. Streptococci of various species are the most common bacteria in the mouth and make up from 30 to 60 percent of the bacteria present. The various species of bacteria in the mouth are each associated with a specific location. The ability of the bacteria to attach to specific tissues governs their site of growth. Bacteria of some species attach to the hard tissue, some to the soft.

The deposits formed by bacteria on the teeth are called *dental plaque.* Organisms in dental plaque are facultative anaerobes and include streptococci, filamentous Gram-positive *Actinomyces, Nocardia,* and *Bacterionema.* The Gram-negative microorganism *Veilonella* also is present in plaque. Some pathogens may also be present in dental plaque. For example, *Streptococcus mutans* is frequently present and releases acid that causes tooth decay. The gingival crevices contain strict anaerobes of the genera *Bacteroides* and *Fusobacterium.*

Digestive Tract

The human stomach is usually sterile. The small intestine contains relatively few bacteria (from 10^3 to 10^5 per milliliter). Those organisms that are present in the small intestine are facultative anaerobes of the genera *Streptococcus* and *Lactobacillus.* The yeast *Candida albicans* may also be present. The microbial population of the small intestine is quite transient. In individuals with digestive disorders the microbial population in the small intestine may resemble that in the colon.

In contrast to the small intestine, the large intestine, or colon, contains many bacteria. Feces contain more than 10^{11} bacteria per gram. Up to one-half of the fecal mass may be bacteria. Most of the bacteria in the large intestine are obligate anaerobes of the genus *Bacteroides.* Facultatively anaerobic Gram-negative rods of the genus *Escherichia* and the Gram-positive rods of the genus *Lactobacillus* make up the bulk of the remaining population.

The microbes of the intestine may synthesize vitamins: These include thiamine, niacin, riboflavin, vitamin B_{12}, folic acid, biotin, and vitamin K. It is only if the diet is deficient in these vitamins that the production by microorganisms contributes significantly to the nutrition of humans.

Genitourinary Tract

The kidneys, ureter, and bladder are normally free of bacteria. Infection, however, is common in these sites in humans. This is probably because the urethra opens near the anal orifice and is thus often contaminated with streptococci, *Bacteroides,* and enterobacteria. Infection through sexual activity is also common.

The female genital tract has a normal flora that changes depending on the female's hormonal status and stage of sexual development. The carbohydrate content of the secretions of the vaginal wall varies during the estrus cycle, and this in turn regulates the pH of the vagina because the carbohydrate is fermented to lactic acid by resident lactobacilli. The lactobacilli are predominantly found on the vaginal epithelial cells, where they are conveniently located to bring about the fermentation. The vagina has a neutral pH in prepubescent females and those past menopause. During these periods the vaginal wall secretes little carbohydrate. The microbial populations in the vagina of the prepubescent and aged female include streptococci and many other bacteria but few of the carbohydrate-fermenting, lactic acid–producing lactobacilli.

KOCH'S POSTULATES AND THEIR LIMITATIONS

Our knowledge of the relationship of microbes to infection and disease is of relatively recent origin. It was only in the nineteenth century that the science of bacteriology was created. Before that time many explanations for disease were given. Miasmas from swamps and bad air, for example, were considered to be causes of disease. In English the name *malaria,* given to the disease caused by a protozoan and spread by mosquitoes, immortalizes this misconception. Malaria is Italian for *bad air.*

Two individuals who were leaders in the development of the field of medical microbiology and in gaining acceptance for the roles of germs in disease were Louis Pasteur of France and Robert Koch of Germany. Pasteur showed that fermentation of grape juice to wine was a microbial process brought about by yeasts, and that wine spoilage was the result of other fermentations by other organisms. He showed that many off-tastes in wines could be prevented by heating the wine moderately to kill heat-sensitive microbes before bottling it. The process, now called *pasteurization* in his honor, is widely used today. Its use has been extended to products other than wine, milk being perhaps the most familiar. Pasteur considered that illness in humans and animals was analogous to spoilage in wine, and much of his subsequent work and our present understanding of infection and disease stem from this insight.

Robert Koch was among the first to offer convincing scientific proof that germs caused disease when, in 1876, he showed that *Bacillus anthracis* was the causative agent of anthrax, a fatal disease in cows, sheep, and humans. Robert Koch's major contribution to our present understanding of the role of microbes in disease stemmed, however, from his systemization of techniques for determining which organisms caused which diseases. The systems he developed for cultivation of bacteria in solid media permit ready isolation and growth of bacteria in pure culture. When the systems are used, the bacterial cultures obtained are from colonies that develop from single organisms fixed in space in a solid medium. They are thus pure cultures of the organism producing the colony. The use of solid-culture techniques thus permits one type of microbe to be isolated from among the complex and confusing mixtures normally present in the environment.

Koch's formulation of a set of rules, now called Koch's Postulates, systemized the criteria for relating the various microbes that were isolated by the new techniques to the particular diseases they cause. Koch's Postulates consist of four rules for determining the relationship of a microbe to a disease (Table 1.2). They are that one must: (1) isolate the disease-causing microorganism from all cases of the disease but not from healthy individuals, (2) grow the microorganism in pure culture, (3) induce the disease with the cultured microorganism in some experimental animal, and (4) reisolate the microorganism from the diseased animal.

These rules have both great utility and severe limitations. The limitations can best be understood if one considers the fluidity and variety of host–parasite relationships. Some hints of this fluidity and variety can be seen from our discussion of normal microbial populations in the preceding sections.

There is little trouble using Koch's Postulates to define the relationship between a highly virulent pathogen and the disease it causes. Such a relationship, however, is the exception and not the rule. Problems arise particularly in application of the rules to microbes of low virulence and to microbes that may be opportunistic pathogens. In the latter groups, one finds many organisms that are a part of the normal microbial population associated with plants and animals,

---

Table 1.2   KOCH'S POSTULATES

---

1. The microorganisms must be present in all cases of a disease and not present in the healthy counterparts of the host.

2. The microorganisms must be isolated from the host and grown in pure culture.

3. The disease must be induced by the inoculation of the pure culture of the isolated microorganisms into a suitable experimental animal.

4. The microorganism must be recovered from the experimentally infected host.

The association of potentially pathogenic microorganisms with healthy hosts makes application of the second part of the first postulate problematic. In such cases one cannot show that the pathogen is always absent from healthy individuals. The best-documented examples of the maintenance of a pathogenic microbe in healthy humans are those for *Salmonella typhi, Corynebacterium diphtheriae,* and *Neisseria gonorrhoeae.* A woman named Mary, later known as "Typhoid Mary," was a cook. Wherever she worked, people developed typhoid fever. It was shown that she shed *S. typhi* in large numbers in her feces. She contaminated her hands when cleaning herself and then contaminated the food she handled. No carrier of *C. diphtheriae* or *N. gonorrhoeae* has ever become as famous as Typhoid Mary, but these organisms can be cultured from the mouths and vaginas, respectively, of some healthy people. These healthy carriers are often reservoirs of infection between epidemics. In recognition of this problem, the requirement that the organisms be absent from healthy individuals now is commonly deleted when the postulates are stated.

The first part of the first postulate, which requires that the organism always be present in all cases of the disease, may not be true of certain diseases. Some causative organisms, for example, need not themselves be present in the host to cause disease. The ingestion of the toxin of *Clostridium botulinum* with food is sufficient to produce the disease botulism. This makes application of the first part of the first postulate inappropriate for this disease.

The first part of the first postulate may be impossible to fulfill in other cases also. One cannot always expect the same organism to be present in all cases of the disease. To explain this anomaly one must recognize that there are only a limited number of ways in which disease may manifest itself. Infection in the lungs by any of many different organisms may produce pneumonia. Hepatitis may be produced by a variety of viruses as well as by other agents. Diarrheas are also caused by many types of organisms. As a consequence, it may not be possible to isolate the same organism from all cases of a given disease.

The second postulate, requiring not only the isolation of the microorganism but its growth in pure culture, may also be difficult to fulfill. Growth in culture has been particularly difficult for some bacteria such as *Mycobacterium leprae,* the cause of leprosy, and the spirochete that causes syphilis, *Treponema pallidum.* Viruses are a particularly difficult case. They cannot be cultivated apart from living cells. Many other obligate parasites also cannot be cultivated without a host cell. In such cases growth of the organism in association with suitable host cells may be accepted as equivalent to pure culture.

Restriction in host range may be a serious handicap to the study of some human pathogens. The third postulate cannot be fulfilled if no suitable experimental host is available. Until recently, for example, no experimental host could be infected with Hanson's bacillus (*Mycobacterium leprae*). This prevented fulfillment of the third postulate for leprosy. Today it is known that the organism will grow in the armadillo. Even when an experimental host has been found in which an organism may grow, the disease produced may not resemble that in the definitive host. These are a few of the factors limiting the utility of Koch's Postulates, or at least making it necessary to consider their application with some discretion.

SUGGESTIONS FOR FURTHER READING

J.-F. Bach, *ed. Immunology*, 2nd edition. John Wiley & Sons, New York, 1982.

F. MacFarlane Burnet and D. O. White. *Natural History of Infectious Diseases.* Cambridge University Press, London, 1972.

E. L. Cooper. *General Immunology.* Pergamon Press, Oxford, England, 1982.

J. P. Kreier and J. R. Baker. *Parasitic Protozoa.* Allen & Unwin, London, 1987.

C. A. Mims. *The Pathogenesis of Infectious Diseases*, 3rd edition. Academic Press, New York/London, 1988.

H. Smith, J. J. Skohal, and M. J. Turner, *eds. The Molecular Basis of Microbial Pathogenicity.* Verlag Chemie Weinhein, Weinheim, Germany, 1980.

W. Trager. *Living Together: The Biology of Parasitism.* Plenem Press, New York, 1986.

P. J. Whitefield. *The Biology of Parasitism.* University Park Press, Baltimore, 1979.

R. H. Whittaker. The Kingdoms and the Protozoans. In *Parasitic Protozoa*, J. P. Kreier, *ed.* Academic Press, New York, 1977.

Chapter 2

Introduction to Host Resistance

DESCRIPTION OF THE RESISTANCE SYSTEMS

The immune system of mammals has a constitutive, or innate, component and an inducible, or adaptive, component. Constitutive mechanisms for host protection develop during ontogeny without contact with any particular parasite or its products and are not specific for any particular parasite. Inducible mechanisms are only developed following exposure to a particular parasite or its products and are specific for the inducing parasite (Figure 2.1). Inducible immunity is fully developed only in vertebrate animals, but constitutive mechanisms occur in all living things. The term *resistance* is often used in place of constitutive immunity since the word *immunity* has a connotation of specificity that, as just noted, is usually not present reptiles are crocodiles and alligators. They have a spleen and lymphoid tissues along the gut. The descendants of the original stem reptiles (Cotylosaurs) such as turtles, snakes, and lizards have a variety of lymphoid tissue. Among the turtles, there are species with lymphoid nodules and lymphoid aggregates similar to those of birds. Lizards and snakes possess lymphoid organs similar to both avian and mammalian lymphoid organs, as well as rudimentary lymphatic ducts. The avian and the mammalian lymphoid systems both evolved from a system present in their common reptilian ancestors.

Birds have a lymphoid system of the same complexity as that of reptiles. The readily discernible lymphoid organs include lymph nodes, a thymus, spleen, bone marrow, and Bursa of Fabricius. Birds also have a unique type of lymph node called a *hemolymph node*, in addition to lymph nodes of the types present in other animals. In birds, as in mammals, the bursa, spleen, and lymph nodes have well-defined centers of lymphocyte division and maturation. Birds reject grafts and produce a vigorous antibody response.

The immune system of mammals has been most extensively studied, and most of our information about immune mechanisms is based on experiments that use cells and antibodies from rodents and primates. The lymphoid systems of the latter two groups are remarkably similar. There are three major groups of mammals: the monotremes (egg laying), the marsupials, and the placental mammals. Although monotremes lay eggs and have some other reptilian characteristics, their lymphatic system and lymphoid organs are very similar to those of placental mammals. The placental mammals and the marsupials have highly organized, extensive lymphoid systems connected by strategically distributed lymphatic ducts that permit drainage and filtration of fluids from all tissues. The system thus provides a mechanism for clearing foreign material from tissues and trapping it in lymphatic tissues. The characteristics of the immune systems of vertebrates of various classes are outlined in Table 2.1.

MANIPULATION OF THE HOST DEFENSE SYSTEMS

The constitutive system is not readily manipulated. It may be enhanced by good nutrition or damaged by malnutrition, stress, fatigue, or injury. As with any genetically determined trait, its characteristics are affected by selection. When previously isolated populations mix and exchange their microbes, the resulting diseases may be devastating and selection for resistance may be severe. The population of Europe was severely affected by syphilis after its introduction from America in 1493, for example, and the Native American population was devastated by newly introduced European and African diseases during the early period of European colonization of America.

The inducible, or adaptive, system is the system manipulated by immunization. Although the capacity of the inducible system to respond to a particular parasite is genetically determined, as noted earlier, the actual expression of the system requires induction by contact with the organism or its products. Inducible immunity can be actively induced or passively transferred. When actively induced,

Table 2.1   THE NATURE OF LYMPHOID ORGANS AND OF IMMUNE RESPONSES OF
VERTEBRATES OF VARIOUS CLASSES

		Functional activity	
Vertebrate class	Lymphoid organs	Graft rejection	Antibody formation
Jawless fishes, *e.g.,* hagfish	No thymus equivalent present	+/−	+
Cartilaginous fishes, *e.g.,* sharks	Thymus equivalent present Spleen present	+	+
Bony fishes	Thymus equivalent present Spleen present Lymphoid cell aggregates present	+	+
Amphibians			
Newts/Salamanders	Thymuslike organ present Spleen present	+	+
Frogs/Toads	Thymuslike organ present Spleen present Lymph nodes present	+	+
Reptiles			
Alligators/Crocodiles	Spleen present Thymus not described	?	?
Lizards/Turtles/Snakes	Bursalike organ present Thymus equivalent present Lymph nodes present	+	+
Birds	Bursa with a defined inner structure present Thymus and spleen present Lymph nodes present	+	+

Mammals	No bursa (bone marrow is the
	  probable bursal equivalent)
	Thymus, spleen, lymph nodes,
	  and lymphatic duct system
	  all present
		+	+

the recipients generate the mediators of immunity themselves, after contact with the parasite or its products. In passive transfer, the mediators of the immunity generated by one individual are transferred to another, for example by serum transfer, and confer on the recipient specific immunity for a short time.

Both active and passive inducible immunity may be conferred naturally or artificially. Natural active inducible immunity often follows infection. Artificial active inducible immunity follows administration of vaccines. Natural passive inducible immunity is passed by means of antibody transfer from the mother to her offspring either across the placenta or via the first milk. Artificial passive inducible immunity is the result of administration of immune serum (see Figure 2.1).

SUGGESTIONS FOR FURTHER READING

J. T. Barrett. *Textbook of Immunology,* 4th edition. C. V. Mosby , St. Louis, Missouri, 1983.

E. L. Cooper. *General Immunology.* Pergamon Press, Oxford, England, 1982.

J. Klein. *Immunology: The Science of Self–Nonself Discrimination.* John Wiley & Sons, New York, 1982.

M. J. Manning and R. J. Turner. *Comparative Immunobiology.* Halsted Press, New York. 1976.

A. I. Oparin. *Genesis and Evolutionary Development of Life.* Academic Press, New York, 1968.

R. T. Smith, R. A. Good, and P. A. Miescher, *eds. Ontogeny of Immunity.* University of Florida Press, Gainesville, Florida, 1967.

R. T. Smith, P. A. Miescher, and R. A. Good. *Phylogeny of Immunity.* University of Florida Press, Gainesville, Florida, 1966.

Chapter 3

Constitutive Host Resistance

INTRODUCTION

Constitutive, or natural, resistance is the result of the actions of a number of systems. These may be differentiated into external and internal systems. Among the external systems are the skin and mucous membranes, which protect by inhibiting entry of microbes into the body, and various antimicrobial substances secreted onto the skin and mucous membranes that inhibit microbial colonization. The internal systems are those that inhibit colonization by microbes that succeed in passing the external systems. These include a variety of antimicrobial substances in the blood and body fluids, and a variety of phagocytic cells. The internal systems come into play following injuries that breach the physical barriers and permit entry of microbes into the body. Constitutive resistance is not specific.

The nature of the constitutive resistance systems varies to some extent from species to species and is also affected by the environment. Important factors in determining the effectiveness of the constitutive resistance systems include nutritional status, injury, and age.

THE EXTERNAL DEFENSE SYSTEMS

The first lines of defense against infection are the external systems. Major components of the external systems are the mechanical barriers, the effectiveness of which is enhanced by various antimicrobial secretions (Figure 3.1). The mechanical barriers to microbial invasion of animals are formidable.

The Skin

The skin covers most of the external surface of the body. It is continuous with the mucosa at the body's orifices. The mucosa lines the lumens of all of the hollow organs that connect to the body's orifices. The skin is the largest organ in the body, weighing up to 5 kg in adult humans. The skin provides a tough, dry surface that is resistant to penetration. In some areas, hair masses protect the skin from injury. The skin is constantly lubricated by sweat and sebum. These glandular secretions contain lactic acid and free fatty acids that inhibit microbial growth. The low pH of the skin surface (about pII 5.5), which is in part determined by the lactic acid and free fatty acids, also provides a poor environment for many pathogenic microorganisms.

The skin normally has microbes growing on it. These organisms, which are adapted to life on the skin, may prevent colonization by pathogens by filling up available space and utilizing attachment sites and available nutrients.

The Mucosa

The mucosa lining the lumens of the hollow organs of the body that connect to the body's orifices provides a barrier in these locations as the skin does for the external surfaces. Since many essential exchanges, such as gas exchange in the

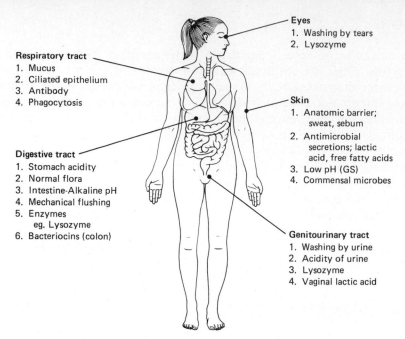

Eyes
1. Washing by tears
2. Lysozyme

Respiratory tract
1. Mucus
2. Ciliated epithelium
3. Antibody
4. Phagocytosis

Skin
1. Anatomic barrier; sweat, sebum
2. Antimicrobial secretions; lactic acid, free fatty acids
3. Low pH (GS)
4. Commensal microbes

Digestive tract
1. Stomach acidity
2. Normal flora
3. Intestine-Alkaline pH
4. Mechanical flushing
5. Enzymes eg. Lysozyme
6. Bacteriocins (colon)

Genitourinary tract
1. Washing by urine
2. Acidity of urine
3. Lysozyme
4. Vaginal lactic acid

Figure 3.1 Many factors mediate natural resistance to penetration of the external surface of humans by parasites. The physical barriers, the skin and mucous membranes, are of primary importance in this resistance. The lumens of the digestive, respiratory, and genitourinary tracts are considered external since the epithelia lining these organs forms a continuous layer with the skin. Some factors enhancing the effectiveness of the physical barriers are listed here.

lungs and nutrient absorption in the intestines, must occur across the mucosa lining hollow organs, these membranes cannot be as effective a barrier as the skin.

The mucosa has several associated systems that aid in preventing microbial colonization and penetration. These include a layer of mucus that is constantly renewed and, in some mucosal surfaces, ciliated cells that move the mucus layer in an ordered fashion to sweep out particles that adhere to it.

The Respiratory Tract

In the respiratory tract the mucus layer and ciliated cells together are called the *ciliary escalator system.* Both the upper and lower respiratory tracts are protected from inhaled particles by the ciliary escalator system. The mucus on the mucosa in the nasal cavity traps many inhaled particles. The turbinates, which act as baffles for the air flow, increase the surface for trapping. The cilia in the nasal mucosa keep the film of mucus moving toward the mouth. The particles trapped in the mucus are swallowed when they reach the mouth. Small particles ($\cong 0.5 \ \mu$m) may escape trapping in the nose and be inhaled into the lower tract. They may be trapped in the mucus in the trachea and bronchioles or enter the alveoli of the lungs, where (see Chapter 7). In vetebrates, a complex system of cells has evolved to recognize foreign substances, synthesize the recognition molecules, and eliminate the foreign substances (see Chapter 8). The cells of this system are to a large degree within the lymphatic tissue.

The composition and functions of the lymphoid system are more complex in the more recently evolved vertebrates. In general, the system becomes more complex as one moves from fish to amphibians, reptiles, birds, and mammals.

During embryonic development the stem cells of the immune systems of vertebrates develop in the bone marrow. These stem cells then differentiate along two major pathways. The cells destined to participate in the cellular aspects of inducible immunity migrate and differentiate in the thymus or in a thymus equivalent. The cells that will produce antibodies—the humoral response—differentiate by migrating through an organ that provides a distinct environment. In birds, this organ is the Bursa of Fabricius. In amphibians, reptiles, and mammals, the precise location of bursal-equivalent lymphoid tissues is not clear; however, as they have the ability to produce antibody, it is probable that they possess a bursal-equivalent organ. The bone marrow is probably the bursal equivalent in these animals.

An inducible system clearly antecedent to that seen in mammals first appears in fish. There are three living classes of fishes. In a limited form, an inducible system is present in the most primitive fishes (Agnatha, or jawless fish), such as the lamprey and hagfish. These fishes have lymphoid tissue which, as noted previously, is an important element of the inducible system. This lymphoid tissue is in the gut walls. The jawless fishes destroy grafts and make a single type of antibody molecule called *IgM*. The second class, cartilaginous fishes (Chondrichthyes), in which sharks, rays, and skates are placed, have a discrete thymus equivalent, a spleen, and another encapsulated lymphoid organ. They also make antibodies and destroy grafts. The third class is the bony fishes (Ostreichthyes), which are now represented by the ray-finned fishes, or teleosts. Teleosts have a spleen, thymus, and several discrete lymphoid cell aggregates and are capable of graft rejection and formation of several types of antibody. Even among the fishes, therefore, development of immune function and increasing complexity of lymphoid tissue accompany evolutionary advance.

Amphibians were the first vertebrates to colonize land. The amphibians, which are derived from a bony fish, carried the inducible system with them into the new environment. Newts and salamanders (Urodela), the more primitive amphibians, have a functional thymus and spleen. Frogs and toads (Anura), which are more advanced, have a thymus, spleen, and lymph glands. These lymph glands are suggestive of mammalian lymph nodes but have a poorly defined internal structure. The spleen is the major antibody-producing organ in amphibians; the thymus functions as a source of the lymphocytes that cause graft rejection and is located just posterior to the eyes.

Reptiles descended from ancient, now-extinct amphibians. They freed themselves from life in water by developing a skin that reduced evaporation and by developing eggs that could hatch on land. Reptiles have an inducible system more like that of mammals than that possessed by amphibians. They possess a thymus with an internal structure similar to that of mammals. The most primitive living

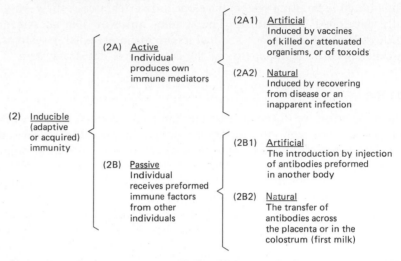

(1) Constitutive (innate) immunity (resistance) develops as the individual develops. It does not require contact with any parasite for full expression.

(2) Inducible (adaptive or acquired) immunity

(2A) Active — Individual produces own immune mediators
 (2A1) Artificial — Induced by vaccines of killed or attenuated organisms, or of toxoids
 (2A2) Natural — Induced by recovering from disease or an inapparent infection

(2B) Passive — Individual receives preformed immune factors from other individuals
 (2B1) Artificial — The introduction by injection of antibodies preformed in another body
 (2B2) Natural — The transfer of antibodies across the placenta or in the colostrum (first milk)

Figure 2.1 There are a variety of mechanisms by which organisms resist parasitization. The constitutive mechanisms (1) develop as the individual develops. The development is under endogenous control. The inducible mechanisms (2) develop only partially under endogenous stimuli and require contact with the parasite or its products for full development. The inducible mechanisms are commonly classified into active (2A) and passive (2B) forms depending on whether the individual develops its own immune mediators or receives those produced by another. Active and passive immunity may each be further divided into artificial (2A1; 2B1) and natural (2A2; 2B2) types. The artificial types are those that result from intervention by physicians or veterinarians.

in natural resistance mechanisms. Constitutive resistance is implemented by a much broader range of mechanisms than is inducible immunity. There are many mechanisms shared by the two types of defense, however, and many of the same cells and serum proteins contribute to both.

Both the constitutive and the inducible systems are under genetic control. They differ in that the constitutive system develops fully under the stimulation of endogenous inducers as the individual develops, whereas the full development of the antiparasitic mechanisms of the inducible system, as noted earlier, requires induction by contact with the parasite or its products.

The constitutive system includes the physical barriers to microbial invasion such as the skin and mucous membranes, antimicrobial substances on the skin and in the body fluids, and various cells that ingest parasites, secrete antiparasitic substances, or in various ways attack parasites. These will be described in detail in Chapter 3. The inducible system utilizes specific antibodies and various types of cells that may specifically attack the invading microorganism. The inducible system is described in Chapters 5 through 10.

EVOLUTION OF HOST DEFENSE SYSTEMS

The inducible immune system developed in vertebrates as they evolved; it is most fully developed in mammals. The system, however, like all systems developed through evolutionary processes, had its origins in preexisting systems; in this case in cells and other components of the constitutive defense system.

Contact Avoidance

The most primitive of the defense mechanisms is contact avoidance. When single-cell suspensions from one species of sponge are placed in culture, the cells will associate into colonies and take on a characteristic sponge morphology. When sponge cells derived from two different species are mixed, the cells will associate with like or self; two distinctly different colonies will form, each comprised of cells of only one species. Similar observations have been made with coral. When two pieces of coral from the same species are placed in close association with one another, they will eventually grow together. However, if two pieces of coral from different species are placed in close apposition, they will continue to grow but contact will be avoided by formation of a gap between the cells of the two species. Some species of coral are more aggressive than others: Such corals will react to the presence of individuals of another species by forming structures that compete with the other species for nutrients. They eventually destroy the individuals of the competing species. The isolation of a parasite in the body by the formation of a connective-tissue wall is a defense mechanism that probably had its roots in contact avoidance.

Phagocytic Defense

Most cells of multicellular animals can ingest particulate materials. Many multicellular animals, however, have cells that specialize in ingesting foreign material that may enter their bodies. These cells are called *phagocytes* and the phenomenon is called *phagocytosis*. Defense by phagocytic cells appeared early in the evolution of multicellular animals. Phagocytes are present in animals of all classes, from sponges through arthropods and vertebrates. Small particulate substances such as bacteria may be taken up by phagocytosis. When soluble material is engulfed, the process is called *pinocytosis*. After ingestion, the engulfed substance is present in a vacuole. A second kind of vacuole, a lysosome, serves as a reservoir for cellular enzymes and other substances that will digest the internalized microorganisms after the two kinds of vacuoles fuse. When the foreign material is too large to be ingested, phagocytic cells may surround the material, forming a capsule that walls off the foreign material from the host cells. Phagocytic defense mechanisms are evolutionarily antecedent to inducible defenses. They have been retained as part of the constitutive defenses by all animals and have been incorporated into the inducible responses as these evolved.

Phagocytosis is often facilitated by soluble substances present in the bodies of multicellular organisms. Many types of multicellular organisms have soluble sub-

stances in the body fluids that provide protection against invaders. A protein has been isolated from snails that will agglutinate bacteria, for example. This agglutinin has specificity for certain carbohydrates that are commonly present on the surfaces of bacteria. Many other invertebrates have proteins in their hemolymph that specifically bind to microorganisms and cause agglutination. The agglutinins also prepare the coated material for ingestion and thus facilitate phagocytosis. Materials that coat a particle and facilitate its phagocytosis are called *opsonins*. These opsonic substances are the evolutionary precursors of the antibodies of the inducible immune system.

Immunological Memory

The array of constitutive defense mechanisms is usually adequate to protect the individual from most microbes; however, some microorganisms are able to evade or overcome the constitutive resistance mechanisms. When this occurs in vertebrates and infection results, the inducible immune response is invoked and may be able to destroy the parasite. It is the nature of the inducible response that once invoked against a particular parasite, it remains developed in some degree and the individual is able to deal more rapidly and effectively with the same parasite on subsequent encounters. This retention of capability to respond is called *immunological memory*, and the subsequent response is referred to as the *anamnestic response*. The development of immunological memory was a considerable advance in the evolution of host defense systems.

Immunological memory is present to a degree in earthworms. Grafts between genetically identical worms are accepted, but those between genetically different worms are rejected. The onset of rejection of a heterologous graft in earthworms is slow and often does not begin until 30 to 150 days after transplantation. Even after onset, the rejection process proceeds slowly, requiring several weeks for complete rejection. Once a graft has been rejected, however, a second graft from the same donor may be rejected more rapidly. The process is specific because the rejection of a graft from an unrelated third-party donor proceeds at the same pace as rejection of the original graft.

The rejection process that has evolved in mammals is similar to that in earthworms but is more vigorous and more highly specific. In mammals, grafts between individuals of the same species are rejected within two weeks and the development of memory results in an accelerated reaction that is complete within seven days.

Lymphoid Cells and Organs

Invertebrates rely primarily on constitutive mechanisms, including ingestion by phagocytic cells, for the destruction of foreign materials that enter their bodies. As noted in the section "Phagocytic Defense," some constitutive agglutinins may aid ingestion. Vertebrates, unlike invertebrates, recognize foreign substances by both inducible and constitutive cellular and humoral mechanisms (see Chapters 5–9). The capacity to adaptively acquire the ability to synthesize antibodies that can bind specifically to newly introduced foreign materials is found only among vertebrates they are ingested by phagocytic cells. The particles trapped in the mucus in the trachea and bronchioles, and those ingested by cells in the alveoli, are moved upward within the mucus secretion, along with the cells, by the mucociliary escalator. The ciliated cells in the lower tract are similar to those that line the upper respiratory tract. The mucus is swept upward at a rate of about 1 cm per hour to the back of the mouth, where it is swallowed. Sneezing and coughing may also aid in removal of material from the respiratory system.

The Mouth

The mouth is normally populated with microorganisms. Some adhere to the teeth and some to the cheeks and gums. Saliva constantly enters the mouth. The tongue cleans the teeth, and swallowing removes the saliva and loosened particles as well as the mucus from the respiratory tract. Organisms that do not adhere cannot persist in this environment.

In addition to the mechanical cleaning systems in the mouth, there are chemical ones. Saliva, for example, contains lysozyme, an enzyme that digests the cell walls of bacteria, especially Gram-positive microorganisms, and thus destroys many pathogens.

As noted in the previous section, microorganisms entering the mouth from the respiratory system are cleared by swallowing. Swallowed microorganisms enter the digestive tract.

The Digestive Tract

The human digestive tract is protected from swallowed microbes by the antimicrobial environment of the stomach. The high acidity (pH = 2.0–3.0) of the human stomach is very effective in killing ingested microbes. The small intestine has an alkaline pH but contains abundant proteolytic enzymes that may inhibit microbial growth. The movement of intestinal contents may keep normal populations down by sweeping microbes out of the small intestine. The large intestine, unlike the stomach and small intestine, characteristically contains many bacteria. Gram-negative microorganisms within the normal flora secrete substances called *bacteriocins* that inhibit the growth of many pathogens. They also prevent the establishment of pathogens by competing with them for food and space. The normal movement of food and feces through the intestinal tract prevents many pathogens from establishing themselves there. Clearance is most effective against organisms that cannot adhere to the mucosa.

The Urogenital Tract

The urogenital tract is protected primarily by mechanical barriers and flushing mechanisms. Sterile urine flushes the urinary tract every five to eight hours, removing nonadherent organisms and preventing the adherence of microorganisms to all but the outermost portions.

The vagina has a tough epithelium, and during the period of sexual activity the epithelium produces secretions rich in carbohydrates, which support a normal population of lactic acid–producing bacteria. The low pH (pH $\approx$ 5.0) produced within the vagina by the lactic acid–producing bacteria is inhibitory to many pathogens.

The Eye

The conjuctiva, the membrane surrounding the eye, is protected chiefly through the flushing action of tears. Tears continually bathe the eye, and fluid movement is enhanced through the action of blinking. When the eye is irritated, tears are produced in large volumes. This enhances the mechanical flushing of the eye. Tears also contain large amounts of lysozyme which, as noted previously, lyses many bacteria.

THE INTERNAL DEFENSE SYSTEMS

Microbes that by one means or another succeed in passing the external barriers and associated defense systems next encounter the second line of defense, the internal systems. These include, as mentioned earlier, a variety of antimicrobial substances in the blood and body fluids and a variety of phagocytic cells. The phagocytic cells are a major factor in this line of defense.

The Morphology and Development of Phagocytic Cells

In mammals there are two classes of phagocytes, the mononuclear and the polymorphonuclear phagocytes. These cells are part of the leukocyte system, which includes, in addition, the lymphocytes important in the inducible system (Figure 3.2).

The mononuclear and polymorphonuclear phagocytes are produced in the bone marrow from a common stem cell (Figure 3.3). The stem cells committed to produce polymorphonuclear leukocytes differentiate into myeloblasts, and those that will produce mononuclear phagocytes differentiate into monoblasts. The sequence for polymorphonuclear leukocyte differentiation requires four cell divisions; each results in a progressive decrease in cell size and an increase in nuclear compaction. The compact nucleus ultimately assumes the characteristic polymorphonuclear shape. The myeloblast gives rise to promyelocytes that divide to produce first myelocyte I cells, then myelocyte II cells. The myelocyte II cells give rise to metamyelocytes. Following the production of the metamyelocyte, no further cell division occurs. The metamyelocytes develop into band cells that become segmented cells and, finally, mature polymorphonuclear leukocytes as they leave the bone marrow and enter the blood. Under conditions of stress, such as is caused by infection, immature forms such as band cells may enter the blood.

The mononuclear phagocyte is derived from the monoblast. The monoblast produces promonocytes that divide three times before becoming monocytes. The maturation of the monocyte into the macrophage requires no further cell division.

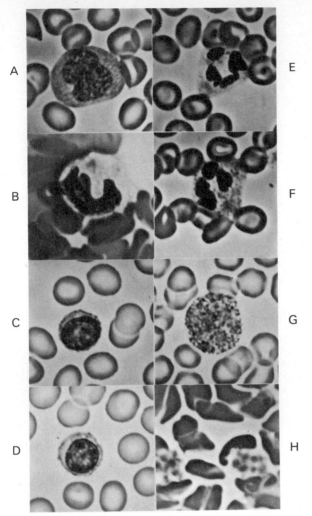

Figure 3.2 Photomicrographs of cells in Giemsa stained blood films. The morphology of the various leukocytes in human blood, including monocytes (2A, B), lymphocytes (2C, D), polymorphonuclear neutrophils (2E, F), eosinophils (2G) and platelets (2H), is shown. Monocytes have a relatively large, often bean-shaped nucleus and extensive cytoplasm. Lymphocytes have a small round compact nucleus and a thin rim of cytoplasm. Polymorphonuclear neutrophils have a multilobulated nucleus, the lobes of which are connected by thin strands of nuclear material. They have a poorly staining cytoplasm. Eosinophils have nuclei similar to polymorphonuclear neutrophils, but the cytoplasm is filled with eosinophilic granules that, in the example shown, almost obscure the nucleus. Platelets are anucleate fragments broken off from pseudopods produced by megokaryocytes that reside in the bone marrow. In the photomicrograph shown, there are two clumps of platelets, each containing from 8 to 12 platelets. The clumping results from handling of the blood during slide preparation. Erythrocytes, roughly circular anucleate cells that in some cases were grossly distorted when the blood film was prepared, are visible in all of the micrographs.

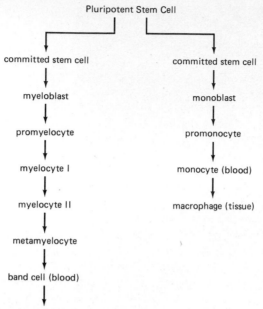

Figure 3.3 Differentiation of polymorphonuclear leukocytes and mononuclear phagocytes. A common stem cell in the bone marrow gives rise to committed stem cells that will form either polymorphonuclear leukocytes or macrophages. When polymorphonuclear leukocytes are produced, the stem cells give rise to myeloblasts that divide and differentiate into promyelocytes, myelocytes I and II, and metamyelocytes. The metamyelocytes mature with no further cell division into band cells, which in turn mature into segmented cells that enter the blood and become mature polymorphonuclear leukocytes.

To form macrophages, the committed stem cell will divide and become a monoblast. The monoblasts differentiate into promonocytes. The promonocytes divide three times and differentiate into monocytes that enter the blood. The monocytes may leave the circulation and enter the tissues to become macrophages.

The monocyte enters the blood and circulates before it enters the tissues to become a macrophage.

Macrophages may be fixed at some site or may be free to wander; they are found throughout the body. Macrophages have a long life span. The maturation of the macrophage is influenced by their tissue environment, and macrophages may take on different characteristics, depending on their anatomical location. This attribute of macrophages has resulted in a confusing nomenclature. For example, macrophages in the endothelial lining of the blood vessels of the liver are called *Kupffer cells*, macrophages in the connective tissue are referred to as *histiocytes*, those in the central nervous system are called *microglial cells*, and those in the skin are called *Langerhan's cells*. The phagocytic cells in the peritoneal cavity, lung, spleen, and lymph nodes are just referred to as *macrophages* and are distinguished by their anatomical location. Macrophages found in the lung, for example, are called *alveolar macrophages,* and those in the abdomen are called *peritoneal macrophages.*

The polymorphonuclear leukocytes are also known as *granulocytes* because of the many granules found in their cytoplasm. The contents of the granules determine the cell's staining properties and help to distinguish the different cells of the granulocytic series. Three types of granulocytes based on staining characteristics have been described. These are neutrophils, eosinophils, and basophils. The stain most commonly used to distinguish these cells is the Giemsa stain, an azure B eosinate. It is prepared by interaction between two basic dyes, azure B and methylene blue, and an acidic dye, eosin. The basophilic, or cationic, components react with the negatively charged molecules of the granules, staining them blue. The acidophilic, or anionic, component reacts with the positively charged molecules, staining them red. The granules of the neutrophil are not ionically charged at physiological pHs and thus do not stain; they assume a gray or neutral tint.

The granules of the neutrophil and eosinophil contain enzymes, whereas those within the basophil contain biologically active amines. The enzymes in the neutrophilic granules are important for the destruction and digestion of microorganisms and other foreign organic materials (Table 3.1). The granules are classified into two types: the primary, or azurophilic, granules, and the secondary, or specific, granules. The terms *primary* and *secondary* refer to the color or appearance of the granules during differentiation rather than to the importance of the granules. The azurophilic granules contain peroxidase, myeloperoxidase, acid hydrolases, neutral proteases, cationic antimicrobial proteins, and lysozyme.

The neutral proteases include elastase, collagenase, and cathepsin G. Enzymes released by neutrophils activate complement and generate kinins (see Chapter 4); the enzymes therefore enhance vascular permeability and chemotaxis indirectly. The specific granules contain lactoferrin and lysozyme.

The polymorphonuclear neutrophil is the most abundant of the white blood cells in humans, comprising about 45–70 percent of the circulating leukocytes. They have a life span of three to five days, are mobile, respond to chemotactic stimuli, and are highly phagocytic. They are among the first cells to accumulate at a site of injury.

Table 3.1   ENZYME CONTENT OF GRANULES AND LYSOSOMES IN NEUTROPHILS AND MACROPHAGES

Neutrophils		Macrophages (lysosomes)
Primary granules	Secondary granules	
Acid hydrolases	Lysozyme	Acid hydrolases
Neutral proteases	Lactoferrin	Neutral proteases
Peroxidase		Peroxidase
Myeloperoxidase		Myeloperoxidase
Cationic proteins		Lysozyme
Lysozyme		

The eosinophils play a major role in defense against helminthic parasites such as *Trichinella* and *Schistosoma.* The basic protein found in the granules of these cells may be the major factor in the killing of these parasites. The eosinophils attach to the surfaces of the parasites, probably with the aid of antibody, and discharge their granules against the parasites' surface, where they cause injury to the parasites' membranes. Eosinophils are much less phagocytic than are neutrophils. These cells make up from one to two percent of the polymorphonuclear leukocytes.

Basophils function as carriers of inflammatory mediators. The granules of basophils contain histamine and other vasoactive compounds. The release of the contents of the granules serves to amplify the inflammatory response (see Chapter 5). Basophils generally account for less than one percent of the polymorphonuclear leukocytes.

Cells of the mononuclear phagocyte lineage initially contain granules; these are lost during differentiation. The mononuclear phagocytes, which comprise from two to eight percent of the circulating leukocytes, contain enzymes similar to those present in neutrophils (Table 3.1). The enzymes are contained within bags made of membrane, called *lysosomes.* The mononuclear phagocyte is long lived and continues to synthesize enzymes throughout its life.

The acid hydrolases of mononuclear phagocytes act at acidic pH and cleave phosphate ester bonds that occur in proteins, polysaccharides, lipids, and nucleic acids. The enzymes are distinguished by their substrates and include fucosidase, 5'nucleotidase, galactosidase, arylsulfatase, mannosidase, N-acetyl-glucosaminidase, glucuronidase, and glycerophosphatase. Other enzymes included in this group are responsible for protein hydrolysis and are called *cathepsins A, B, C,* and so on. Neutral proteases include cathepsin G, whose substrates are cartilage, proteoglycans, fibrogen, and casein, and the enzymes elastase and collagenase. The latter two enzymes have been shown to play an important role in the destruction of normal tissue that may occur during an inflammatory response. The peroxidase enzyme catalase protects the phagocytes from the toxic effects of the hydrogen peroxide produced following the binding and phagocytosis of foreign substances.

Chemotaxis

Phagocytic cells are attracted to an area of infection or tissue damage by microbial and host-derived chemotactic factors. The host-derived chemotactic factors include components of the complement, clotting, fibrinolytic, and kinin systems that are activated either directly, by contact with microbes, or indirectly by the actions of proteolytic enzymes released by the invading microorganisms on damaged cells (see Chapter 4). The complement component C5a is a chemotactic factor.

Phagocytosis

Many of the antimicrobial substances in the blood and body fluids function by facilitating phagocytosis. Some antimicrobial substances, such as those of the complement system, act both by facilitating phagocytosis and by directly inducing damage to the membranes of the microbes. The direct antimicrobial actions of complement will be described fully in Chapter 9, in the section entitled "Complement-mediated Effector Mechanisms."

Phagocytosis by single-cell animals is a feeding process. In multicellular organisms, the feeding process has increased significance as it is a function of specialized cells that protect from infection and remove foreign material from the body. These specialized cells, or phagocytes, scavenge foreign material, including microbes, that may enter the body. They do this based on recognition mechanisms in their membranes and with the aid of constitutive and inducible opsonins. In addition to their role as scavenger cells, the phagocytes participate in the inflammatory response and initiate and regulate the inducible immune response that develops in vertebrates following the breaching by parasites of the physical barriers to infection.

Opsonization

Once the phagocytes have arrived, they must bind to the foreign object through membrane receptors for phagocytosis to occur. The phagocyte may recognize inert particles through electrostatic bonds and hydrophobic interactions that do not form with the hydrophilic surfaces of the animal's own cells. Some inert materials, such as carbon particles, are only ingested after being coated with serum proteins. The specificity for recognition of the particles as foreign in such cases is a function of the serum protein. These serum proteins also have sites recognized by receptors on the phagocytes and thus serve as a bridge between the phagocyte and its target (Figure 3.4).

The process of preparation of a particle for ingestion by coating with serum protein is called *opsonization*. Opsonins are substances in the serum that coat particles and cause them to be engulfed by phagocytic cells. The most important of the opsonins in serum are antibodies, the C3b component of the complement system, and fibronectin (see Chapter 4).

Antibodies are components of the inducible immune response and will be considered fully in Chapter 7. The complement system is involved in both the constitutive and the inducible systems. The complement system is a group of serum proteins that activate each other sequentially following activation of the initial component by contact with permissible surfaces of microbes or other foreign material, or by contact with immune complexes in the body. When involved in the constitutive defense, complement is activated through the alternate pathway. When involved in the inducible response, activation is through the classical pathway. In the latter case, combination of antibody with the microbe or other target initiates activation of C1; in the former, direct binding of the constitutive serum protein—the complement component C3—with the microbe or other target initiates the process (Figure 3.5).

The surfaces of many nonpathogenic microorganisms contain components that initiate the complement cascade by the alternate pathway. It would perhaps be better to say that many microorganisms are nonpathogenic because they activate complement through the alternate pathway and are thus opsonized and phagocytized by constitutive mechanisms.

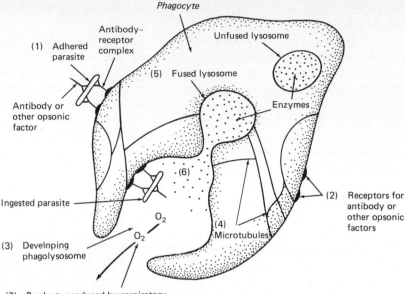

Figure 3.4 Binding of an opsonized bacterium (1) to receptors on the surface of the phagocyte (2) results in initiation of phagocytosis (3) and the respiratory burst. Ingestion proceeds with the aid of microtubles (4), by a series of actin-binding reactions. Fusion of the phagosome with granules and lysosomes (5) results in the release of enzymes into the phagolysosome (6). Some enzymes and other substances may escape from the developing phagolysosome under some circumstances (7) as when the particle is too large to be ingested, for example.

By definition, pathogenic microorganisms are those that have the ability to evade or negate the various constitutive defense mechanisms. This is illustrated by the case of the pneumococcus. The antiphagocytic components covering the microbe's surface protect it. After antibody is produced as part of the inducible response, it binds the antiphagocytic components. The microbe is thus opsonized and then may be phagocytized. The inducible response thus negates the mechanism used by the microbe to evade the host's constitutive defense. It is probable that complement, acting as a constitutive opsonin following activation by the alternate pathway, is the older mechanism of defense, having evolved earlier than the inducible system.

Fibronectin is a high molecular weight serum protein that facilitates binding of most particles to phagocytic cells. It is thus an important constitutive opsonin. The opsonic activity of fibronectin is actually an attribute of fibronectin fragments produced by proteolytic enzymes. These enzymes are active at sites of injury and microbial invasion, and thus activate the opsonic fibronectin system at the sites where it is needed. Since the formation of antibody after infection requires time, the constitutive opsonins C3b and fibronectin, which are always present in serum, are probably the most important opsonins active soon after injury. Other serum

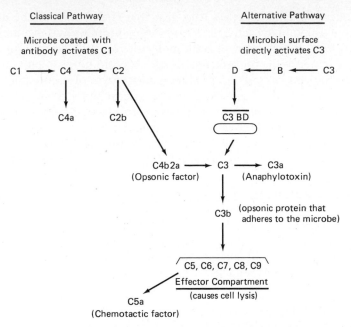

Figure 3.5 In this diagram the two major pathways for activating the complement system are shown, along with the common components that make up the effector compartment. Factors B and D of the alternative pathway are distinct from C1, C4, and C2 of the classical pathway. C3 is common to both pathways. During activation by the classical pathway, C1 binds to the antibody-coated microbe and activates C4 and C2 simultaneously. The C4b,2a complex serves as a C3 convertase to activate C3. In the alternative pathway, C3 binds directly to the microbe's surface as a complex with factor B and is activated. Factor B binds factor D. A complex of factors B, D, and activated C3b is thus generated on the microbe's membrane and converts additional C3. C3b and 34b are opsonic; C3a and 34a are ana-phylatoxins. The components C5 through C9 are activated in numerical order and form a very large complex of factor C9 that is inserted into the microbe's membranes and results in the lysis of the bacterium or other microbe that has entered the body. One of the products of activation of C5 is C5a, a strong chemotactic factor.

proteins, such as the acute phase reactants, including C-reactive protein, may also be constitutive opsonins.

Ingestion

After attachment of an opsonized particle to the phagocyte, the phagocyte will surround the particle by forming pseudopods. The extent to which the phagocyte surrounds the opsonized particle is directly proportional to the extent of opsonization. The pseudopods move along the particle in a zipperlike fashion from one opsonizing molecule to the next until the particle is completely surrounded by pseudopodia which then fuse.

The exact mechanism by which the pseudopods surround the particle is only partially understood. Nonetheless it is clear that the contact of the particle with the phagocyte's membrane activates actin-binding proteins in the cytoplasm. These proteins promote the assembly of actin molecules and the gelation of the actin in the cytoplasm underlying the attachment site. Myosin binds to polymerized actin, and then the molecules contract, producing movement of pseudopods around the particle being engulfed. Orientation of the microfilaments and their points of attachment to the cell membrane determine the form and direction of pseudopodial extension. The pseudopod moves around the particle by a series of reactions initiated by additional membrane–particle contact (Figure 3.4). Once a microbe or other particle is within the cell, it is surrounded by the cell membrane that lines the phagocytic vacuole or phagosome.

For protection to result, it is of course not enough for the phagocyte just to ingest a microbe; it must also kill it. The killed microbe or other ingested particle must then be disposed of. The killing of ingested microbes and the destruction of ingested material is carried out by a variety of mechanisms. The mechanisms by which phagocytic cells kill microorganisms can be classified as either oxygen-dependent or oxygen-independent.

Oxygen-dependent Killing of Microbes

In the oxygen-dependent reactions, adherence of a particle to the phagocyte's surface initiates a series of biochemical changes within the phagocyte that are collectively called *the respiratory burst* (Figure 3.6). The final result of these changes is production of superoxide, singlet oxygen, hydrogen peroxide, and hypochlorite in the phagolysosome; these oxidize proteins and lipids in the microbe, thereby causing its death.

The first event in the series of events that constitute the respiratory burst is the activation of the oxidase that catalyzes the transfer of one or two electrons from NADPH to oxygen and results in the formation of superoxide and hydrogen peroxide. During the course of this reaction, highly reactive oxygen intermediates are formed. These are superoxide ions, peroxide ions, and hydroxyl radicals. Singlet oxygen has two unoccupied electron orbits in its outer valence orbit. It is the reduction of oxygen by the acquisition of electrons in this outer valence orbit that produces the superoxide and peroxide ions. The hydroxyl radicals are formed when the superoxide ions react with hydrogen peroxide.

During the course of the reactions involved in the respiratory burst, oxygen is energized and an atomic rearrangement occurs. As a result of this, the valence electrons move from their normal orbits to orbits at a higher energy state. These energized forms of oxygen are unstable, and when their electrons return to the ground state, energy is released as photons, which can be detected as emitted light. The resulting emitted light, or chemoluminescence, is a sensitive indicator of the occurrence of the respiratory burst.

As noted previously, among the metabolites of oxygen that are known to participate in microbial killing are hydrogen peroxide, which occurs in millimolar concentrations within the phagolysosome, and hypochlorite. Hydrogen peroxide has only moderate antimicrobial activity by itself. The major contribution of hy-

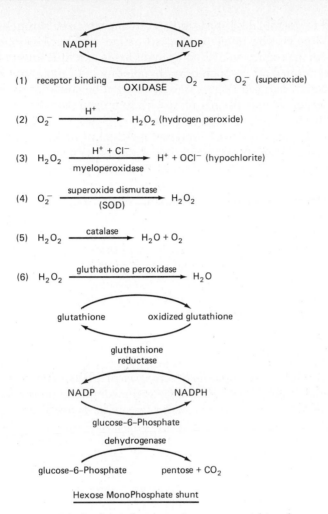

Figure 3.6 O_2-dependent reactions occur within phagocytes during the respiratory burst. The respiratory burst is initiated by binding of an opsonized particle to a phagocyte. This binding may initiate ingestion and activation of an oxidase enzyme, resulting in the production of superoxide within the developing phagosome; NADPH is converted to NADP in this process: (1) the superoxide is converted to hydrogen peroxide (2) within the phagosome by addition of a hydrogen ion. Fusion of lysosomes or granules with the phagosome introduces myeloperoxidase and halides (I_2, Cl_2, or Br_2) into the phagosome (now called a *phagolysosome*). The introduced enzymes and halides produce hypohalite (OCl^-), which will cause halogenation of microbial proteins and lipids and will kill the microbe (3). Reactions 4 through 6 are a mechanism to inactivate any H_2O_2 that may escape from the phagolysosome and thus protect the cell. In (4) superoxide is dismutated to H_2O_2, which is acted on by catalase (5) to form H_2O and O_2. Reaction (6) results in inactivation of H_2O_2 by oxidation of glutathione.

drogen peroxide to microbial killing is indirect. It appears to be through the generation of hypohalites via the myeloperoxidase–halide system. Myeloperoxidase is known to catalyze the reduction by hydrogen peroxide of halide ions to hypohalite. The hypohalites formed are hypochlorite, hypoiodite, and hypobromite, depending on the halide ion reduced (Figure 3.6). These halide compounds may directly affect microorganisms or may further react with hydrogen peroxide to form singlet oxygen, which is also a strong oxidizing agent.

Several mechanisms have been proposed for the killing of bacteria and other microbes by products of the myeloperoxidase–halide–hydrogen peroxidase system. These mechanisms include halogenation of microbial proteins, with subsequent loss of structure and function of the protein; the oxidative decarboxylation of amino acids, with the generation of toxic aldehydes; and the oxidation of thiol groups in enzymes, which may result in inactivation of enzymes that are vital to microbial function.

Oxidation or halogenation of carbon bonds present in unsaturated fats and lipids may also occur. Lipids are essential components of the cell walls and membranes of all cells, including those of bacteria. The oxidation of lipids can lead to alterations in membrane structure and function, and can be as serious to microbial survival as is damage to microbial proteins.

Oxygen-independent Killing of Microbes

The oxygen-independent antimicrobial activities of phagocytes result from the actions of materials from lysosomes and from the components of granules in the phagocyte cytoplasm. Fusion of the phagosome with cytoplasmic granules and lysosomes results in introduction into the phagosome of materials that cause acidification. The result is the lowering of the pH of the phagolysosome containing the microorganisms from neutrality to a pH of from 3.0 to 6.0. Some microorganisms are directly killed by the low pH or by the organic acids in the phagolysosome. The acidification of the phagosome also provides the optimal environment for the action of enzymes such as myeloperoxidase and the acid hydrolases that digest microbes.

Another oxygen-independent antimicrobial mechanism acts through lysozyme. Lysozyme acts by attacking the beta 1–4 glycosidic linkages that join the N-acetyl muramic acid and N-acetyl glucosamine in the bacterial cell wall. In most intact bacteria, these bonds are buried in the cell wall and are not generally accessible to the enzyme. However, the action of a combination of hydrogen peroxide and vitamin C in the acidic environment within the phagolysosome exposes these bonds and facilitates the action of lysozyme.

Many polycationic proteins that have antimicrobial activity have been described. Both large (50,000 daltons) and small polycationic proteins (10,000–25,000 daltons) are present in phagolysosomes. These inhibit respiration and the synthesis of protein, DNA, and RNA, and increase the permeability of bacterial cell membranes. The sensitivity of microorganisms to cationic proteins varies with the microbial species.

Lactoferrin, a protein that occurs in the phagocyte's granules, has a strong affinity for iron. It competes with the microorganisms for iron, a growth requirement of bacteria. Lactoferrin is usually secreted by the neutrophil into the extracellular environment where it acts, and is rarely found in the phagosome.

Destruction of Ingested Microorganisms

The destruction of the microorganisms killed by the various means in the phagocytes and the destruction of other ingested biodegradable material are carried out by enzymes. These enzymes, which are similar to enzymes of the digestive tract, generally are present in the lysosomes of the phagocytes. The fusion of the lysosomes with the phagosomes results in the exposure of the phagocytized material in the vacuole to the enzymes. The fusion of the lysosomes with the phagosome and the subsequent activation of the enzymes only within the phagolysosome protects the phagocyte's cytoplasm from damage by the enzymes. Some of the enzymes may escape from the phagosome through the membrane channel formed when fusion of the pseudopods is occurring, or the enzymes may be liberated as a result of cell death. These extracellular enzymes are probably responsible for the tissue injury that may occur during inflammatory reactions. They may also, as noted previously, activate the fibronectin system.

SUGGESTIONS FOR FURTHER READING

P. Davies, P. J. Bailey, M. M. Goldenberg, and A. W. Ford-Hutchinson. "The role of arachidonic acid oxygenation products in pain and inflammation." Ann. Rev. Immunol. *2:*335, 1984.

S. K. Durum, J. A. Schmidt, and J. J. Oppenheim. "Interleukin 1: An immunological perspective." Ann. Rev. Immunol. *3:*263, 1985.

D. T. Fearon and W. Wong. "Complement ligand receptor interactions that mediate biological responses." Ann. Rev. Immunol. *1:*243, 1983.

R. M. Friedman and S. N. Vogel. "Interferons with special emphasis on the immune system." Adv. Immunol. *34:*97, 1983.

F. A. Kuehl and R. W. Egan. "Prostaglandins, arachidonic acid and inflammation." Science *210:*978, 1980.

G. L. Larsen and P. M. Henson. "Mediators of inflammation." Ann. Rev. Immunol. *1:*335, 1983.

H. Z. Movat. *The Inflammatory Reaction.* Elsevier, Amsterdam, The Netherlands, 1985.

C. W. Parker. Mediators: Release and Function. In *Fundamental Immunology,* W. E. Paul, *ed.* Raven Press, New York, 1984.

B. Samuelson. "Leukotrienes: Mediators of immediate hypersensitivity." Science *220:*568, 1983.

R. Snyderman and M. C. Pike. "Chemoattractant receptors on phagocytic cells." Ann. Rev. Immunol. *2:*257, 1984.

E. R. Unanue and B. Benacerraf. *Textbook of Immunology,* 2nd edition. Williams & Wilkins, Baltimore, 1984.

Chapter 4

The Inflammatory Response

A Bridge between the Constitutive and Inducible Systems

INTRODUCTION

Inflammation is a complex series of events that is a part of the response of all multicellular organisms to the introduction into their tissues of living and nonliving foreign agents. The word *inflame* means literally "to set on fire"; its use here refers to all of the changes that occur during the local and systemic responses to tissue damage. The inflammatory response should be thought of as a protective response; however, it may cause some tissue damage.

Unlike most of the other constitutive host resistance factors, many of those involved in inflammation are inducible. They differ from most of those of the inducible response, however, in not having memory—that is, a second contact with the same inducer does not produce a stronger response than did the first—and, in lacking specificity for particular microorganisms, inflammation provides protection against a variety of organisms, not just the one inducing it.

The initial inflammatory events take place at a local site but may trigger events that cause a systemic response. The initial early response to tissue damage occurs within minutes of injury.

The five cardinal signs of acute inflammation are redness, or erythema; swelling; pain; heat; and loss of function. These signs are caused primarily by processes related to vascular change. Vasodilation causes heat and erythema. Exudation of blood plasma and leukocytes causes swelling. Pressure on nerve endings in swollen tissue and the effects of some prostaglandins cause pain. Loss of function may result from buildup of extravascular fluids and cells at the inflamed site. Function may also be restricted as a result of pain.

Some of the mediators of the inflammatory response participate in specific immune reactions and therefore will be described in more detail in later chapters. The inflammatory reactions help initiate the inducible response and are amplified by it. The inflammatory response, however, has been conserved in its original form in vertebrates of all species. The response itself, by mobilizing leukocytes and bringing plasma to the inflamed site, protects the animal; thus its role is not limited to the initiation of the inducible response.

Although many soluble factors, blood proteins, and cells participate in the inflammatory response, the main purpose of all of the factors is to cause phagocytic leukocytes and blood plasma to leave the circulation and enter the damaged tissue. The phagocytes in the tissue carry out an array of activities at the inflamed site, the central one being phagocytosis to rid the area of microorganisms and damaged tissue and thus to set the stage for healing. The plasma carries opsonins to aid the phagocytes in clearance of microbes, and other substances to aid in repair of tissue. All of the events between the initial damage and the final restoration of the integrity of the tissue may be considered parts of the inflammatory response.

LOCAL INFLAMMATORY EVENTS

Effects of Vasoactive Amines on the Microcirculation in the Inflamed Area

There are dramatic changes in both the microcirculation and the distribution of blood cells at sites of tissue damage. The injury itself elicits a neurological response that, within seconds of injury, causes contraction of smooth muscle in blood vessels and a temporary decrease in blood flow to the area. The injury also causes the release of histamine and serotonin from tissue mast cells, which store these substances in granules. Both histamine and serotonin are amines that have potent effects on smooth muscle. Within minutes of injury, these substances cause the smooth muscle of capillaries and arterioles to relax, resulting in increased blood flow, which causes the wound temperature to increase by 3–5°C and the tissue to become red, which is the first visible sign of inflammation.

Dilation of the capillaries and, especially, the postcapillary venules due to the actions of the vasoactive amines on smooth muscle causes the gaps between the endothelial cells that line the vessels to become enlarged. The enlarged gaps permit leakage not only of plasma, but also of leukocytes. The leukocytes actively emigrate through the openings (Figure 4.1).

Effects of Prostaglandins and Leukotrienes on the Inflamed Area

In addition to the vasoactive amines histamine and serotonin, there are other vasoactive hormones released at the site of an inflammatory response. They include the prostaglandins and leukotrienes. The prostaglandins and leukotrienes are lipid hormones. They are derived from arachidonic acid that is cleaved from the membrane phospholipids by phospholipase A2 (Figure 4.2). The phospholipase is activated by substances that damage cell membranes. After release, the arachidonic acid is oxygenated by one or the other of two enzyme systems. These are the cyclooxygenase system, the actions of which result in the production of the prostaglandins; and the lipooxygenase system, the actions of which result in the production of the leukotrienes. A large number of different prostaglandins have been described. The major prostaglandins produced are PGE1, PGE2, PGE2a, prostacyclin (PG12), and Thromboxane A2. The leukotrienes produced include LTB4, LTC4, LTD4, LTE4, and LTF4.

The prostaglandins were so named because they were originally identified in that portion of human seminal fluid produced by the prostate gland. However, the production of prostaglandins is not limited to reproductive organs. They are produced by most cells, including the phagocytic leukocytes. The leukotrienes derive their name in part from the leukocytes that produce them and in part from their chemical structure, which is that of a triene, that is, a polyunsaturated fat.

One of the important events that occurs during an inflammatory response is the infiltration of leukocytes into the inflamed site. One of the leukotrienes, LTB4, is strongly chemotactic and attracts neutrophils and mononuclear phagocytes. Most of the other leukotrienes are relatively weak chemotactic agents in comparison to LTB4.

Prostaglandins and leukotrienes, together with the vasoactive amines histamine, serotonin, and bradykinin, play an important role in causing the pain characteristic of inflammation. They do this in part by inducing swelling that causes pressure on nerve endings, but they may act directly, also. The vasoactive amines described earlier in this section act synergistically with the prostaglandins to directly induce pain. Whereas prostaglandins of the E series can induce a sensation of pain alone, the prostaglandin PGE2 usually acts together with histamine and bradykinin to intensify the sensation. The prostaglandin acts by sensitizing pain receptors. A combination of various leukotrienes, or prostaglandins alone, also may elicit pain. Pain is an important factor in our response to injury or infection. It

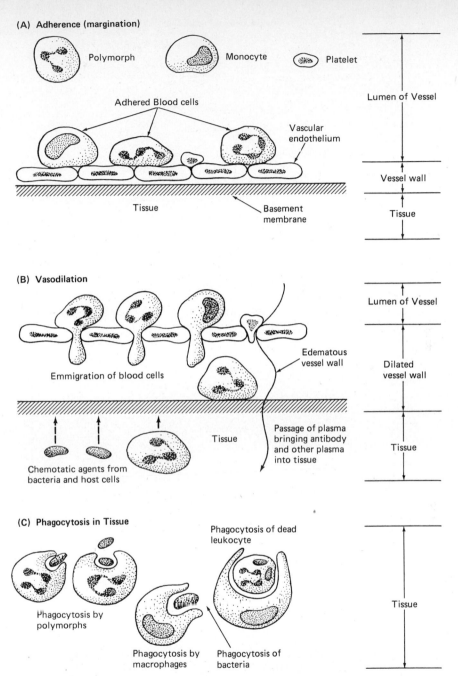

Figure 4.1 Changes within the postcapillary venules at an inflamed site and some of their consequences. (A) Adherence (margination) of platelets, neutrophils, and monocytes to vascular endothelial cells. (B) Vasodilation and increased permeability of vascular walls to leukocytes, and emigration of neutrophils from the blood into the tissue in response to chemotactic agents. (C) Clearance of microorganisms and damaged tissue from the inflamed site by phagocytosis. (Figure reproduced from *Immunology III*, J.A. Bellanti, W. B. Saunders Co., Philadelphia, with permission.)

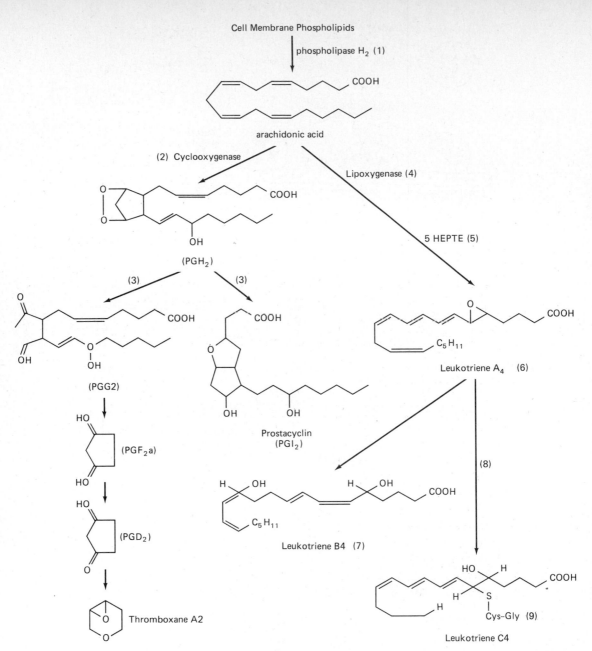

Figure 4.2 An outline of the production of arachidonic acid metabolites from cell membrane phospholipids. The arachidonic acid is released from the membrane by action of phospholipase H_2 (1). When the released arachidonic acid is oxygenated by cyclooxygenase, (2) PGH2 is formed. Prostaglandins PGG2, PGF2a, PGD2, and Thromboxane A2 are formed by enzymatic reactions from PGH2 (3). When the arachidonic acid is oxidized by lipoxygenase (4) 5-HPETE is formed (5). The leukotrienes are derived from 5-HPETE, which serves as the precursor for leukotriene A4 (6). Leukotriene B4 (7) is formed from A4 by a different enzymatic reaction than that which converts A4 to C4 (8). Leukotriene C4 is formed by the addition of glutathione. Leukotriene D4, E4, and F4 are formed by a series of reactions that only affect the amino acid substitution on the -S-Cys residue (9). *Slow-reacting substance-A* is another name for a mixture of leukotrienes C4, D4, and E4.

causes us to protect the painful area and to reduce activities that may aggravate the damage. Without pain, use of the affected part may continue until severe damage occurs.

The synergistic actions of prostaglandins, leukotrienes, and vasoactive amines in the inflamed site not only increase pain, they also affect vascular permeability. The effects on vascular permeability may be different depending on which prostaglandins and leukotrienes are present.

The synergistic interactions between PGE2, PG12, and histamine increase vascular permeability during inflammation. The leukotrienes LTC4 and prostaglandin PGE2, acting jointly, also increase vascular permeability. The leukotrienes LTC4 and LTD4 produce vasoconstriction. The enhancement of permeability by the combined actions of prostaglandins, leukotrienes, and vasoactive amines results in great enhancement of the inflammatory response with increase in infiltration of plasma and leukocytes into the site of tissue damage. The vasoconstriction, on the other hand, reduces the inflammation. As the degree of inflammation produced depends in part on the relative concentration and types of prostaglandins and leukotrienes at the sites of inflammation, these hormones play a significant role in the regulation of the response.

Mediation of Inflammation by Blood Proteins

There are several major blood protein systems that are activated by injury. The activation of these systems results in a cascade of chemical reactions that generate soluble mediators of inflammation. These systems include the kinin system, the complement system, the clotting system, and the fibrinolytic system (Figure 4.3). Each cascade consists of a set of reactions that develop in an ordered sequence. The components of the systems are plasma proteins. Some of the components, when activated, are enzymes and have as their substrates the next component within the series. The purpose of these cascades is to amplify the local response and to initiate events further from the site. The local events include all those already described as characteristic of inflammation: an increase in blood flow to the site of inflammation, the attraction of leukocytes, and an increase in blood vessel permeability (Table 4.1). These systems not only generate products that enhance inflammation, but also generate products that serve as feedback inhibitors to control the extent of activation. This is necessary to prevent the reactions from becoming too extensive.

The mediators of inflammation are all present in the blood plasma in inactive form. The initial event triggering activation is common for the clotting system, the kinin system, and the fibrinolytic system, but not for the complement system. When plasma enters damaged tissue, the first component of these blood-borne systems to be activated is Hageman Factor. Activation results from contact with, and binding to, collagen in the damaged tissue. Collagen is present throughout the body since collagen fibers make up the matrix of the body's tissues.

Hageman Factor is usually described as the first component (Factor XII) of the clotting system, but since activated Hageman Factor (HFa) also initiates the activation of the kinin and the fibrinolytic systems, it could be considered the first component of these systems also.

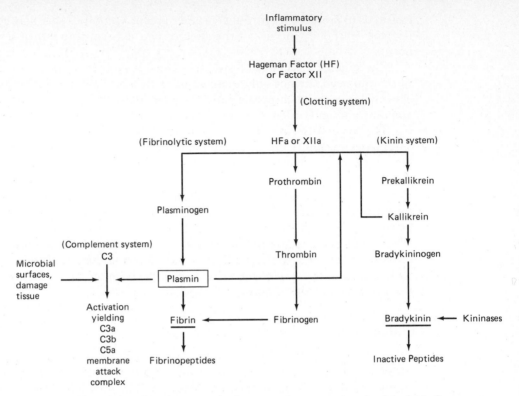

Figure 4.3 The relationships between the four protein systems involved in the inflammatory response. The systems are identified in the parentheses. An *a* after the name identifies an activated factor or product. Only the major reactants are shown. Fibrin and bradykinin are the major products of the clotting and kinin systems. Plasmin is an important product of the fibrinolytic system because it not only lyses fibrin clots but also contributes to activation of the various other systems. The complement system releases chemotactic substances (C3a, C5a), opsonins (C3b, C4b), vasodilators (C2b, C4a, C3a, C5a), and the membrane attack complex (C5-9) that causes lysis of membranes to which it attaches. The clotting system yields fibrin for formation of clots to limit bleeding and stop the spread of infection. When acted on by plasmin of the fibrinolytic system, the clots yield fibrinopeptides that are vasodilators. The kinin system yields bradykinin, which is a vasodilator and is chemotactic, and kininases that inactivate bradykinin.

The clotting cascade that results in the formation of clots consists of a sequence of reactions that convert prothrombin into thrombin, which then converts fibrinogen into fibrin, forming the dense mesh or web of stable fibers characteristic of clots. This fiber web traps platelets and other blood cells and microorganisms, inhibiting bleeding and the spread of microorganisms from the site of injury.

For proper healing to occur, clots must be removed. This is done by enzymatic digestion. An important enzyme in this process is plasmin. Plasmin exists in the plasma in its inactive form, plasminogen. Plasminogen is activated in inflamed tissue by products of the kinin system; it in turn activates the complement system and Hageman Factor.

Table 4.1   IMPORTANT MEDIATORS OF INFLAMMATORY EVENTS THAT ARE GENERATED FROM BLOOD PROTEIN

Mediator	Source	Increased vascular permeability	Chemotactic for phagocytes
Bradykinin	Kinin system	+	+
Kallikrein	Kinin system	−	+
Fibrinopeptides (fibrin split products)	Fibrinolytic system	+	+
C3a	Complement system	+	−
C5a	Complement system	+	+

As noted previously, plasmin is a proteolytic enzyme, one function of which is to lyse clots. Plasmin slowly degrades the fibrin network that is the result of the clotting reaction and thus allows phagocytic cells access to the microbes trapped in the clot, paving the way for replacement of the clot by scar tissue or cells. Some of the products of plasmin digestion of fibrin are short polypeptides called *fibrinopeptides.* These are vasodilators that bring more plasma and leukocytes into the area while the clot is being resolved. When plasmin acts on Hageman Factor, it converts it to a prekallikrein activator. The latter protease converts prekallikrein into kallikrein, which in turn converts the precursor protein kininogen into bradykinin. Bradykinin is an extremely potent vasodilator that is also chemotactic for phagocytic cells and thus further amplifies the reaction. Various kininases are also produced as the inflammatory reaction progresses. These break bradykinin down into inactive peptides and thus control the extent of activation by this pathway (Figure 4.4).

Components of the complement system enter the tissues with the infiltrating plasma. The complement components make up 10 percent of the globulin fraction of the serum. The complement system is a multicomponent system consisting of many enzymes and binding proteins. There are two distinct pathways for activation of the complement system. One is called the *classical pathway* and consists of nine numbered components, of which the first (C1) is triggered by binding to antibody when it is present in an immune complex. The second pathway is the *alternative pathway* that is triggered by the binding of the third component (C3) of complement to a variety of membranes or membrane-bound substances, including carbohydrates on cell walls of some bacteria, by some viruses and by the damaged tissue found at inflammatory sites. As antibody is not generated for several days after infection and is thus not available to form complexes immediately, the complement activation that occurs early in the inflammatory reaction is through the alternative pathway.

Both pathways of complement activation are similar from C3 onward. The alternative pathway invoked as part of the constitutive defense was certainly developed earlier in the evolution of vertebrates than was the classical pathway, which is initiated by antibody and is thus part of the inducible system.

The activation of the complement cascade results in the generation of media-

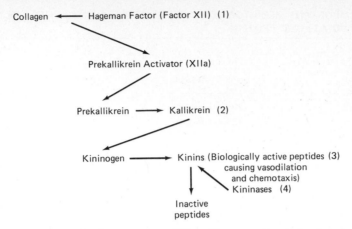

Figure 4.4 The kinin system: When Hageman Factor in the plasma comes in contact with collagen in the tissue, it becomes activated (1). Following a series of subsequent interactions (2) kinins including bradykinin (3) are produced. These hormones are released in the tissues and cause further vasodilation and transvasation of more plasma. The chemotactic characteristics of kinins such as bradykinin cause leukocytes to enter the inflamed tissue. The kininases (4) are enzymes that degrade kinins and thus reduce inflammation. Regulation of inflammation is a result of a shifting balance between production and destruction of the various agents that mediate inflammation.

tors of inflammation, some identical and some distinct from those of other systems (Table 4.2). The system provides a number of proteins that can facilitate the phagocytosis of microbes and thus enhance immunity. The effector compartment of the complement cascade begins with the deposition of C3 onto cell membranes in the form of a split product of C3, designated C3b. When C3b is deposited on the membrane of a microbe, the microbe's susceptibility to ingestion by phagocytic cells is enhanced. The small molecules split from complement components during activation; C4a, C3a, and C5a are all anaphylatoxins, which means they cause the

Table 4.2   BIOLOGICALLY ACTIVE COMPONENTS GENERATED BY ACTIVATION OF THE COMPLEMENT SYSTEM

Complement component	Activity
C2b	Vasodilation
C4a	Causes release of vasodilating amines (anaphylatoxin) from granulocytes
C4b	Opsonization (causes adherence of microbes to leukocytes)
C3a	Causes release of vasoactive amines from granulocytes (anaphylatoxin), induces chemotaxis
C3b	Opsonization (causes adherence of microbes to leukocytes)
C5a	Causes release of vasoactive amines from granulocytes (anaphylatoxin), induces chemotaxis

release of histamine from cells and, as a result, smooth muscle contraction. Histamine, as noted earlier, increases vessel permeability. The small split component of C5, C5a, is a very potent chemotactic factor for polymorphonuclear leukocytes and macrophages. The mechanism whereby the complement components interact and activate each other will be described in detail in the context of activation of complement by immune complexes in Chapter 9.

That the actions of the complement system are important among the protective mechanisms invoked during inflammation is apparent, as individuals lacking complement are more susceptible to infection, particularly by Gram-negative bacteria, and to immune complex disease than are normal people.

The kinin and complement cascades are considered to be more important to host defense than the clotting and fibrinolytic systems. The latter are considered to be more important as homeostatic mechanisms than as host protective mechanisms. One must consider, however, that formation of clots may contribute to host defense by errecting a fibrin barrier to the spread of microbes. This fibrin barrier may be greatly strengthened by subsequent transformation into scar tissue. The actions of fibrinolytic factors such as plasmin may dissolve the clot. Further enzymatic action may result in liquidation of the injured tissue. The liquified material is called *pus* if it contains many infiltrated leukocytes. Pus may be either resorbed or discharged to the outside. If pus formation occurs inside an area walled off by fibrosis, the result is formation of an abscess. Microbes may survive inside an abscess, but at least their effects are then only local. Infection with some microorganisms, such as staphylococci, commonly results in formation of abscesses. Infection with others, such as streptococci, commonly results in a spreading infection with little tendency to abscess formation.

Blood Cell Movement into the Inflamed Area

In the inflamed area, the endothelial linings of the capillaries and venules change under the influence of the various soluble mediators in such a way as to promote the adherence of platelets, polymorphonuclear neutrophils, and monocytes. Platelet adherence to the endothelial lining of the altered capillary or venule is prominent early in the response. Platelet adherence requires thrombin (a clotting system factor) and divalent cations (Mg^{2+}, Ca^{2+}). The first platelets to adhere release adenosine diphosphate, which causes other platelets to attach, aggregate with each other, and release serotonin, histamine, and factors that promote clotting. Clotting takes place both within the vessels and outside of the circulation at the inflamed site. If platelets are depleted from a laboratory animal, the inflammatory response is greatly diminished.

Following platelet aggregation, the number of leukocytes, especially polymorphonuclear leukocytes and monocytes that adhere to the vessel walls, greatly increases. The process of attachment of leukocytes to endothelial cells at sites of inflammation is called *leukocyte margination.* It is rapidly followed by leukocyte emigration out of the small junctures between the endothelial cells. After the passage through the gaps between the endothelial cells, the leukocytes pass through the basement membrane of the vessel to enter the tissue. This entire process requires activity on the part of the monocytes and polymorphonuclear leukocytes since the openings between the endothelial cells are much smaller than the diameter of the leukocytes. The leukocytes move as if with purpose into the inflamed tissue. The direction is provided by the chemotactic factors released in the inflamed tissue. These chemotactic factors are so named because they attract the phagocytic cells. The process of active passage of leukocytes through the vascular walls into tissues is termed *diapedesis.*

Although inflammation may result in tissue destruction, the final result is healing through the formation of new connective tissue. This is accomplished by enzymatic digestion of dead tissue, phagocytic removal of microbes and dead cells, the growth of capillaries into the damaged site, synthesis of collagen by fibroblasts, and regeneration of cells including mucosal and epithelial cells.

SYSTEMIC CONSEQUENCES OF THE INFLAMMATORY REACTION

Induction of Fever

Several important consequences of the inflammatory response are systemic. Fever is one hallmark of the systemic inflammatory response. During the localized inflammatory response, macrophages release a pyrogenic (fever-inducing) substance called *endogenous pyrogen* that acts on the portion of the hypothalamic region of the brain that controls body temperature. Endogenous pyrogen is a hormone or a mixture of hormones, and is very closely related to the macrophage product called *interleukin-1 (IL-1)*, which acts on lymphocytes to augment specific immune responses. IL-1 was one of the first products of macrophages to be shown to augment specific immune responses and to induce fever. IL-6, a more recently described interleukin, is also a component of endogenous pyrogen.

Another group of hormones that are generated during inflammation and induce fever are the prostaglandins discussed earlier. The relationship of prostaglandins to fever was first suspected when it was discovered that fever-reducing drugs such as aspirin inhibit prostaglandin production. Later it was shown that the injection of PGE1 or PGE2 causes fever. Like IL-1, prostaglandins of the E series appear to work through the hypothalamic region of the brain to raise body temperature.

Stimulation of Production of Blood Cells by Colony-stimulating Factor

During an acute inflammatory reaction, in addition to production of Il-1, prostaglandins, leukotrienes, and vasoactive amines, there is greatly increased production of a group of substances, termed *colony-stimulating factor (CSF),* that is required for the production of granulocytes or monocytes from bone marrow precursor cells. The increase in CSF in serum during inflammation presumably initiates production of the polymorphonuclear leukocytes and monocytes needed to replenish losses that occur during the inflammatory response.

Table 4.3 ACUTE PHASE REACTANTS INDUCED BY INFLAMMATION AND THEIR BIOLOGICAL ACTIVITIES

Acute phase reactant	Inflammatory activity
C3	Anaphylatoxin, opsonin
a_1-antitrypsin	Inhibits trypsin and thus reduces tissue damage
a_1-antichymotrypsin	Inhibits chymotrypsin and thus reduces tissue damage
Haptoglobulin	Salvages iron from hemoglobulin
Transferrin	Blocks use of iron by microbes
Fibrinogen	Causes clotting
C-reactive protein	Activates the complement system, opsonin

Induction of Acute Phase Reactants

Within 6 to 12 hours of the initiation of an inflammatory response, there is a marked increase in the synthesis by liver hepatocytes of a group of plasma proteins that are called *acute-phase reactants.* This diverse group of plasma proteins includes some that are substrates of the local inflammatory response (for example, C3 and fibrinogen) and others, such as α 1 antitrypsin, that serve as protease inhibitors to limit tissue damage. C-reactive protein (CRP) is the prototype acute phase reactant of humans and displays Ca^{2+}-dependent binding to some bacteria— for example, pneumococci—and to damaged membranes. The binding of CRP to a bacterium facilitates its phagocytosis by macrophages and polymorphonuclear leukocytes. CRP also activates complement by the classical pathway, but inhibits its activation by the alternative pathway. Since "CRP-like" proteins are widely distributed among both invertebrates and vertebrates, it is probable that these proteins represent the forerunners of the recognition structures that evolved into antibody molecules. Since CRP and some related proteins have been retained by vertebrates through evolution, they must perform a useful function. They probably serve as nonspecific host resistance factors and may also function to aid tissue repair. Table 4.3 lists several acute phase proteins.

SUGGESTIONS FOR FURTHER READING

P. Davies, P. J. Bailey, M. M. Goldenberg, and A. W. Ford-Hutchinson. "The role of arachidonic acid oxygenation products in pain and inflammation." Ann. Rev. Immunology *2:*335, 1984.

C. A. Dinarello and S. M. Wolff. "Molecular basis of fever in humans." Am. J. Med. *72:*799, 1982.

F. A. Kuehl and R. W. Egan. "Prostaglandins, arachidonic acid and inflammation." Science *210:*978, 1980.

I. Kushner, J. E. Volanakis, H. Gewurz. "C-reactive protein and the plasma protein response to tissue injury." Annals N.Y. Acad. Sci. *389:*482, 1982.

G. L. Larsen and P. M. Henson. "Mediators of inflammation." Ann. Rev. Immunol. *1:*335, 1983.

C. W. Parker. Mediators: Release and Function. In *Fundamental Immunology,* W. E. Paul, *ed.* Raven Press, New York, 1984.

B. Samuelson. "Leukotrienes: Mediators of immediate hypersensitivity." Science *220:*568, 1983.

Chapter 5

The Inducible System

History of Development of Immunology as a Component of Host—Parasite Interaction

INTRODUCTION

In the fields of human and veterinary medicine the study of immunology has overshadowed the study of other aspects of host–parasite interaction. This is certainly the result of the dramatic accomplishments in disease prevention and treatment that resulted from the manipulation of the immune systems of humans and domestic animals with vaccines and immune serum.

IMMUNIZATION

One of the earliest procedures of immunization used was variolation. This procedure involved the deliberate inoculation of people with material from persons with mild cases of smallpox. The objective was to induce mild disease and, as a result, immunity. Variolation was probably developed in China and was based on the observation that people who had recovered from even a mild case of smallpox were seldom infected a second time. The procedure was introduced into England from Turkey by Lady Montague in 1718. This dangerous procedure was replaced in 1796 by Jenner, who substituted infection with the very mildly pathogenic cowpox virus for immunization against smallpox.

With the identification of pathogenic bacteria as causative agents of specific diseases in the 1880s by Louis Pasteur in France and Robert Koch in Germany, the stage was set for the rational development of immunization procedures. Quite soon after the identification and isolation of pathogenic organisms, attempts were made to use them to develop vaccines against infectious diseases. Pasteur, in particular, worked on use of the isolated organisms to induce immunity. He recognized that identification and isolation of causal pathogens were absolutely necessary if prophylactic immunization was to be possible; he further recognized the necessity of selecting nonpathogenic or weakly pathogenic strains of the pathogens for use as safe immunizing agents. Such nonpathogenic but immunogenic varieties of pathogenic microorganisms are today said to be *attenuated.* Pasteur successfully immunized chickens against chicken cholera in 1880 with living but nonpathogenic microorganisms. Pasteur also developed attenuated varieties of pathogens for use as vaccines against anthrax (1881) and rabies (1885).

Pasteur recognized that the induction of immunity by infection with attenuated pathogens was a process similar to that used by Jenner when he immunized against smallpox by infecting with cowpox. In Latin the word for cow is *vacca,* and thus Pasteur called the process *vaccination* in honor of Jenner's achievement.

Not all of the early attempts to immunize against disease were successful. Robert Koch proved in 1882 that the tubercle bacillus (*Mycobacterium tuberculosis*) was the etiologic agent of tuberculosis. He attempted to immunize with material from cultures of the organism. The material he injected was spent medium from cultures of human tubercle bacilli. No immunity resulted from the injection, but a febrile reaction and swelling at the site of injection occurred 24 to 48 hours later in people harboring the tubercle bacillus.

This reaction was later shown to be diagnostic for tuberculosis and is now widely used as a diagnostic aid. The type of material Koch used is now called *old tuberculin*. Today we use an extract of old tuberculin called *purified protein derivative (PPD)* to test for tuberculosis. In Koch's honor the diagnostic reaction is called the *Koch phenomenon*. Later attempts to immunize against tuberculosis using attenuated strains of the organism such as the Bacillus of Calmette-Guerin (BCG) have met with little success. Thus the problem was not that Koch used a nonliving preparation as the immunogen, but rather resided in the nature of immunity to tuberculosis.

THE NATURE OF INDUCIBLE IMMUNITY

Once it had been demonstrated that immunity could be induced by infection, many scientists became interested in determining how hosts controlled infection and how immunity was generated. Some scientists believed that immunity was largely cell based, whereas others considered humoral factors to be of prime importance. Our present understanding of the basis of immunity is summarized in Table 5.1.

The Russian zoologist Eli Metchnikoff, in particular, made important contributions to our understanding of how hosts control infection. He was a strong advocate of the cellular theory of immunity. He suggested as early as 1884 that leukocytes, through their phagocytic abilities, played a major role in disease resistance. He made this claim on the basis of his experiments with starfish larvae, in which he observed phagocytic cells surrounding splinters that he had introduced into the almost transparent bodies of the animals. Pasteur invited Metchnikoff to the Pasteur Institute in Paris, where for the next 28 years he worked to verify his cellular theory of immunity.

The field of cellular immunology has developed and changed since Metchni-

Table 5.1   CLASSIFICATION OF DEFENSE REACTIONS

Effector mechanism[a]	Type of response	Outcome of defense response
Cellular	Engulfment	Uptake of foreign material (phagocytosis)
	Cytotoxic	Destruction of infected cells or nonself cells by contact
Humoral	Agglutination	Clumping of organisms and phagocytosis
	Precipitation	Clumping of soluble molecules and phagocytosis
	Neutralization	Inactivation of toxins
		Blocking of infection by viruses and other intracellular parasites
	Complement fixation	Lysis of parasites
		Phagocytosis of parasites

[a]Some cellular and some humoral responses are noninducible and some are inducible. if noninducible, there is no increase in the factor following exposure to antigen; if inducible, there is increase.

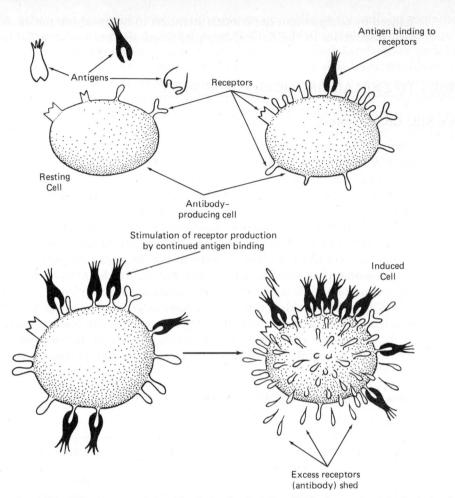

Antigen binding to receptors

Antigens — Receptors

Resting Cell

Antibody-producing cell

Stimulation of receptor production by continued antigen binding

Induced Cell

Excess receptors (antibody) shed

Figure 5.1 Illustration of the side-chain theory of antibody formation based on the drawings in the original paper by Paul Ehrlich (1897). The antigen (toxin) binds to the side-chain (receptor) that is specific for it and is located on the cell surface. The binding was thought to prevent the normal physiological function of the receptor, resulting in the overproduction of the receptors which in turn are released as antibody into the blood. The theory correctly predicted the binding of antigen to the antibody-like receptors on lymphocytes.

cepted clonal selection theory of antibody formation by 60 years and is largely compatible with it.

At the turn of the century there were thus two opposing theories to explain how hosts controlled infection and developed immunity. The respective adherents of each theory gathered experimental data to support their viewpoints. In 1908 the Nobel prize in medicine was jointly awarded to Metchnikoff and Ehrlich in recognition of their contributions to our understanding of host defense against infection. The joint award shows clearly the early recognition that the cellular and humoral components of the immune response are simply separate manifestations of one system.

The Clonal Selection Theory

The studies by Ehrlich and others demonstrated that infection resulted in production of a serum factor, called by Ehrlich *antibody*, which increased the ability of a host to control infection. As it was recognized that biological molecules are produced by cells, interest was generated in the cellular basis of antibody synthesis. The cells secreting antibody have only recently been identified, however. Early studies indicated that antibody-synthesizing cells were found in the lymph nodes and spleens of immunized animals, but whether they were Metchnikoff's phagocytes or lymphocytes, another cell type prominent in those tissues, was not determined. Attempts to induce antibody synthesis *in vitro* by culturing lymphocytes with antigen were mostly unsuccessful until the mid-1960s. Progress in this area until 1960 was best summarized on page 86 by Sidney Raffel in his text, *Immunity:*

> Cells of the reticuloendothelial system are probably not involved in the process–this despite the fact that they come very naturally to the minds of immunologists as possible antibody producers because of their propensity for taking up foreign substances introduced into the body. Lymphocytes have a better claim to some role in the process of antibody formation, if not the central one of actual synthesis. If this turns out to be a valid conclusion, it would be doubly welcome, first for clarifying the mystery of antibody origin and second for answering the question as to what useful purpose these ubiquitous cells serve.

In the 10 years after 1960 it was shown that some types of lymphocytes were indeed the cells that synthesized antibody. In addition, other classes of lymphocytes, which contribute to the development of immunity in other ways, were identified.

The realization that a variety of types of lymphocytes contribute to the immune response was derived from experiments that indicated that lymphocytes from both the bone marrow and the thymus were required for antibody synthesis. Additional experiments indicated that macrophages were also required to initiate antibody production, but did not themselves produce it.

By the end of the 1960s it was accepted that some types of lymphocytes differentiated into plasma cells, which are the cells that secrete antibody. However, there was no satisfactory answer to the question of how these cells could make antibody against the vast array of antigenic determinants to which the system responded. Most antigens are complex and have many determinants. A *determinant* (or *epitope*) is the site on an antigen to which antibody binds. The nature of antigens is described in Chapter 6. The immune response may be directed toward one or all of the determinants.

On the basis of ideas described by Jerne as early as 1955, both Burnet and Talmadge in 1957 separately proposed the clonal selection theory. This theory states that an immunocompetent organism contains many different clones of lymphocytes, with each clone derived from a single parent cell. They further proposed that the lymphocytes that comprise a clone each display receptors for a single antigenic determinant. These cells, once triggered by the binding to their receptor of the appropriate determinant, increase in numbers and then produce antibody with the same specificity as the receptor (Figure 5.2).

The clonal selection theory thus simply states that the antigen induces proliferation of a subset of preexisting lymphocytes from among the lymphocytes in the organism. The cells of the clone that is induced not only bind the antigen, but increase in numbers and produce antibody to the antigen. The differentiation of the lymphocyte into an antibody-producing cell is the result of interaction with

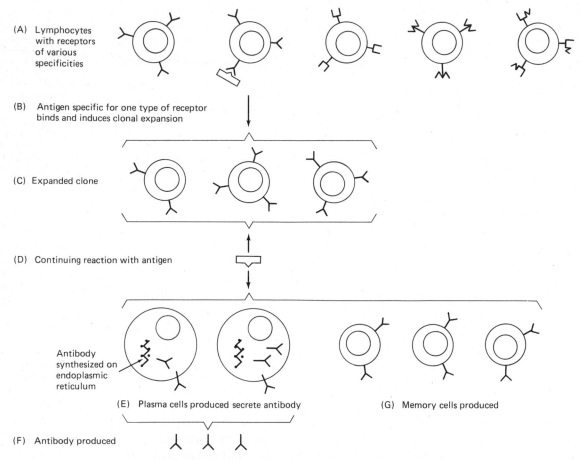

(A) Lymphocytes with receptors of various specificities

(B) Antigen specific for one type of receptor binds and induces clonal expansion

(C) Expanded clone

(D) Continuing reaction with antigen

Antibody synthesized on endoplasmic reticulum

(E) Plasma cells produced secrete antibody

(G) Memory cells produced

(F) Antibody produced

Figure 5.2 The clonal selection theory of antibody production. A pool of lymphocytes having receptors for various antigens exist in the body (A). Antigen specific for one type of receptor (B) induces expansion of clones of lymphocytes with appropriate receptors (C). The continuing action of antigen (D) induces production of plasma cells that are rich in endoplasmic reticulum (E) and will secrete antibody (F), and produce memory cells (G) ready to respond if the antigen is encountered again.

many other cells; however, the initial event is the binding of a particular antigen to the appropriate lymphocyte (Figure 5.3). This scenario is similar to that proposed in Ehrlich's side-chain theory.

As evidence indicating that lymphocytes are not all of one class was obtained and it was discovered that some lymphocytes mature in the thymus and others in the bone marrow, the clonal selection theory was extended. Burnet, in particular, continued to develop the clonal selection theory. He proposed that the various clones were developed during the fetal period and that their production was the

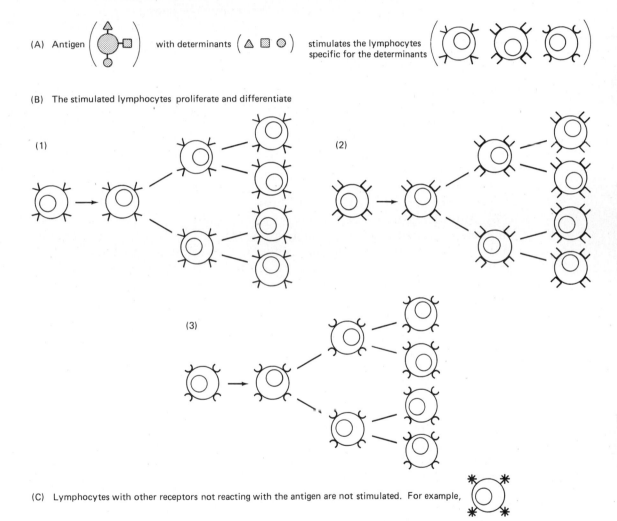

Figure 5.3 The selection of lymphocyte clones by antigenic determinants on an antigen. The distinct determinants (A) each stimulate clones with receptors for just one of the determinants (B). The response eventually results in the elaboration of polyclonal antibody to the antigen that can be recovered from the serum of the organism. The unselected clones (C) remain dormant within the lymphoid tissues.

result of somatic mutation. He also proposed that clones with specificity for self-antigens were developed but were deleted. In fact, Burnet and others had already shown that tolerance to nonself antigens could be induced by exposing the fetus to the antigen. Upon maturation, the immune system failed to respond to the foreign antigen. At present a variety of explanations are offered for self-tolerance, including deletion of clones capable of responding to self and suppression of self-clones by suppressor T-cells.

Since it had been demonstrated that a variety of cell types are involved in the immune response, further progress required an examination of the contributions of each cell type to the development of the immune response.

SELF-RECOGNITION IN IMMUNOLOGY

The introduction of the concept that antigen is recognized in the context of self-recognition was a further advance in the clonal selection theory. It is now known that the response to an antigen begins when an appropriate thymic lymphocyte encounters the antigen on the surface of an antigen-presenting cell. The antigen receptor on the thymic lymphocyte recognizes foreign antigen only in the context of a simultaneous recognition of self-antigens. The self-antigens that must be present for an antigen to be recognized are membrane proteins of the Ia group and are coded by the genes of the major histocompatibility complex (MHC) (Figure 5.4). Antigen recognition is restricted by self-recognition both for initiation of an immune response by helper T-lymphocytes and for that portion of the effector phase of the immune response that is mediated by cytolytic lymphocytes. Graft rejection is an exception to the rule that foreign antigens are recognized by T-cytolytic lymphocytes only with simultaneous recognition of self–MHC antigen. Individuals will reject grafts that have only nonself–MHC antigens.

The most dramatic demonstration that foreign antigens are only recognized if there is also self-recognition is the observation that cytolytic lymphocytes from mice immunized with a virus only recognize viral antigens expressed on the surfaces of cells from mice of the same inbred strain. This limitation on recognition is referred to as *MHC restriction.*

The reason for self-recognition along with recognition of nonself is not obvious. However, the MHC gene products that restrict antigen recognition by helper lymphocytes are different from the products that restrict antigen recognition by cytolytic lymphocytes. One function of the system therefore may be to prevent cytolytic lymphocytes from destroying the antigen that is displayed on cells required for initiation of the immune response.

GENETICS OF THE IMMUNE RESPONSE

The clonal selection theory states that antibody specificity is genetically determined. The period of 1976–1982 saw the partial resolution of the problem of how an animal can maintain in its genome the huge repertoire of genes that are required

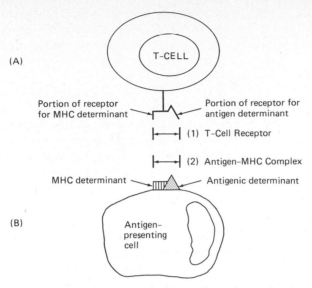

Figure 5.4 T-cell recognition of antigen only occurs when the antigen is associated with the Ia molecules coded for by the major histocompatibility complex (MHC). This type of recognition is called *associative recognition*. The T cell has a receptor (1) complementary to the complexed MHC determinant and the antigenic determinant (2).

to program recognition of all the antigen specificities that the system recognizes. Scientists in several laboratories have used the analytical techniques of molecular genetics to show that with gene recombination and somatic mutation during development, the number of genes available—probably more than 10^7—is sufficient to permit development of the multitude of clones of lymphocytes necessary for the recognition of the many specificities that are, in fact, recognized.

HORMONAL SUBSTANCES INDUCED IN IMMUNITY

Among the more exciting discoveries of recent years has been the discovery that lymphocytes that have bound antigen produce polypeptides that act on nearby cells. Macrophages that contact antigen have also been shown to be capable of producing such substances. These substances are called *interleukins* because they carry signals between leukocytes; they have been shown to be differentiation factors. Interleukin-1, a macrophage product, induces differentiation of antigen-responding T-cells so that they can respond to interleukin-2 by dividing. Interleukin-2 and interleukin-3, which are both produced by thymus-derived lymphocytes, act as growth factors for many types of stem cells, including those for other thymus-derived lymphocytes. Other products of thymus-derived lymphocytes facilitate the differentiation of bone marrow–derived lymphocytes into antibody-secreting cells. The major factors that were identified in this latter group were B-cell growth factor (BCGF) and T-cell replacing factor (TRF). They were collectively called *B-cell stimulating factors (BSF)* by their discoverers. Such discoveries brought the studies of host–parasite interaction and cell biology together.

IMMUNOCHEMISTRY

One of the greatest contributions of immunochemistry to our understanding of the role of inducible immunity in host–parasite interaction in vertebrates was the elucidation of the nature of antibody. Despite studies that demonstrated antibody function as early as the 1800s, it was not until 1929 that Tiselius and Kabat found that all antibody activity was confined to the gamma-globulin fraction of serum. This led to the realization that antibody is gamma globulin. We now use the hybrid term *immunoglobulin (Ig)* as the official designation for antibody molecules.

Once it had been determined that antibody molecules are globulins, the question remained as to how antibody specificity was carried by these molecules. Studies of the nature of the globulin molecule were needed. By 1960 several biochemists had unraveled the amino acid sequence and polypeptide structure of human antibody molecules and shown that antibody specificity was determined by the amino acid sequence in the antibody receptor region. This observation put to rest permanently the instructive theories of antibody formation that proposed that antigens somehow determined folding of the polypeptide antibody molecule and in this way determined antibody specificity.

The development of immunochemistry contributed to the development of the understanding of immunology in other ways, too. It put immunology on a firm experimental basis through the development of methods for quantitating antigens and antibodies. Experimentation at the Rockefeller Institute in the 1930s led to development of quantitative precipitation methods for measuring antigen and antibody, and to the discovery that carbohydrates of bacteria may be antigenic. At the same time, scientists at the Rockefeller Institute discovered how antigen and antibody react to form insoluble complexes.

Karl Landsteiner, a founder of the science of immunochemistry, discovered the human AB0 blood cell antigens in the 1930s. Beginning in 1917, Landsteiner and his students investigated antibody specificity. They determined that antibodies could distinguish between structurally similar organic compounds. They found that antibodies to small nonantigenic organic compounds could be generated if the nonantigenic compounds were attached to large protein molecules that they called *carrier molecules.* The small compounds they studied were called *haptens* by Landsteiner. Many important principles of immunological specificity were established by Landsteiner and his students using these *hapten-carrier* conjugates as antigens.

As a result of these developments, the study of the immunological aspects of the host–parasite interaction now has a firm biochemical, genetic, and cellular base. We know perhaps more about the nature of the immunological changes induced in vertebrates by infection than we do of the mechanisms controlling host–parasite interaction in the nonimmune host, but even in this area our understanding of host–parasite interactions is expanding rapidly.

SUGGESTIONS FOR FURTHER READING

W. Bulloch. *The History of Bacteriology.* Oxford University Press, London, 1938.

F. MacFarlane Burnet. *The Clonal Selection Theory of Acquired Immunity (Books One and Two Combined).* The University Press, Cambridge, England, 1969.

P. Ehrlich. *Collected Papers of Paul Ehrlich, Vol. 2.* Pergamon Press, New York, 1957.

K. Landsteiner. *The Specificity of Serological Reactions.* Harvard University Press, Boston, 1945.

E. Metchnikoff. *Immunity in the Infectious Diseases.* Macmillan, New York, 1905.

S. Raffel. *Immunity,* 2nd ed. Appleton-Century-Crofts, New York, 1961, page 86.

A. M. Silverstein. "Cellular vs. humoral immunity: Determinants and consequences of an epic 19th century battle." Cell. Immunol. *48:*208, 1979.

A. M. Silverstein. "Development of the concept of immunologic specificity." Cell. Immunol. *67:*396; *71:*183, 1982.

A. M. Silverstein. The History of Immunology. In *Fundamental Immunology,* W. E. Paul, *ed.* Raven Press, New York, 1984.

A. M. Silverstein and A. A. Bialasiewicz. "A history of theories of acquired immunity." Cell. Immunol. *51:*151, 1980.

A. M. Silverstein and G. Miller. "The royal experiment on immunity: 1721–1722." Cell. Immunol. *61:*437, 1981.

Chapter 6

The Inducible Defense System

Antigens

INTRODUCTION

The word *antigen* was coined from the words *antibody* and *generator.* Thus an antigen was originally considered to be a substance that induces production of antibody. In practice, immunologists have defined an antigen as a substance that induces an immunological response in an immunocompetent animal and that can be shown to react with the products produced by the immunocompetent animal in some detectable way. This definition broadens the meaning of the word to accommodate the nonantibody-mediated immune reactions that are induced by antigens.

An antigen is thus defined in terms of what it does. The definition says nothing about what an antigen is. Our present knowledge of what antigens are is derived from the study of the characteristics of substances shown to be antigenic by their introduction into immunocompetent animals. Analysis of materials that induce an immune response has shown most of them to be proteins or complex carbohydrates; lipids and nucleic acids may also be antigens when associated with proteins. As all living systems are made up largely of proteins, carbohydrates, lipids, and nucleic acids, most of the components of living systems can be shown to be antigens by being injected into some animal.

An *antigenic determinant* is the region of an antigenic molecule that fits into the combining site of an antibody or a T-cell receptor. The word *determinant* is usually used synonymously with the term *epitope.* The term *epitope,* however, is more commonly used when the determinant is defined by a monoclonal antibody. The word is also commonly used to refer to the antigenic site on the surface of the native molecule. Complex molecules such as proteins often have many determinants. The portion of the antigenic determinant that governs the specificity of the antigen is termed *immunodominant.* Most haptens are immunodominant.

Antigenic determinants are relatively small portions of a larger molecule and do not induce antibody formation by themselves. They do act as haptens. The size of a determinant corresponds to the size of a combining site on an antibody molecule: for proteins it is from 6 to 10 amino acids; for polysaccharides it is about 5 sugars.

Some immunologists prefer the terms *immunogen* and *immunogenicity* to *antigen* and *antigenicity.*

CHARACTERISTICS OF ANTIGENS

As an antigen is any injected material that will induce an immunological response in an immunocompetent animal and can be shown to react with the products of that response in some detectable way, a description of the characteristics of antigens is in a sense a summary of characteristics shared by a fairly heterogeneous population of substances.

A list of the characteristics of antigens usually includes the statement that they are foreign to the animal in which they are antigenic. In addition, substances that are antigenic are biodegradable and are complex, which usually requires them to be of high molecular weight.

Foreignness

An important function of the immunological system of vertebrate animals is to protect the animal from infection. Infection can be considered to be the invasion of the body of the animal by another living agent. The objective of the invasion and occupation from the standpoint of the invader is the utilization of the resources of the invaded animal, or host. To survive, the invaded or, to use the medical term, *infected* animal must prevent the injury to itself that could result from the invasion of its body and the utilization of its resources. To protect itself, the host must be able to recognize and destroy the invader or, if it cannot destroy it totally, it must at least limit its growth and spread through the body.

Vertebrates are large, complex, multicellular animals. They can in a sense be considered colonies of cells, the individual cells of which are highly integrated and tightly controlled. A defense against an invader can only be made if the system can distinguish the invader from itself. The ability to distinguish between self and the invader and then to take action against the foreign agent is the measure of immunocompetence.

Because parasites are constructed of proteins, lipids, carbohydrates, and nucleic acids as are their hosts, recognition by the host of the parasite and its products as foreign depends upon recognition of fine points of difference between the molecules of the parasite and the host.

Self-recognition or, perhaps, failure of the immunological system to respond to self is programmed into the system as the fetus develops. For the present discussion, it is sufficient to realize that for a molecule to be immunogenic, it must differ in some respect from all the molecules of the immunocompetent animal into which it is introduced. Thus a molecule is not normally an antigen to the animal from which it is derived, but may be an antigen in some other animal.

In general, the more distantly related the species are, the more differences their molecules will have and the more strongly they will react to introduction of molecules of the other species.

It is a fact, however, that tissues cannot be freely transferred from one member of a species to another member of the same species. Molecules of one individual of a species that are antigenic in another member of the same species are called *isophile antigens,* or *isoantigens.* A well-studied example of such antigens is the blood group system. The histocompatibility system, of which the blood group system is a special case, prevents ready transfer of organs such as hearts, kidneys, and skin among individuals of the same species.

A moment's reflection makes it obvious that histocompatibility did not arise to prevent tissue transfer among members of the same species. The development and maintenance of the complex histocompatibility system is almost certainly a result of selection for ability to control infection. Histocompatibility is determined by histocompatibility molecules present in the membranes of cells of animals. The system that controls tissue transfers in mice is called the *major histocompatibility complex (MHC).* In humans, immune responses to leukocytes in blood given during therapeutic transfusions provided a means to study histocompatibility. Thus, the analogous system in humans is called the *human leukocyte antigen (HLA) system.*

The presence of a number of genes, each of which has a number of alleles that are reassorted during sexual reproduction, assures a unique histocompatibility display in each individual of the species (see Chapter 11). Because this system assures that each individual has a unique pattern of "self" markers determined by random segregation during gamete production and fusion, no parasite can evolve a molecular configuration identical to the histocompatibility display of all individuals of the species and thus evade recognition as foreign by all members of the species.

Although in general it is true that immunocompetent individuals do not respond to their own components, it is unfortunately not always true. It is to be expected that a complex system will sometimes fail. Response to self is called *autoimmunity,* and the self materials to which the response occurs are called *autoantigens.* Chapters 10 and 11 are specifically concerned with autoimmunity and histocompatibility.

Some self materials to which an individual may respond are developed in isolation during embryogenesis. Once produced, they do not normally break down and leave their sites of synthesis during the life of the individual. The lens of the eye and much brain tissue are in this category. If as a result of injury molecules are released from such normally sequestered organs, they may be treated as foreign because the immune system did not encounter them during the time when self-recognition was developed.

Slightly altered self molecules may also be treated as foreign. The subsequent response may produce products that react with the unaltered molecules as well as with the altered ones. Drugs given for therapy may initiate autoimmune responses by this mechanism. Blackwater fever, an autoimmune response to one's own red cells in persons repeatedly infected with malaria and treated with quinine, is such a condition.

Some microorganisms may produce molecules similar to those of the host but sufficiently different to be treated as foreign. Here, too, the products of the immune response may react with the related host molecules. Rheumatic fever is probably initiated by infection with streptococci. The autoimmune reaction against heart and joint tissue that follows is a result of the similarity of molecules in the parasite to those in the tissue.

Failure of the regulatory systems of the immunological response may also occur, resulting in severe autoimmune disorders.

Biodegradability

As noted earlier, the immune system is a major system for protection against infection in vertebrate animals. Phagocytosis and digestion of the invading organisms were developed early in the evolution of multicellular animals as a defense against infection. The more sophisticated systems of higher vertebrates are built on the earlier systems and are shaped by their nature. Nonbiodegradable materials may be walled off and isolated by a connective tissue capsule that forms around them and by calcification of the enclosing wall of connective tissue; however, the phagocytes cannot process indigestible materials and initiate an immune response with them. The requirement for biodegradability is a result of the fact that the antigen-presenting cells, which are responsible for initiation of most immune responses, can only initiate the induced immune response if they can present partially digested fragments of the antigenic molecules to other cells involved in the system. A few antigens called *T-independent antigens* do not require processing by antigen-presenting cells, but these are few in number and represent a special case.

Complexity and Molecular Weight

It is clear from empirical observation that molecules must be fairly large and complex to be immunogenic. One of the smallest proteins shown to be immunogenic in rabbits is human glucagon. It has a molecular weight of 3500 daltons and is a straight chain polypeptide containing 29 amino acids.

Insulin has a molecular weight of approximately 5700 daltons and contains 51 amino acids. Porcine insulin, which differs from human insulin in only 3 amino acids, will sometimes cause an immunologic response in humans to whom it may be given as part of the therapy for diabetes. This problem can be avoided by use of human insulin produced by genetically modified bacteria. Human insulin is identical in all humans and is thus treated as self by all humans.

THE HAPTEN-CARRIER CONCEPT

Karl Landsteiner (1868–1943), an immunochemist best known for his studies of blood groups in humans, advanced our understanding of antigens and antigenicity by developing the hapten-carrier concept. Landsteiner developed this concept from his studies of immune responses to proteins to which various chemical groups (called *haptens*) were attached. He called the protein molecules *carriers.* Arsanilic acid and dinitrophenol were typical of the haptens he used. Then, as now, bovine or equine albumin was a commonly used carrier, and the rabbit was the animal immunized. The structures of these haptens and the modes of their attachment are shown in Figure 6.1.

The immunization of a rabbit with equine albumin to which dinitrophenol is attached results in the production of antibodies specific for dinitrophenol and for various regions of the albumin molecule. There may be some antibodies with specificity for the region of attachment of the hapten to the carrier, also. Absorption of the immune serum with the carrier molecule similarly linked to a different hapten will remove the antibodies specific for the carrier and the attachment site. The remaining antibodies are specific for the hapten and can then be studied.

It has been determined that antibodies specific for virtually any relatively small molecule can be produced if they are attached to a suitable carrier molecule.

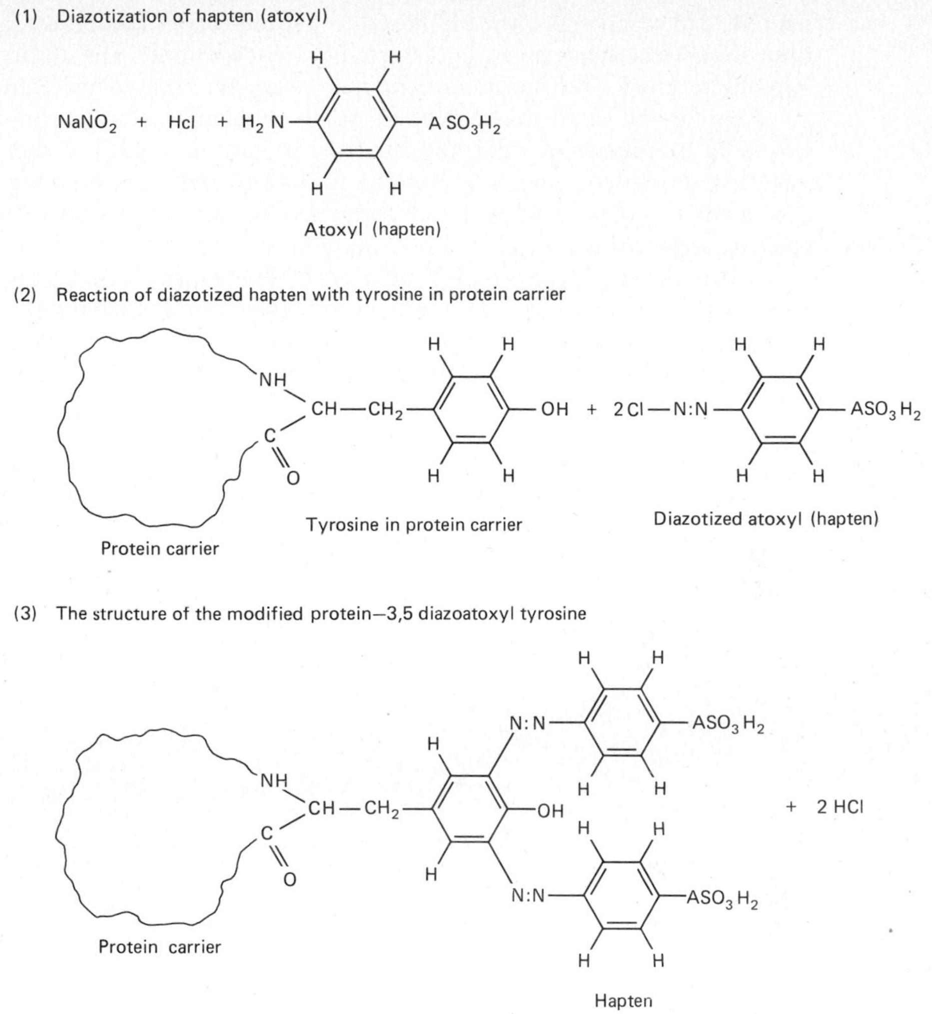

(1) Diazotization of hapten (atoxyl)

$$NaNO_2 \;+\; Hcl \;+\; H_2N \text{—} \text{[benzene ring with H, H top; H, H bottom]} \text{—} ASO_3H_2$$

Atoxyl (hapten)

(2) Reaction of diazotized hapten with tyrosine in protein carrier

Protein carrier   Tyrosine in protein carrier   Diazotized atoxyl (hapten)

$$\cdots NH\text{—}CH\text{—}CH_2\text{—}\text{[ring]}\text{—}OH \;+\; 2\,Cl\text{—}N{:}N\text{—}\text{[ring]}\text{—}ASO_3H_2$$

(3) The structure of the modified protein—3,5 diazoatoxyl tyrosine

Protein carrier   Hapten   + 2 HCl

$$N{:}N\text{—}\text{[ring]}\text{—}ASO_3H_2$$

$$N{:}N\text{—}\text{[ring]}\text{—}ASO_3H_2$$

Figure 6.1 A common method of attaching haptens to a carrier molecule is by diazotization. In this process the hapten is first modified by reaction with $NaNO_2$ in HCl (1). As a result a reactive diazo group replaces an NH_2 group on the hapten. The diazotized hapten is then allowed to react with an appropriate protein. The diazotized hapten reacts with the aromatic ring of any tyrosines in the protein (2), yielding the modified protein (3).

Antibodies raised in this way are used today for detection and quantification of many hormones and drugs.

Antibodies to a hapten will bind to the hapten, but as free haptens will have just one antibody-combining site, no cross linking and thus no visible reaction will occur. The combining sites of the antibodies will, however, be blocked, and the antibodies will not be able to react with haptens on a carrier molecule. Thus haptens can react with antibody raised to hapten-carrier complexes, and the reaction of the free hapten can be detected by, for example, the ability of the free haptens to block precipitation of the hapten-carrier complexes (Figure 6.2).

Haptens, as noted previously, are small molecules; they are too small to be antigenic in their own right and, in fact, it may be readily demonstrated that injection of haptens does not normally induce an immune response. A hapten is thus a small molecule incapable of inducing an immune response but capable of reacting with antibody induced by injection of a hapten-carrier complex.

It may be that there is no real difference between an aromatic ring attached to a protein by a chemist, for example, and the same aromatic ring that is a part of an amino acid. Thus any site on an antigen to which an antibody reacts may be considered a haptenic site. The term *epitope* may be used to refer to a specific

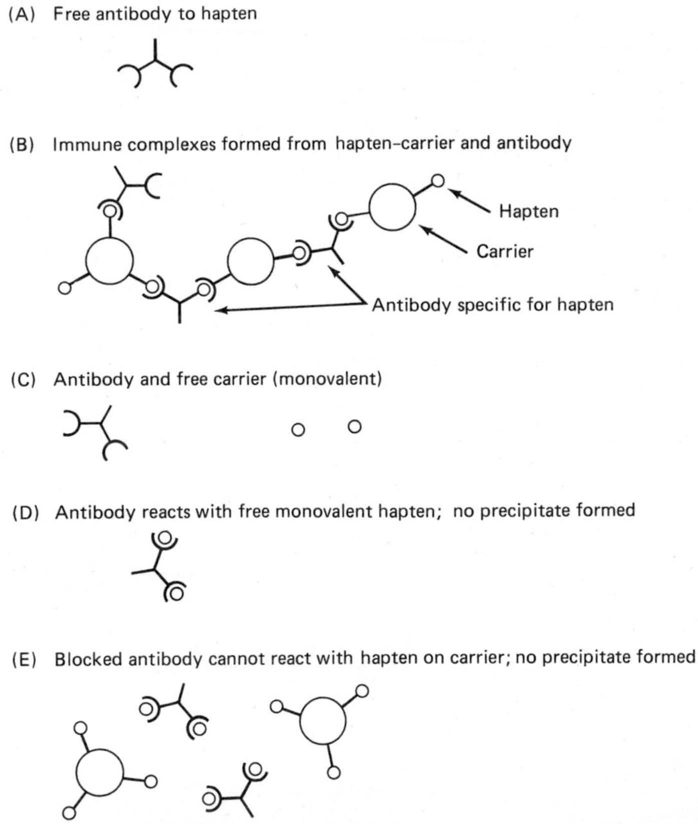

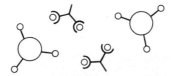

(A) Free antibody to hapten

(B) Immune complexes formed from hapten–carrier and antibody

Hapten

Carrier

Antibody specific for hapten

(C) Antibody and free carrier (monovalent)

(D) Antibody reacts with free monovalent hapten; no precipitate formed

(E) Blocked antibody cannot react with hapten on carrier; no precipitate formed

Figure 6.2 The reaction of haptens with antibody can be detected by using free haptens to block the reaction of the antibody with the hapten-carrier complex. Antibody (A) to the hapten will react with the hapten-carrier complex to form a lattice, yielding a visible precipitate (B). If the antibody first reacts with free monovalent carrier molecules (C), then the reactive sites on the antibody are filled (D) and the antibody cannot react with the multivalent hapten-carrier to produce a visible precipitate.

portion of an antigenic molecule recognized by an antibody or T-cell receptor, regardless of whether it is an intrinsic part of the molecule or was added by a chemist in a laboratory.

SITES ON ANTIGENS RECOGNIZED BY THE PRODUCTS OF THE IMMUNE RESPONSE

Landsteiner's studies of haptens and carriers led to the realization that antibodies react with small portions of the antigen and permit estimates of the size of the reactive sites and their nature.

The sites that are recognized (that is, the epitopes) may be conformational or sequential (Figure 6.3). A conformational site is any surface configuration deter-

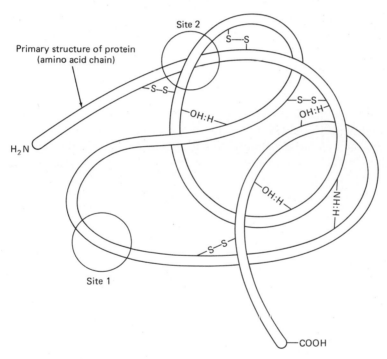

Figure 6.3 Nature of conformational and sequential epitopes on antigenic molecules. The amino acid chains composing proteins are wound back upon themselves like balled string. The epitope may be a section of the chain not involving amino acids in adjacent chains (site 1). This is a sequential epitope. The site may be formed by areas where a portion of the chain is linked to adjacent portions of the chain (site 2). Sites formed in this way depend on the folding of the primary chain and are called *conformational sites.* As they depend on the folding of the chain, they are lost if the molecule is unfolded. Unfolding is one type of denaturation, a process in which the conformation of the molecule is lost. The chains may be held together by covalent disulfide (-S-S-) bonds, hydrogen (-OH:H-) bonds, or other noncovalent types of bonds.

mined by the tertiary configuration of the molecule. Conformational sites of proteins may be determined by adjacent sections of amino acid chains that are brought into proximity by the folding of the chains. Thus conformational sites are lost with denaturation of molecules, a process that affects tertiary structure. Conformational sites may be considered to be analogous to the surface topography of the earth, which results from continental drift and the resultant crushing together of many rock strata.

Sequential sites are sites determined by the sequences of amino acids or sugars in the polymeric chains that make up the large organic molecules that are capable of serving as antigens. In antigenic proteins these sites are sequences of amino acids; in carbohydrates they are sequences of sugars. Sequential sites are not much affected by denaturation, which is a chemical process in which the secondary, tertiary, and quaternary structures of the polymeric molecules are changed.

In techniques such as Immuno-blotting, in which the antigens may be denatured by the detergents used to make them soluble, the antibodies to conformational sites may not be detected; the antibodies to sequential sites do react with the denatured antigen.

It is possible to cut up polymeric antigens using enzymes and to use the fragments as haptens by attaching them to carrier molecules. Antibodies raised to such antigen fragments (which could perhaps be called *antifrags*) have provided material for study of many aspects of antigenicity, including the size of the epitope. The size of the site for sequential determinants may be estimated by determining the minimum size of the polypeptide or polysaccharide that most efficiently blocks the binding of the antibody to the intact antigen. Studies of this nature indicate that epitopes of carbohydrates consist of about 5 sugars and of proteins of from 6 to 10 amino acids. For conformational epitopes, one can consider that the size of the epitope is approximately the size of the antigen-binding region on the antibody molecule. This has been estimated to be 15 nm long by 6 nm wide in one case and 20 nm long by 15 nm wide in another. The size differs from antibody to antibody. By comparison, a human red cell is about 7 μm in diameter and a staphylococcus about 1 μm in diameter. There are 1000 nm in 1 μm.

CROSS REACTIVITY OF ANTIGENS

Immunological reactions may be considered to be sensitive tests for detection of molecular structure. A given antibody, for example, will react with an epitope on the antigen that was used to induce the immune response. Immune sera, however, will often react not only with the antigen that was used to immunize the animal, but also with other antigens. Such cross reactivity may have a number of different causes.

Complex Antigens

Antigens used for immunization may actually be complex mixtures of many antigenic molecules. Such is the case if the antigen consists of a preparation of microbes, for example. Immune sera raised to preparations of one species of Salmonella will often react, usually to a lesser degree, with preparations of other species of Salmonella and even to preparations of more distantly related enterobacteria. In such cases it can be shown that some of the molecules in the different species of organism are identical and some differ. The immune serum raised contains a mixture of antibodies with specificity for the various molecules in the organisms. Cross reactivity may thus be the result of the presence of common molecules in complex antigens of related species.

In some cases cross reactivity may occur between antigen preparations from distantly related or unrelated species. For example, antiserum raised to Rickettsia will agglutinate a strain of *Proteus vulgaris* (0X19). As Proteus are easier to obtain than Rickettsia, Proteus preparations are used as antigens in serological tests to detect Rickettsial infections. The test, named after its discoverers, is called the Weil-Felix reaction.

Another reaction of this type is the Forssman reaction. An antigen in guinea pig kidney induces production in rabbits of an antibody that agglutinates sheep erythrocytes. Sera of people with infectious mononucleosis also contains agglutinins for sheep red cells as well as agglutinins for bovine red cells. Adsorption of sera from people with infectious mononucleosis with guinea pig kidney removes agglutinins for sheep erythrocytes, but not for bovine erythrocytes. These reactions are used in the diagnosis of infectious mononucleosis.

The serological reactions used for the diagnosis of rickettsial infection and mononucleosis are examples of *heterophile reactions* and are typical of a fairly common class of cross reactions. A *heterophile antigen* is thus defined as an antigen that is common to members of unrelated species.

Shared Epitopes

In the previous section it was pointed out that in complex antigens such as preparations of microbes, cross reactivity may result from the presence of a variety of molecules in the preparation, some of which are shared. As immunological reactivity is directed against small regions of molecules (epitopes), however, and not against the whole molecule, cross reactivity may occur because some epitopes on a given molecule may be similar and others distinct. By this mechanism, immune sera raised to a preparation containing only a single type of molecule may react with preparations of different molecules if some epitopes are shared.

When an intact immunocompetent animal is injected with an antigenic substance, the immune sera produced in fact contain a variety of antibodies directed against the various epitopes present on the various molecules in the preparation; they are produced by lymphocytes derived from a number of lymphocyte clones. Such antisera are described as *polyspecific* or *polyclonal.* It is also possible to produce monospecific or monoclonal antibodies. A given plasma cell secretes antibody specific for only a single epitope. In 1975 Kohler and Milstein developed technology that permits selection of a single antibody-secreting cell and production of a population from the selected cell. In this technique the lymphocytes, which have limited ability to reproduce, are fused with an actively reproducing neoplastic cell. The resulting hybrid may reproduce and produce clones. These clones secrete antibodies that are monospecific; that is, directed against a single epitope.

The presence of many distinct epitopes on a molecule can be shown by producing many monoclonal antibodies to a complex type of molecule and determining whether they bind to the molecule independently or block each other's binding. Studies of this type are called *epitope mapping studies.* In these studies one antibody is labeled, possibly with a radioisotope or enzyme. The antigen may be fixed on the walls of a test tube. The unlabeled antibody and the labeled one are allowed to react singly or in combination with the antigen in the test tubes. If the unlabeled antibody binds to the same epitope as the labeled one, then when mixtures of the two are allowed to react, the unlabeled antibody will compete for the epitope and less radioactivity will be bound than if the two antibodies bind to separate sites (Figure 6.4). If one has monoclonal antibodies to polypeptides of known sequence and if they react with a natural antigen, one can use the information from such reactions to map the amino acid sequence of the antigen.

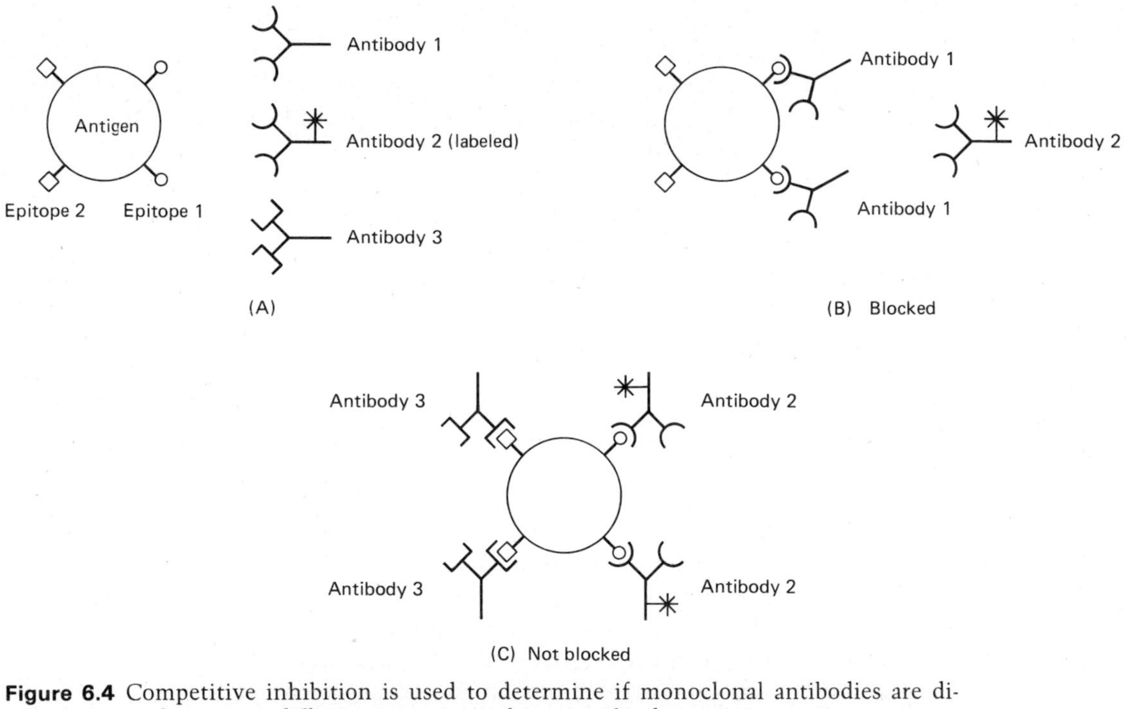

Figure 6.4 Competitive inhibition is used to determine if monoclonal antibodies are directed against the same or different epitopes. In this example, the antigen contains two types of epitopes (A). Unlabeled antibody 1 is specific for the same epitope as labeled antibody 2 and will block reactions of antibody 2 with its epitope (B). Antibody 3 is specific for a different epitope on the antigen and does not interfere with the reaction of antibody 2 with the antigen.

Similarity of Epitopes

In the previous sections antigenic cross reactivity was explained in terms of the presence of a variety of epitopes in antigen preparations. The epitopes were either on different molecules in the antigen preparation or possibly on the same molecule. Landsteiner, however, demonstrated that preparations that are reactive with a single hapten (epitope) will sometimes react with structurally similar haptens. In Landsteiner's day the technology for production of monoclonal antibody had not been developed; he produced monospecific, polyclonal antibodies by absorption of the antibodies with related antigens. Perhaps the simplest way to produce monospecific polyclonal antibodies today is to produce antibody by injection of a hapten-carrier complex into rabbits. The resultant immune serum is then passed through a column to which the hapten is bound (but not the carrier). The column is flushed to remove unbound antibody, and the antibody that had bound to the hapten is eluted by passage of a low pH or other solution, such as one containing a high salt concentration that causes reversible denaturation of antibody. Upon denaturation the antigen–antibody bond is broken and the denatured antibody can be flushed from the column. After dialysis to remove the denaturing agent, the renatured monospecific antibody can be studied. Landsteiner showed that such antibodies could discriminate between ortho, meta, and para forms of aminobenzene sulfonic acid. Although some cross reactivity occurred in all cases, reactions with the homologous system were the strongest. A variety of different groups could be substituted on the aromatic ring, or the side groups could be deleted and the reactions would still occur (Figure 6.5). This type of reaction can be thought of in terms of a hand in a glove. The absence of a finger interferes less with putting on a glove than does placing the fingers in odd positions.

ROUTES OF ADMINISTRATION OF ANTIGENS

To manifest immunogenicity, the potential antigen must enter the tissues of the immunocompetent animal. This may occur by artificial means or by natural ones. Injection by subcutaneous, intramuscular, or intravenous routes (that is, parenteral routes) all serve to introduce antigenic materials into the body. Natural routes of entry usually involve infection. A microorganism invades the tissue and grows there, and thus introduces its components into the tissue. This is the most common natural route of entry of antigens into the body.

Antigens may enter the body by inhalation or, less often, by ingestion. Most of our foods are potentially antigenic. If they are injected into tissues, they certainly invoke an immune response. Digestion precedes assimilation of most foods. Proteins and polysaccharides are reduced to their constituent monomers before absorption. These low molecular weight products of digestion are not antigenic. It also appears that there are mechanisms in the digestive tract that prevent many potentially antigenic foods from causing an immune response if they do enter the body through the gut wall (these sometimes fail, causing us to develop food allergies).

(A) Haptens

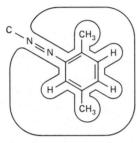

Hapten 1

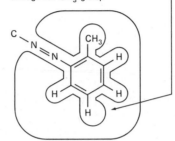

Hapten 2

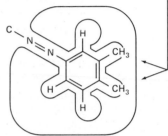

Hapten 3

(B) Haptens in antibody-reactive sites

Hapten fits well into antibody-reactive site

Hydrogen atom fits into site large enough for CH₃ group

Large CH₃ groups do not fit into sites designed for hydrogen atoms

Hapten 1 in antibody site
(Homologous reaction)

Hapten 2 fits into antibody site
(Heterologous reaction)

Hapten 3 does not fit into antibody site
(No reaction)

Figure 6.5 Serologic cross reactions are based on similarity of epitopes. The absence of the bulky CH_3 group on hapten 2 does not interfere with entry of the hapten into the site specific for hapten 1. The presence of two bulky CH_3 groups prevent hapten 3 from fitting into the antibody site complementary to hapten 1.

ADJUVANTS

Adjuvants are substances added to antigen preparations to enhance their immunogenicity. They may or may not be immunogenic in themselves. They are frequently irritating and cause mild inflammation, thus attracting the cells of the immunological system to the site of antigen deposition. Some adjuvants bind the antigen tightly, slowly releasing it after injection and thus prolonging the antigenic stimulation. Most vaccines used in human and veterinary medicine contain adjuvants. Alum is the most commonly used adjuvant in human medicine. It probably acts by binding and then slowly releasing the antigen.

SUGGESTIONS FOR FURTHER READING

J-F. Bach and R. S. Schwartz. Antigens. In *Immunology,* 2nd edition, J-F Bach and R. S. Schwartz, *eds.* Wiley Medical Publishers, New York, 1982.

B. Benacerraf. Studies of Antigenicity with Artificial Antigens. In *Regulation of the Antibody Response,* B. Cinander, *ed.* Charles C. Thomas, Springfield, Illinois, 1971.

J. A. Berzofsky. "Intrinsic and extrinsic factors in protein antigenic structure." Science *229:*932, 1985.

E. S. Golub. The Nature of Antigens. In *Immunology: A Synthesis.* Sinauer Associates, Sonderland, Massachusetts, 1987.

G. Kohler and C. Milstein. "Continuous cultures of fused cells secreting antibody of predetermined specificity." Nature *256:*495, 1976.

R. A. Learner. "Antibodies of predetermined specificity in biology and medicine." Adv. in Immun. *36:*1, 1984.

O. Makela and I. J. T. Seppala. Haptens and Carriers. In *Immunochemistry,* D. M. Weir, *ed.* Blackwell Scientific Publications, London, 1986.

M. Sela. Overview: Antigens. In: *Immunochemistry,* D. M. Weir, *ed.* Blackwell Scientific Publications, London, 1986.

E. R. Unanue and B. Benacerraf. Antigens. In: *Textbook of Immunology.* Williams & Wilkins, Baltimore, 1984.

Chapter 7

The Inducible Defense System

Antibody Molecules and Antigen—Antibody Reactions

MELANIE S. KENNEDY
JANICE BLAZINA

Department of Pathology
College of Medicine
The Ohio State University

INTRODUCTION

The production of antibodies is a part of the immune system's response to antigenic stimulation. In this chapter we will describe the molecular structures of antibodies, the reactions of antibodies with antigens, and the genetic control of antibody production.

Human serum contains a variety of constituents, many of which are proteins. On the basis of electrophoretic mobility, serum proteins can be separated into albumin and alpha 1, alpha 2, beta, and gamma globulin fractions (Figure 7.1).

Antibodies are blood proteins, all of which are a part of the gamma fraction of serum. In addition to those found in blood, some types of antibodies are fixed to body cells or tissues, or exist in body secretions.

Antibodies circulating in the blood are called *humoral antibodies*, whereas those fixed on cells in tissues are referred to as *cell-bound antibodies*. Humoral antibodies react with antigens to produce precipitation, agglutination, and neutralization among other reactions in the body or in test tubes in the laboratory. Cell-bound antibodies facilitate phagocytosis and cause hypersensitivity reactions, including *allergies*.

Antibodies, or immunoglobulins, are produced by plasma cells, the progeny of B-lymphocytes. Antibodies are produced in response to antigenic stimulation and are recognized by their ability to combine specifically with the antigenic substances that elicited their formation. Identification of an antibody depends upon development of a method of detecting its reaction with the appropriate antigen.

The terms *immunoglobulin* and *antibody* are not identical in meaning; use of the term *antibody* implies reactivity against a specific antigen, whereas the term *immunoglobulin* is a chemical description that applies to all protein molecules that carry antibody activity and to certain proteins related by molecular structure. Therefore, although all antibodies are immunoglobulins, it is at least possible that

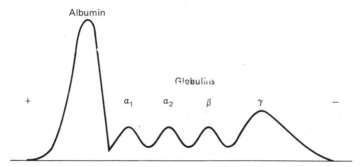

Figure 7.1 Proteins in serum may be separated by electrophoresis. Albumin migrates toward the positive pole, or anode, most rapidly under the conditions normally used for electrophoresis. The globulins migrate more slowly than albumin. Of the various globulins, alpha globulin migrates most rapidly and gamma most slowly. Antibody is found in the gamma globulin fraction of the serum.

not all immunoglobulins are antibodies. One would have to test every immuno-globulin against every possible antigen to prove that some immunoglobulins lacked specificity, an obvious impossibility.

ANTIBODY MOLECULES: THE BASIC IMMUNOGLOBULIN STRUCTURAL UNITS

Immunoglobulin molecules are symmetrical structures. In solution they become Y-shaped after binding to antigen. They consist of four polypeptide chains. There are two identical heavy (H) chains and two identical light (L) chains in each molecule. The heavy chains have domains designated CH1, CH2, and CH3 (Figure 7.2). The heavy and light chains are held together by covalent disulfide bonds and by noncovalent hydrophobic bonds. Heavy chains are composed of 446 or more amino acid residues [molecular weight (M.W.) from 50,000 to 75,000 daltons], whereas light chains have 213 or 214 residues (M.W. 20,000–25,000 daltons). Some antibody molecules exist as monomers, whereas others are composed of more than one of these basic structural units.

Variations that occur in the basic four-chain structure involve chain length, amino acid sequence, and carbohydrate content. These variations determine struc-tural features affecting biological activity and antigenicity. The differences that affect the chemical, physical, and biologic properties of immunoglobulins are found primarily in the heavy chains and can be used to categorize the five major classes, or isotypes, of immunoglobulins: IgG, IgM, IgA, IgD, and IgE. The heavy

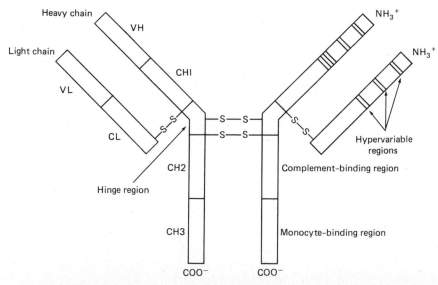

Figure 7.2 Schematic diagram of an antibody molecule. The molecule is made up of heavy (VH, CH1, CH2, and CH3) chains and light chains (VL, CL), each with several domains. The chains are held together in part by disulfide bonds.

chains of the immunoglobulin (Ig) molecules are designated by Greek letters as gamma (γ), mu (μ), alpha (α), delta (δ), and epsilon (ϵ), respectively.

Within some of the classes, subclasses with distinctive heavy chains and differing functional properties occur; in humans there are four subclasses of IgG and two each of IgA and IgM. The two immunologically distinct types of light chains, which differ only in amino acid sequence, are common to all classes of immunoglobulins and are referred to as kappa (κ) and lambda (λ). Any given Ig molecule always contains either kappa or lambda chains but never a mixture of the two.

Various chemical, electrophoretic, and immunologic techniques have been used to gain knowledge about the immunoglobulins. Reduction with subsequent alkylation breaks antibody molecules into their constituent light and heavy chains, and proteolytic enzymes cleave them into fragments.

Each heavy or light chain has a variable, or V, region at the amino-terminal end and a constant, or C, region at the carboxyl-terminal end. The amino acid sequences in the variable regions differ more than the amino acid sequences in the constant regions. The two regions of the Ig molecule, constant and variable, are produced by separate genes.

The polypeptide chains do not simply remain as linear arrays of amino acids after synthesis but are folded and held by intrachain disulfide bonds. The folding produces compact globular regions known as *domains* (Figure 7.3). The light chains have only two domains, one variable and one constant, labeled VL and CL,

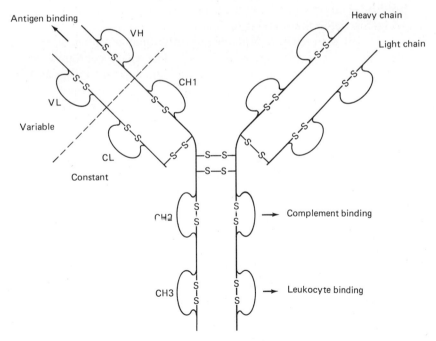

Figure 7.3 The polypeptide chains of the immunoglobulin molecules fold upon themselves to form loops. The folds are held in place in part by disulfide (-S-S-) bonds between parts of the chains. Each domain is created by one of the loops.

respectively. The domains of the heavy chains of IgG, IgA, and IgD include a variable region designated VH and three constant region domains designated CH1, CH2, and CH3. IgM and IgE have a fourth domain in the constant region, CH4. Certain biological functions of immunoglobulins are associated with certain domains. The configuration of the variable domains determines the specificity for antigen. CL and CH1 may aid in orienting the variable regions in combining with antigen. The binding site for the first component of complement, which is the site responsible for complement activation by the classical pathway, is located in CH2. The CH3 domain is the site responsible for binding of antibody molecules to Fc receptors of phagocytes.

The differences in the amino acid sequences in the variable regions of antibody molecules of different specificities are responsible for the specificity of the antibody. Variability of some regions of the variable domains is somewhat limited: In these regions certain amino acids do not differ, and differences at other sites are limited to only a few amino acids. On the other hand, other areas of the variable domains are hypervariable. These are called *complementarity-determining regions.* Three such hypervariable areas are found on light chains and three or four on heavy chains, each containing from 5 to 10 amino acids. Differences in amino acid sequence in the hypervariable regions are responsible for the large number of unique antigen-binding sites that exist. The remaining, less variable, portions of the variable domains provide the framework for alignment of the hypervariable regions in the antigen-combining site. These serve to enclose the hypervariable regions by holding them in close proximity and forming the structure complementary to the antigenic determinant (Figure 7.4).

The fit with antigen depends not only upon complementarity of structure but also upon complementarity of charge. The exact configuration of the antigen-binding site may differ slightly from one molecule to another and yet the immunoglobulins may have the same specificity. The variable region itself forms a unique epitope and may serve as an antigen. This site is responsible for the idiotype of the immunoglobulin.

There is some variation in amino acid sequence in the constant regions. These variations are genetically determined and thus inherited. They are responsible for the differences that determine Ig allotypes and are called *allotypic markers.* The markers in humans are Gm on gamma heavy chains, Am on alpha heavy chains, and Km (or InV) on the K light chains. Three Km (on IgD and IgE), two Am (on IgA), and over 20 Gm (on IgG) allotypes have been defined. Inheritance of these markers is autosomally controlled. In some cases the molecular basis of the allotype is known. As an example, the KM(1,2) allotype has leucine at position 191 in the CL domain of the K light chains, whereas the Km(3) allotype has valine there. These allotypic markers are isoantigens. They are among the epitopes that are recognized by the body of an individual who mounts an antibody response to a foreign immunoglobulin. Typing for these markers is used in paternity testing and in studies of population genetics.

The area of the heavy chains between the first and second constant region domains is the hinge region. This region, which has numerous proline residues and contains the interheavy chain disulfide bonds, allows the Ig molecule to flex into

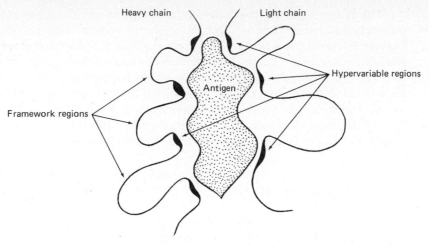

(Only 3 of the heavy chain hypervariable regions
may actually participate in binding antigen.)

Figure 7.4 Diagrammatic representation of an antigen surrounded by the antigen receptor of the antibody molecule. The variable portions of both the heavy and light chains participate in forming the receptor site. The hypervariable regions are those that have contact with the antigen; the rest of the variable regions provide a framework for the hypervariable regions.

various shapes in order to place each of its antigen-combining sites on separate antigens. It is thought that the molecule maintains a T-shape (Figure 7.5) when not combined with antigen (to maximize its ability to contact antigen) but assumes a Y-shape after contacting antigen.

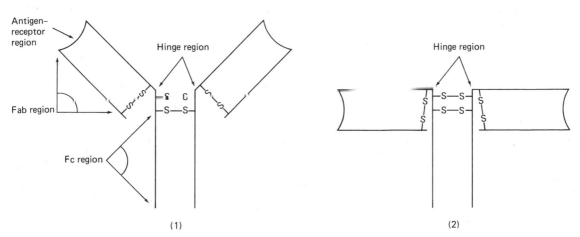

Figure 7.5 The antibody molecule is flexible. Flexibility is greatest in the hinge region. When combined with antigen, the molecule may be **Y** shaped (1); when uncombined, it may be **T** shaped (2).

The hinge region of the antibody molecule is more flexible than the other segments and is therefore susceptible to the actions of enzymes and chemicals. Enzymatic treatment with papain breaks the heavy chain at the amino-terminal side of the interheavy chain disulfide bonds, yielding three pieces of nearly equal size: two identical Fab (antigen-binding or antibody) fragments and the Fc (constant or crystallizable) fragment (Figure 7.6). Each of the two Fab fragments consists of an intact light chain and the amino-terminal half (or Fd fragment) of the heavy chain, linked by a single interchain disulfide bond. The Fc fragment contains portions of heavy chains, only. It can be crystallized but cannot combine with antigen.

The Fab and Fc fragments of the Ig molecule have distinct functions. The Fab fragment binds to antigen because it contains the antibody's binding site. Fab fragments, the binding sites of the antibody, combine with antigen to form soluble complexes that do not precipitate. The Fc portion does not bind to antigen, but on it are sites that determine effector functions of antibody molecules, such as complement fixation, binding to phagocytes, transplacental transfer, binding to mast cells, and secretion into body fluids.

Pepsin, in contrast to papain, cleaves the Ig molecule on the carboxyl-terminal side of the interheavy chain disulfide bonds, yielding a single bivalent fragment called $F(ab')_2$ (M.W. 110,000 daltons); the remainder of the molecule is digested into smaller fragments. The $F(ab')_2$ fragment has the capability of combining with antigen and precipitating. However, neither Fab nor $F(ab')_2$ fragments have all of the biologic properties of intact antibody molecules because they lack the Fc portion.

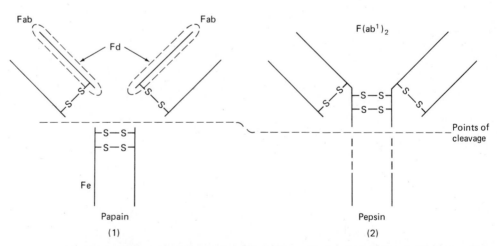

Figure 7.6 Enzyme cleavage with pepsin splits the antibody molecule, yielding two Fab portions and an Fc portion (1). Cleavage by pepsin splits the molecule at a different point, yielding a single $F(ab)_2$ fragment and a fragment that is a portion of the Fc region. Reduction splits the disulfide bonds, yielding two Fd fragments from each Fab fragment.

GENETICS OF ANTIBODY DIVERSITY

As mentioned earlier, the plasma cells are the cells that actually produce and secrete antibody. Mature B-cells have Ig molecules on their surfaces, and each plasma cell produces Ig molecules that have specificity identical to that of the immunoglobulin bound on its membrane. Humans can make millions of different kinds of B-cells, each with the ability to produce an antibody that has a unique specificity.

Since they are proteins, antibodies are coded for by a DNA blueprint. If each antibody were coded for by a separate strip of DNA, a huge amount of DNA would be needed to allow production of the antibodies of the many different specificities that may be made. In addition, the variety of antibodies possible would be fixed by the encoded information. There is not, in fact, a gene for each antibody; rather, the gene for antibody in each lymphocyte results from a process of gene rearrangement that permits generation of antibody molecules of great diversity using only limited amounts of DNA. The rearrangement occurs when lymphoid tissue is formed during embryogenesis.

The fact that the constant and variable portions of the antibody molecule are under separate genetic control allows additional economy of DNA utilization. Since the functions of the constant regions remain constant regardless of antibody specificity, it is only the variable region genes that require great diversity. Because many different variable genes can be produced and any one of them can combine with a more limited number of constant genes, antibodies of many different specificities can be made using a relatively small amount of DNA.

The mechanics of the processes whereby the economy of DNA utilization is achieved are fairly complex. Each strand of the DNA responsible for an antibody, as for any protein, is formed of groups of nucleotides known as *exons* (structural gene segments) and *introns* (intervening sequences) (Figure 7.7). However, during translation only the exon segments provide the information used in making the actual protein. In each pre–B-cell (after development from a stem cell and before expression of surface Ig) the cellular DNA is spliced and rearranged internally (Figure 7.8). First, a heavy chain gene is formed through combination of pieces of DNA on chromosome 14. The heavy chain DNA strip in chromosome 14 consists of four segments that program different parts of the antibody molecule. These are known as V (variable), D (diversity), J (joining), and C (constant); from each of these sections many possible DNA choices may be made. During lymphocyte differentiation one segment of DNA from each of the four categories is chosen, spliced out, and arranged in the order VDJC. Once the four segments of DNA are selected, they are then transcribed to a single, unique strip of messenger RNA (mRNA), which is translated into the unique Ig heavy chain the lymphocyte will be able to produce.

After the heavy chain gene is produced and transcribed, light chain production occurs. Kappa chains are coded for by DNA on chromosome 2, lambda chains by DNA on chromosome 22. For production of light chains, a process of gene rearrangement similar to that just described for heavy chain production is used. For

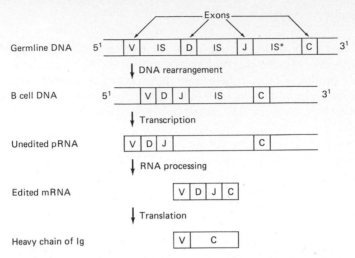

Figure 7.7 Diagrammatic representation of the process by which germline DNA is processed and messenger RNA is produced during development of a mature B-cell. The germline DNA is rearranged and transcribed into RNA; the RNA is edited before any polypeptides are produced.

light chains, however, the process involves selection from only three categories: V (variable), J (joining), and C (constant). Once the three segments of DNA are selected they are joined, transcribed into mRNA, and translated into a unique light chain. The unique light chain combines with the unique heavy chain of the cell, and antibody is formed. Once the gene-assembly process is complete and the B-cell has committed itself to production of a particular antibody, the cell expresses the antibody on its surface. Although before clonal expansion each B-cell has genes for antibody of only one specificity, there exist many B-cells, each with a different antibody-determining gene. The number of possible antibodies is equal to the product of the numbers of gene choices within each category for both the light and heavy chains.

In addition to the antibody diversity resulting from choice of particular DNA sequences, some modification of the specific DNA sequences occurs. If during the rearrangement process two nucleotides from a codon of one V segment of DNA are spliced to one nucleotide of a codon from a J segment to form a new codon, an entirely new triplet may be produced and a different amino acid is thus incorporated into the chain. This process makes an even greater number of antibodies possible. During transcription of the DNA to RNA, the entire sequence is encoded, or transcribed, into precursor RNA. The precursor RNA is spliced and edited into mRNA during a period known as *RNA processing.* This mRNA provides the template on which the antibody molecules are produced. These processes allow an animal to produce lymphocytes with entirely new combinations of DNA that program production of antibody with new specificities. As a consequence, the immune system is able to respond to newly arisen parasites that contain antigens never before encountered (see Chapter 14 for additional discussion).

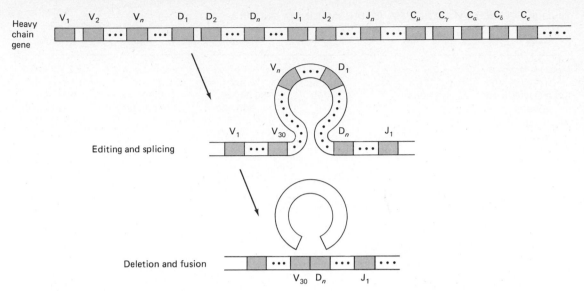

Figure 7.8 Diagram showing method by which the B-cell produces a gene for the production of a heavy chain in humans. A part of the DNA of chromosome 14 is rearranged internally. After rearrangement, deletion and fusion of the DNA segment produces the unique heavy chain gene.

CHARACTERISTICS OF IMMUNOGLOBULIN CLASSES

The five classes of immunoglobulins differ in molecular size, half-life in the plasma, carbohydrate content, and biologic activity (Table 7.1). The serum levels of IgG, IgA, and IgM vary with several factors, one of which is age. The levels of these immunoglobulins are lowest soon after birth, peak during adolescence, and decline gradually with aging.

The IgG molecule (M.W. 150,000 daltons) has a sedimentation coefficient of 7S and, as noted earlier, is composed of two heavy (M.W. 50,000 daltons) and two light chains (M.W. 25,000 daltons) linked by disulfide bonds. Approximately 65 percent of IgG molecules have kappa light chains and 35 percent have lambda. IgG is the most abundant of the immunoglobulins and the most important in humans. It is found in concentrations of 600–1800 mg/dl in serum. About 40 percent of IgG is intravascular and 60 percent is in the interstitial fluid. Because of its ability to diffuse between intravascular and extravascular spaces and its high precipitating capacity, IgG is effective in neutralizing bacterial toxins in both blood and tissues. It is active against infectious agents that are disseminated in the blood, principally the Gram-positive bacteria. It neutralizes viruses and binds to microorganisms, enhancing their phagocytosis. It is therefore an opsonizing antibody. It is synthesized during the latter part of the primary response and is the major antibody synthesized during the secondary immune response. The half-life of IgG varies inversely with its serum concentration and is about 21 days, the longest of all the immunoglobulins.

Table 7.1 CHARACTERISTICS OF HUMAN IMMUNOGLOBULINS

Class	IgG	IgM	IgA	IgD	IgE
Molecular formula	$\kappa\,2\,\gamma\,2$ or $\lambda\,2\,\gamma\,2$	$(\kappa2\mu2)^5$ or $(\lambda\,2\mu2)^5$	$(\kappa2\alpha2)1{-}2$ or $(\lambda2\alpha2)1$ or 2	$\kappa\,2\,\delta\,2$ or $\lambda\,2\,\delta\,2$	$\kappa\,2\,\epsilon\,2$ or $\lambda\,2\,\epsilon\,2$
Molecular weight (daltons)	150,000	900,000	160,000 or 500,000	150,000 to 200,000	190,000 to 200,000
Valency for antigen binding	2	10	2 or 4	2	2
Sedimentation coefficient	7S	19S	7S-11S	7S	8S
Carbohydrate content	3%	12%	7–8%	12–13%	12%
Heavy chains					
Class	γ	μ	α	δ	ϵ
Subclasses	4	2	2	—	—
Molecular weight	53,000	70,000	58,000	65,000	72,000
Allotypes	Gm	—	Am	—	—
Light Chains					
Type	κ or λ	κ or λ	κ or λ	κ or λ	κ or λ
Molecular weight	22,500	22,500	22,500	22,500	22,500
Allotypes	Km (Inv)	Km (Inv)	Km (Inv)	KM (Inv)	Km (Inv)
J chain	—	present	present	—	—
Secretory piece	—	—	present	—	—
Present in epithelial secretions	no	no	yes	no	no
Serum level (mg/dl)	600 to 800	50 to 210	70 to 500	0.1 to 4.0	0.01 to 0.9
Percent of total Ig	70–80	5–10	10–15	1	0.01
Half-life (days)	21–35	5–8	6–11	2–3	2–3
Synthesis (mg/kg body weight/day)	20–40	3–17	3–55	0.4	?
Percent intravascular	45	76	42	75	52
Electrophoretic mobility	Gamma	Between β and γ	Slow Beta	Between β and γ	Slow Beta
Inactivation by sulfhydryl compounds	no	yes	partial	no	?
Blood group activity described	yes	yes	yes	no	no
Usual serological behavioral as RBC antibody	nonagglu-tinating	saline agglu-tinating	nonagglu-tinating	—	—
Placental passage	yes	No	no	no	no
Complement fixation					
Classic	$++$[a]	$+++$	—	—	—
Alternate	—	—	$+$	—	—
Binding to macrophage					
FC receptor	$+$	—	—	—	—
Binding to mast cells and basophils	—	—	—	—	$+$

[a]The numbers of plus signs indicate the relative extent of activation of each pathway.

The differences in the four subclasses of IgG are related to differences in amino acid sequence. Subclass differences were originally demonstrated by immunological means and thus reflect different antigenic structures. The differences, however, do not just determine antigenic characteristics but also determine important biological characteristics of the various subclasses of IgG. For example, IgG3 has the greatest ability to activate complement of any of the IgG subclasses, IgG1 has less, IgG2 even less, and IgG4 does not activate complement. Of the IgG classes, only IgG1 and IgG3 have the capacity to bind to the surface receptors of macrophages and to neutrophils. Organisms opsonized with IgG of these subclasses are thus readily phagocytized. The subclasses of IgG are present in decreasing amounts in the order IgG1 > IgG2 > IgG3 > IgG4. All four subclasses of IgG are transported across the placenta and provide the passively transferred humoral immunity of the newborn human.

IgM has a molecular weight of 900,000 daltons and a sedimentation coefficient of 19S. It is a pentamer of five 7S subunits joined by disulfide bridges in a circular configuration. An additional polypeptide chain, the J (joining) chain (M.W. 15,000 daltons), which differs antigenically and in amino acid composition from the heavy and light chains, polymerizes the subunits. IgM is the largest molecule of any antibody of the five classes. Because of its size, it is restricted primarily to the vascular compartment. Its restriction to the vascular compartment and the fact that it is the first antibody to appear after a primary antigenic stimulus suggest it may have a role in defense against bacteremia. IgM is the most efficient activator of complement since only one bound IgM molecule is needed to lyse cells. On the other hand, IgG requires two or more adjacently bound molecules to activate complement. IgM has a greater role in protection against infection with Gram-negative bacteria than with Gram-positive ones. IgM has two subclasses, but no unique effector functions are known for them.

IgA is the second-most abundant serum Ig. Its principal function is to protect mucous membranes from infection. It is an important first line of defense. It is synthesized by plasma cells in the submucosa of the respiratory, gastrointestinal, and genitourinary tracts, and in excretory glands, and is found in high concentrations in the lymphoid tissues and in secretions such as saliva, sweat, tears, nasal fluid, and milk. It is also present in serum. IgA provides protection to newborns, who ingest it with the first milk or colostrum. Monomeric IgA accounts for 90 percent of IgA in serum; the majority of IgA in exocrine secretions is dimeric. IgA is the most potent of all the immunoglobulins against viruses.

IgA may occur as a monomer or as a polymer of two to five subunits. In serum, IgA exists primarily as a monomer (90 percent) with some polymeric forms, mostly dimers and trimers. As it does with IgM, the J (joining) chain binds the IgA subunits together. In epithelial secretions, secretory IgA is a dimer, consisting of two monomeric IgA's, a J chain, and a nonimmunoglobulin glycoprotein called the *secretory component* (M.W. 85,000 daltons). After their release from the plasma cells, the IgA dimers pass through the epithelial cells to reach the mucosal surface; during this process they are bound to the secretory component. The secretory component is produced by the epithelial cells and is needed for transport across the epithelial cells; it is also responsible for making the IgA molecule resistant to attack by proteolytic enzymes.

In humans, IgE binds to basophils and their tissue counterparts, mast cells, and circulates in serum at very low levels. IgE has a role in many allergic disorders, such as bronchial asthma, hay fever, and anaphylaxis, which are probably extreme forms of basically protective inflammatory responses. IgE may also contribute to defense against parasitic infestation. Allergens stimulate IgE production by lymphocytes and plasma cells, particularly in areas such as tonsillar tissue and Peyer's patches of the gastrointestinal tract. IgE attaches by its Fc portion to membrane receptors on mast cells and basophils, leaving its combining sites free to bind to antigen. When reexposure to the same allergen occurs, the allergen is bound to the IgE on the cell, and vasoactive mediators, such as histamine, are released. The clinical effects of the mediators include respiratory tract constriction and increased vascular permeability and vasodilation, resulting in difficulty in breathing, edema, and skin rashes. Another result of allergic reactions is the production of increased amounts of secretions by cells on mucosal surfaces.

IgD, like IgE, circulates in trace amounts in serum. It has a short half-life (2.8 days), possibly because of its susceptibility to proteolytic degradation. Its known function is to serve along with IgM as an antigen-binding receptor on the surface of B-lymphocytes. IgD probably plays a critical role in differentiation of B-cells or in the initiation of the immune response.

For a summary of the characteristics of the immunoglobulins, see Table 7.1.

ANTIGEN–ANTIBODY REACTIONS

To recognize that an antibody exists, a corresponding antigen must be identified. To do this, a method of detecting the reaction of antibody with antigen is necessary. A variety of methods have been devised for this purpose. Primary reactions, which depend only on antibody binding to the antigen, are the basis of immunofluorescence and radioimmunoassay procedures. Secondary reactions that depend on formation of a lattice yielding insoluble immune complexes and possibly on postbinding conformational changes within the antibody molecule for completion of the reaction are the basis of precipitation, agglutination, and complement fixation reactions.

Precipitation is one of the oldest methods for detecting antigen–antibody interaction and remains widely used today. In 1935 Heidelberger described the precipitin curve (Figure 7.9). Precipitation results from the formation of an insoluble complex when soluble antibody reacts with soluble antigen, yielding a three-dimensional latticelike structure. When the number of antigenic sites is roughly equivalent to the number of antibody-binding sites available, a zone of equivalence, or of optimal proportions, results. At the zone of equivalence, precipitation is maximal. The chemical interaction between antibodies and antigens involves such forces as hydrogen bonding, electrostatic attraction, hydrophobic bonding, and electron cloud bonding. In the mixture of antigen with an antiserum, several different antibody molecules can bind to each antigen molecule and cause lattice formation. If antibody is in excess, the lattice does not form; if antigen is in excess, a precipitate may form but then will redissolve.

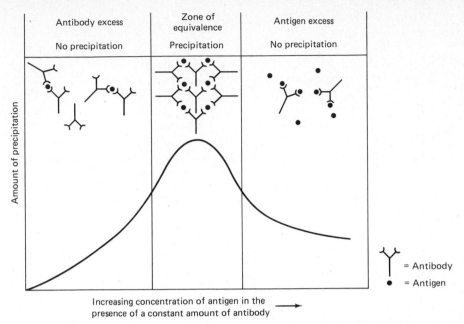

Figure 7.9 Maximum precipitate forms at the zone of equivalence, where the proportions of antibody and antigen are optimum to produce a large lattice that is insoluble. The amounts of precipitate in antibody or antigen excess are smaller than at the zone of equivalence. In these zones many complexes too small to be insoluble and precipitate are formed.

Agglutination is an assay based upon the same principles as precipitation. It is widely used for blood typing. Agglutination, like precipitation, occurs in two stages. Antibody first reacts with antigenic determinants that are parts of larger structures such as red cells or bacteria (sensitization), and then forms bridges between antigenic determinants on adjacent cells to yield grossly visible clumps (agglutination). When antibody is in excess, a phenomenon known as the *prozone* may occur. In blood group work, for example, reactions of high titer antibodies with their antigens may be weak or negative when undiluted serum is used but become strong with diluted serum. This is because outside of the zone of equivalence a lattice does not form and clumping cannot occur. The process of formation of a lattice during agglutination is similar to the process that occurs in precipitation. Precipitation reactions can be converted to agglutination reactions by absorption of the soluble antigen onto erythrocytes, polystyrene or latex spheres, bentonite, or starch granules. Latex particles coated with IgG, for example, are used as the antigen in agglutination tests for diagnosis of rheumatoid arthritis.

Immunoprecipitation may be carried out in an agarose gel matrix. The earliest technique, that of Ouchterlony, or double diffusion precipitation, is a qualitative test. In this test a visible line of precipitate forms between wells, one containing specific antibody and the other the antigen. If samples are placed in adjacent wells cut in a gel, the precipitin lines that form may reveal immunological identity, partial identity, or nonidentity between the samples in the wells (Figure 7.10).

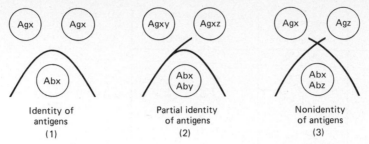

Figure 7.10 Diagrammatic representation of a double diffusion precipitation reaction in gel. If the antigens in the two antigen-containing wells (Agx) are identical (1), a single line forms. If the two antigens are partially different (Agy, Agz), a spur forms (2). If the two antigens are completely different (Agx, Agz), the two precipitation lines simply cross (3).

Immunoelectrophoresis (IEP) is a separation of antigens by their electrophoretic mobility as well as by diffusion. Other procedures that are modifications of the precipitation reaction include two-dimensional IEP, crossed IEP, and countercurrent IEP. These are all qualitative procedures.

There are also a number of quantitative assays based on the principle of precipitation of antigen–antibody complexes in gels. In radial immunodiffusion (RID) and rocket electrophoresis, antibody is incorporated into an agarose gel. Quantification is based on the distance antigen migrates into the antibody-containing gel from the point of application. In RID the precipitate forms a ring around the sample well. The antigen diffuses into the antibody-containing agar; precipitation occurs when the antigen–antibody proportions are optimal. A series of antigen standards of known concentrations are used to obtain a calibration curve and to determine the amount of antigen in the sample (Figure 7.11). In rocket immunoelectrophoresis the antigen is forced into the gel by an electric current (Figure 7.12). Rocket immunoelectrophoresis is a rapid method suitable for measuring antigens that

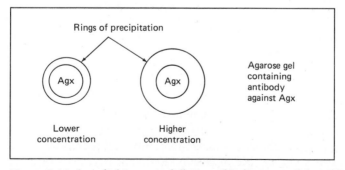

Figure 7.11 In radial immunodiffusion, the diameter of the ring of precipitation around the antigen (Agx)–containing well is proportional to the antigen concentration. The procedure can therefore be used to determine the concentration of an antigen in a solution of the antigen.

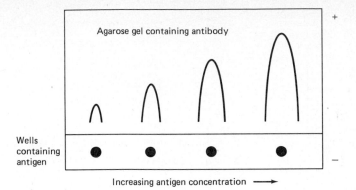

Figure 7.12 In rocket immunoelectrophoresis the antigen is forced into the antibody-containing agarose gel by an electric current. The size of the peak of precipitation is proportional to the amount of antigen placed in the well. If standards containing known amounts of antigen are run simultaneously, samples can be evaluated to determine antigen concentration by comparison of the size of the precipitation peaks produced by the unknown samples and the peaks produced by the standards.

move toward the positive pole on electrophoresis. Both rocket immunoelectrophoresis and radial immunodiffusion techniques are used in assays for serum proteins. IgG, IgA, and IgM can be quantified by RID; however, this method is too insensitive to detect IgE in the very low concentrations at which it occurs in serum.

The principle of immunoprecipitation is also used in turbidimetric and nephelometric assays. In these assays the antigen–antibody complexes are measured in suspension by the percentage of light transmitted or by the degree of light scatter, respectively. These assays are useful for the precise measurement of the amounts of a wide variety of proteins in the serum, including the immunoglobulins and complement components.

Some clinically significant proteins occur at concentrations too low to be detected by immunoprecipitation methods. In 1960 Yalow and Berson introduced radioimmunoassay (RIA), which is a sensitive and specific technique. This method permits measurement of very low concentrations of any material to which an antibody can be raised. Sensitivity results from the low levels of radioactivity that can be measured. The specificity of the assay is determined by the specificity of the antibody to which the radioisotope is coupled. A more specific antibody is usually required for RIA than for precipitation assays.

Radioimmunoassays are of two types: competitive RIA and sandwich RIA. In the competitive RIA (Figure 7.13), radiolabeled antigen is added to the sample being tested for unlabeled antigen. An antibody specific for the antigen is added. After washing the precipitate to remove unbound radiolabeled antigen, the radioactivity in the precipitate is measured with a gamma counter. The percentage of label in the precipitate is inversely proportional to the amount of unlabeled antigen present in the sample. In this form of the RIA, competition between labeled and unlabeled antigen forms the basis of the test.

Competitive binding procedures can also be based on competition between

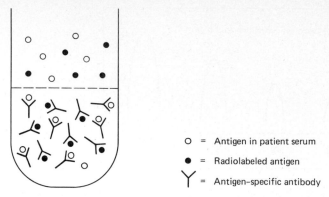

Figure 7.13 In competitive radioimmunoassay a radiolabeled antigen is added to the sample. This radiolabeled antigen directly competes with the unlabeled antigen for the antibody added. The amount of labeled antigen in the precipitate is inversely proportional to the amount of unlabeled antigen in the sample.

labeled and unlabeled antibodies. Determination of the proportion of a known amount of labeled antibody bound in the precipitate permits calculation of the amount of unlabeled antibody. For use in these tests, antibody must be labeled with a suitable radionuclide without destroying its specificity.

The sandwich RIA generally uses a solid phase to which specific antibody is fixed (Figure 7.14). First the specimen (for example, patient serum) is added, and then a radiolabeled antibody specific for the suspected antigen. After a washing to remove unbound antibody, the radioactivity retained is counted with a gamma counter. The amount of radiolabel that is bound is directly proportional to the amount of antigen in the sample.

The sandwich technique is useful because with it one can detect either anti-

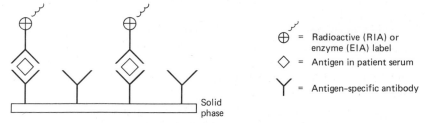

Figure 7.14 The sandwich radioimmunoassay uses a solid phase to which specific antibody is attached. The specimen that may contain antigen is added and allowed to react; then the surface is washed to remove any unbound antigens. Radiolabeled antibody is then added. After time is allowed for reaction, the unbound labeled antibody is washed away and the bound label is counted. The amount of label that is bound is directly proportional to the amount of antigen in the sample. The same basic procedure is used in the enzyme-linked immunosorbentassay; the only differences are the substitution of an enzyme for the radiolabel and the use of a chromogenic substrate and color detection instead of a radioisotope counter for determining the amount of binding that occurs.

body or antigen. If antigen is used to coat the solid phase, then antibody can be detected by use of a labeled second antibody, such as antihuman globulin, directed against the antibody of concern. If antibody is used to coat the solid phase, then antigen can be detected. In this case the radiolabel is linked to antibody. Tests for hepatitis B antigen in serum use the sandwich technique. Unlabeled antibody to hepatitis B antigen is fixed to a solid phase and the serum to be tested is added. If the antigen is present in the serum, it combines with the antibody on the solid phase; when radiolabeled antibody is added, it will attach to the bound antigen. After the unbound radiolabeled antibody is washed away, the amount of radiolabeled antibody is determined and is a measure of the amount of antigen that was present in the serum.

Both monoclonal and polyclonal antibodies are used in immunoassays. RIA is widely used in clinical chemistry, particularly for determination of hormone levels and for monitoring drug levels during treatment.

The enzyme-linked immunosorbent assay (ELISA) was first introduced in 1971 by Engvall and Perlmann. The term *enzyme immunoassay (EIA)* is an alternative generic term for this type of test and is used to cover the many variations in the protocols of the actual assay. Enzymes such as alkaline phosphatase or peroxidase can be linked to antibody without destroying cither the antibody's specificity or the enzyme's activity. The enzyme acts as a label that makes detection possible. Both monoclonal and polyclonal antibodies can be utilized. Enzyme labels are cheaper, simpler to measure, and far more stable than radioactive labels. For these reasons, ELISA or EIA assays have in many cases replaced RIA and have done so while maintaining sensitivity and specificity. Many of the assays for hepatitis A and B in use today are based on ELISA.

Enzyme immunoassays are used to measure either antigen (direct) or antibody (indirect). For direct EIA, a specific antibody is absorbed onto the walls of an appropriate plastic tube and the sample, which may contain antigen, is added (Figure 7.14). After washing to remove unbound material, an enzyme-labeled (enzyme-linked) antibody is added. After incubation and washing, a substrate for the enzyme is added. The substrate must be one that yields a colored product when acted on by the enzyme. The amount of color generated by the reaction in a fixed time is directly proportional to the amount of antigen in the sample being tested. The indirect EIA is used to detect antibody in serum. The antibody in the serum sample is bound on an antigen that has been absorbed onto the walls of the tube in which the reaction is run. An enzyme-linked antibody specific for the antibody in the serum sample being tested is added. The amount of color generated after a chromogenic substrate has been added is measured. This method is currently used by blood centers to screen blood for antibody to the human immunodeficiency virus (HIV).

Fluorescent assays are frequently used for the detection of antibodies in serum or antigens in tissue or cells. Fluorescent antibody tests such as the indirect immunofluorescent antibody assay (IFA) are similar in principle to the indirect EIA. For detection of antigens, a tissue section or cell culture fixed to a slide serves as the antigen. The antigen in the tissue or cell is detected by its reaction with an antibody to which a fluorescent emitter such as fluorescein isothiocyanate (FITC) or rhodamine is attached. An ultraviolet light source is used to excite the FITC, which fluoresces or gives off light at a longer wavelength with a lower energy than that of the exciting incident light.

An ultraviolet microscope or other instrument designed to detect fluorescence permits detection of the bound fluorescent antibody. After the fluorescent-labeled antibody reacts with cellular antigens, for example, the antibody-coated cell becomes visible upon exposure to ultraviolet light, usually by emitting a yellow-green light. Immunofluorescent antibody assay allows rapid and easy detection of autoantibodies to a variety of antigens in tissues.

The direct FA test for antigen in cells or tissues uses a specific antibody labeled with a fluorescent dye as a detection system (Figure 7.15). In the indirect FA test, a fluorescent-labeled antiglobulin is used to detect unlabeled antibody that is bound to the antigen. The indirect test is more flexible and generally yields a brighter fluorescence than does the direct test. A third procedure, the sandwich test, detects antibody in the cytoplasm of cells. Antigen is the first reagent, then fluorescent-labeled antibody is added, and the antigen is sandwiched between the two antibodies. Cell surface markers, such as surface antigens of T-lymphocytes and immunoglobulins present in and on B-lymphocytes, are also frequently detected by fluorescent assays.

Both monoclonal and polyclonal antibodies have been used in fluorescent assays. The choice of which to use depends upon the requirements of the particular assay and the nature of the analysis. For assays in which the most important consideration is specificity, such as separation of T- and B-lymphocytes, monoclonal antibodies are used. On the other hand, in screening assays where sensitivity

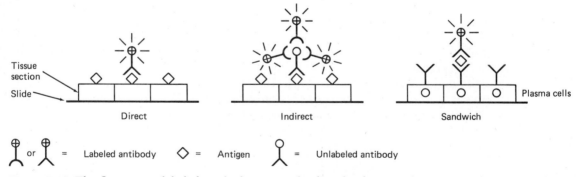

Figure 7.15 The fluorescent labeled antibody test can be done by direct, indirect, or sandwich procedures. The direct test uses a labeled antibody to detect antigen in a tissue section, blood film, or other specimen. The indirect test is used to detect antigens in similar situations but can also be used to detect antibodies. The detection system uses a labeled antigamma globulin. Where antibody binds on the antigen, the labeled antiglobulin will bind. The sandwich procedure has a more limited use than the other procedures. It is used to detect antibody on, for example, plasma cells. The cell is exposed to antigen, then to labeled antibody to the antigen. The antigen will only bind to cells with bound antibody of the correct specificity, and this in turn determines which cells will bind the labeled antibody.

is of utmost concern (that is, tests where it is important not to miss any possible positives), polyclonal antibodies are used.

The technique of neutralization can be used to detect the reaction of antigen and antibody when no precipitation occurs. A special type of neutralization is used in blood group work. Soluble blood group substances can be added to a serum containing multiple antibodies to remove one or more of them. This allows easier identification of the remaining antibodies. Neutralization is also widely used in work with viruses. A dose of virus known to be lethal for cells in culture is mixed with the serum to be tested for antibody against the virus. The mixture is added to the cell culture and the culture is observed. If neutralizing antibody is present in the serum sample, the virus is neutralized and will not kill the cells. Neutralization of toxin by antitoxin is also used. For example, toxin neutralization occurs *in vivo* when an individual exposed to *Clostridium tetani* is injected with antitoxin as part of the prophylaxis of tetanus.

Complement fixation resulting in lysis is also a valuable laboratory technique (see Chapter 9 for the complement activation sequence). Antibody can be detected by its ability to bind complement in the presence of an appropriate antigen. Red cells coated with antibody are used as indicator cells. If antibody is present, the complement is bound to the antigen–antibody complex formed and is not available to bind to the antibody-coated red cells, and the red cells do not lyse (Figure 7.16). Complement fixation is the basis of the lymphocytotoxic tests for detection of histocompatibility antigens (HLA). In this technique, living lymphocyte suspensions are exposed to antisera and complement. If the lymphocytes possess antigen corresponding to the antibody used, complement is fixed and the cells are lysed. Cells damaged by the fixed complement are penetrated by an added stain, commonly eosin or trypan blue, and undamaged cells are not. By this reaction, cell surface antigens can be identified.

Lysis, *in vivo* and *in vitro*, requires antibody, antigen, and complement. The complement does not have to be from the same species of animal as the antibody, however. Complement is fairly unstable and is less stable than antibodies. Because

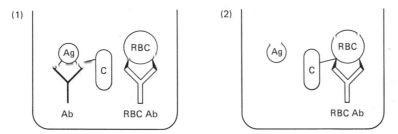

Figure 7.16 These diagrams indicate the basis of the complement-fixation test. If antibody is present in the serum being tested, it binds to the antigen. The complement that is available is then bound and is not available to lyse the red cell indicator system (1); if antibody is not present in the serum being tested, the complement is not bound in the test system and is available to lyse the antibody-coated red blood cells in the indicator system (2).

of this, fresh sera will often lyse bacteria (bacteriolysis) or red cells (hemolysis), but aged or heated serum may only cause agglutination. The lytic reactions due to fixation of complement are an important part of the immune defense mechanisms.

Most laboratories use a combination of these techniques, depending upon the nature of the samples received and the results desired. For example, a blood center processing blood from donors may use EIA to test for hepatitis B antigen and antibody to HIV, agglutination to determine blood type, and complement fixation to determine HLA type.

SUGGESTIONS FOR FURTHER READING

J. A. Bellanti. *Immunology III.* W. B. Saunders, Philadelphia, 1985.

J. B. Henry. *Clinical Diagnosis and Management by Laboratory Methods,* 17th edition. W. B. Saunders, Philadelphia, 1984.

E. J. Holborow and W. G. Reeves. *Immunology in Medicine,* 2nd edition. Grune & Stratton, New York, 1983.

P. L. Mollison, C. P. Englefriet, and M. Contreras. *Blood Transfusion in Clinical Medicine,* 8th edition. Blackwell Scientific Publications, Oxford, 1987.

S. L. Robbins and R. S. Cotran. *Pathological Basis of Disease,* 2nd edition. W. B. Saunders, Philadelphia, 1979.

I. M. Roitt. *Essential Immunology,* 5th edition. Blackwell Scientific Publications, Oxford, 1984.

I. M. Roitt, J. Brostoff, and D. K. Male. *Immunology.* Gower Medical Publishing, London, 1985.

D. P. Stites, J. D. Stobo, H. H. Fudenberg, and J. V. Wells. *Basic and Clinical Immunology,* 5th edition. Lange Medical Publishers, Los Altos, California, 1984.

N. W. Tietz. *Fundamentals of Clinical Chemistry,* 2nd edition. W. B. Saunders, Philadelphia, 1976.

F. K. Widman. *Technical Manual of the American Association of Blood Banks,* 9th edition. Arlington, 1985.

Chapter 8

The Inducible Defense System

The Induction and Development of the Inducible Defense

DIANE W. TAYLOR

Department of Biology
Georgetown University

INTRODUCTION

As you learned in earlier chapters, the immune system is composed of cells, tissues, and organs working together for the maintenance of health. Unlike other easily identifiable biological systems—for example, the digestive or respiratory systems, which have a unitary structure—the immune system consists of components scattered throughout the body. The cells of the immune system recognize and destroy invading pathogens or nonself antigens. As you may remember from Chapter 2, the hallmarks of the inducible immune system are recognition, specificity, and memory. The cell responsible for these properties is the lymphocyte. This chapter will provide information on how lymphocytes recognize and respond to antigens, factors that influence lymphocyte differentiation, and how lymphocytes interact with each other to bring about immunity. In an immune response, lymphocytes usually interact with a second cell type, the macrophage.

CELLS OF THE INDUCIBLE IMMUNE SYSTEM

The Lymphocyte

Morphologically, the lymphocyte usually appears in the peripheral blood as a small round uninucleate cell approximately 7 to 8 μm in diameter. The nucleus occupies the bulk of the cell, with a small amount of basic cytoplasm surrounding it (Chapter 3, Figure 3.2). The lymphocyte that is commonly observed in blood films, for example, is in the resting stage (G_o) of the cell cycle. The cytoplasm contains a few mitochondria, a small number of ribosomes, little or no endoplasmic reticulum, and an interphase nucleus. However, upon activation by antigen, lymphocytes increase in size (≈ 12 μm), undergo morphologic changes, and are termed *lymphoblasts* (or *blasts*). Because most lymphoblasts ultimately secrete products (for example, antibodies or interleukins) or transport intracellularly produced molecules to cell surfaces (for example, the interleukin-2, or IL-2, receptor), lymphoblasts have many of the morphologic characteristics of secretory cells. The Golgi apparatus becomes prominent, and there are large amounts of rough endoplasmic reticulum and polyribosomes. Activated cells usually undergo cell division, during which chromosomes and spindle fibers are evident. Electron micrographs of resting, dividing, and activated lymphocytes showing these attributes are shown in Figure 8.1.

Although they are indistinguishable one from the other when examined by light or electron microscopy, lymphocytes can be divided into subsets that have different immunologic functions. A summary of the attributes of the major lymphocyte subsets is shown in Table 8.1. Those lymphocytes responsible for producing antibodies (Chapter 7) are B-lymphocytes. They are called *B-cells* because they were first identified in the Bursa of Fabricius of chickens. Upon activation, B-cells undergo cell division, and some differentiate into antibody-producing cells, called *plasma cells.* The other major group of lymphocytes require the presence of the thymus for their development and are called *T-cells.* T-cells can be divided into several subsets with different biological functions. Major subsets include T-helper (T_H) cells that provide "help" for antibody production and cell-mediated immune responses; T-suppressor (T_S) cells that prevent or turn off an immune response; cytotoxic T-cells (T_{CTL}, or T_C) that lyse abnormal, histoincompatible, and virus-infected cells; and delayed type hypersensitivity (T_{DTH}, or T_D) cells that mediate delayed type hypersensitivity reactions.

Lymphocytes of the various subsets generally have different glycoproteins on their surfaces, commonly called *surface markers* or *surface antigens.* The immunologic importance of some of the surface markers has been established, but the functions of others are less clear. Surface markers distinguish T-cells with different immunologic roles. The major T-cell subsets and the corresponding surface markers found in mice and in humans are shown in Table 8.1. The life span of lymphocytes is uncertain. Estimates of their life span range from a few weeks to 20 years.

The Macrophage

From Chapter 4, "The Inflammatory Response," you learned about the role of macrophages and related cells in phagocytosis. Macrophages also function as "accessory" cells in the inducible immune response. They internalize foreign antigen by phagocytosis or pinocytosis, process it within endosomal vesicles, and reexpress it on their surfaces. This process will be described in detail later. Thus, macrophages are frequently called *antigen-presenting cells, antigen-processing cells (APC),* or *antigen-binding cells (ABC).* Many cells of the macrophage lineage function as APC. These include monocytes in the blood, histocytes in the connective tissue, macrophages in the spleen, alveolar macrophages in the lungs, glial cells in the central nervous system, and dendritic cells (which are APC even though they are not strongly phagocytic) in the lymph nodes.

Morphologically, macrophages (from the Latin word meaning "big-eaters") are large (10 to 50 μm) cells that are pleomorphic in shape and have a characteristic bean-shaped nucleus (Chapter 3, Figure 3.2). They possess lysosomes that contain numerous enzymes required for antigen degradation and for killing of intracellular pathogens. The presence of esterase is diagnostic for macrophages, but they also contain the following bioactive molecules within their lysosomes: lipase, acid

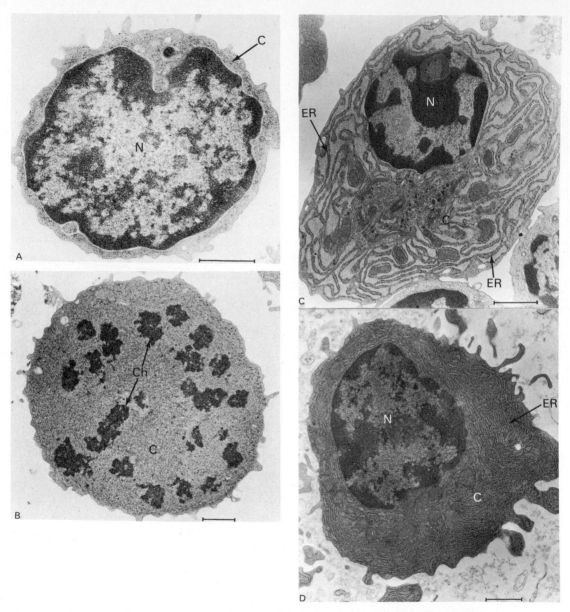

Figure 8.1 Electron micrographs of lymphocytes: (a) A resting lymphocyte. The nucleus (N) occupies most of the cell. There is a thin rim of cytoplasm (C). This could be either a B- or T-cell. (b) Upon antigenic stimulation, cell division occurs and individual chromosomes (Ch) are observed. With further differentiation, B cells become plasma cells. (c) Typical mouse and (d) human plasma cells. The presence of a massive amount of endoplasmic reticulum (ER) in the cytoplasm of the lymphocyte is the distinguishing characteristic of the cells that are actively synthesizing and secreting antibody. Bar represents 1 μm. (Photos courtesy of G. B. Chapman.)

Table 8.1 LYMPHOCYTE SUBSETS

Subset	Major surface markers[a]		
B-cells	$_s$IgM, $_s$IgD, receptors for C3b and F$_C$, Class II (Ia) molecules		
Plasma cells	Ig of isotype secreted increased levels of Class II (Ia) molecules		
	Mice		**Humans**
T-cells			
Immature	Thy 1, TL, Qa		CD 1, CD 4, CD 8[b]
Thymocytes	Lyt 1, Lyt 2,3		
T$_H$	L3T4		CD 4, CD 3,
	High level Lyt 1		Receptor for SRBC[c] or CD2
T$_{CTL}$	Low level Lyt 1		CD 8, CD 3
T$_{DTH}$	High level Lyt 1		CD 4, CD 3
	L3T4		
T$_S$	Lyt 2,3, I-J or Lyt 1, 2, 3, I-J		CD 8, CD 3

[a]All nucleated cells in the body possess Class I surface markers; thus, Class I markers are present on both B- and T-cells and do not serve to differentiate lymphocyte subsets.

[b]A variety of monoclonal antibodies have been produced against cell surface markers on human T-cells. Since some of the monoclonal antibodies recognize the same surface marker, a standardized nomenclature has been devised such that antibodies binding to the same molecule are combined into a numbered cluster of differentiation (CD) group.

[c]Mature human T-cells possess a receptor for a determinant (CD2) expressed on sheep red blood cells (SRBC) and therefore adhere to SRBCs.

phosphatase, catalase, muramidase (lysozyme), ribonuclease, galactosidase, and cytochrome oxidase. In addition, macrophages produce immunoregulatory compounds such as interleukin-1 (IL-1) and interferons (IFN).

Like lymphocytes, macrophages have a number of unique cell surface markers. These include receptors for the Fc domain of antibody, the C$_{3b}$ component of complement, and IL-1. They also have Class II molecules coded for by the major histocompatibility complex, which will be described in the next section.

GENETIC REGULATION OF THE IMMUNE SYSTEM

Numerous genes located on various chromosomes code for molecules essential to the immune system (Table 8.2). These include genes coding for antigen receptors on B-cells and T-cells, genes coding for the heavy and light chains of antibody molecules, and genes coding for the T-cell receptor (TCR). These are the genes that code the information that permits recognition of antigen and of self. A number of independent genes have been identified that code for immunoregulatory molecules, called *cytokines,* that are produced by macrophages (monokines) and lymphocytes (lymphokines). Some of these are listed in Table 8.3.

In addition, a major complex of genes, located on chromosome 17 in mice and

Table 8.2   CHROMOSOMAL LOCATION OF GENES CODING FOR IMPORTANT
IMMUNOLOGICAL MOLECULES

| | Chromosome number | | Gene products |
	Mouse[a]	Humans	(M.W., in daltons)[b]
Ig heavy chain	12	14	50,000–70,000
Ig kappa chain	6	2	23,000–25,000
Ig lambda chain	16	22	23,000–25,000
T-cell receptor			
Alpha chain	14	14	"approximately" 40,000–50,000
Beta chain	6	7	"approximately" 40,000–50,000
MHC complex	17	6	Class I: 45,000
			Class II: 28,000 and 23,000
β2-microglobulin	2		
Interferon-γ	10	12	12,000
ly 1	19	—	40,000–60,000
			(dimer)
ly 2,3	6	—	
CD 4	—	—	62,000
CD 8	—	—	76,000 (dimer)

[a]Mice have 20 pairs of chromosomes.

[b]Molecular weight of glycoprotein form.

chromosome 6 in humans, codes for the major histocompatibility or tissue transplantation molecules. This region is referred to as the *major histocompatibility complex (MHC)* in mice and as the *human leukocyte antigen complex (HLA)* in humans. It is becoming common today to refer to the HLA complex in humans as the MHC. Figure 8.2 shows the major regions of the histocompatibility complex. Genes located in regions K and D in mice and A, B, and C in humans code for proteins present on almost every nucleated cell of the body. They are called *Class I proteins.* There are numerous alleles in the population for each gene locus, and alleles are codominantly expressed. That is, every cell in humans possesses two Class I A proteins, one of which is coded for by a gene received from the father (allele 1) and one of which is coded for by a gene received from the mother (allele 2). Thus a single human cell expresses six different Class I antigens: A_1, A_2, B_1, B_2, C_1, C_2. In humans, 23 specificities at A, 49 at B, and 8 at C have been defined (undoubtedly more exist). If the alleles were equally represented in the population, then the chances of finding two individuals (other than identical twins) with the same MHC–Class I antigens, would be $\frac{1}{23} \times \frac{1}{23} \times \frac{1}{49} \times \frac{1}{49} \times \frac{1}{8} \times \frac{1}{8}$, or approximately 1 in 81,000,000. Differences in MHC proteins play a major role in transplantation immunity (Chapter 11).

Each Class I protein consists of two noncovalently linked polypeptides. The one coded by the Class I gene has an Mr of 45,000 and five general regions (Figure 8.2). The segments of the first three regions are exposed on the surface, to which they are anchored by a hydrophobic segment inserted in the cell membrane. The

Table 8.3 IMPORTANT REGULATORY AND EFFECTOR CYTOKINES

Name	Alternative name	M.W. (daltons)	Source	Target	Function
Afferent-enhancing cytokines					
IL-1	LAF, TRFm,	Mice: 15,000 Humans: 18,000	Macrophages B-cells	T- & B-cells Other cells (see text)	multifunctional growth and inducing factor (see text)
IL-2	TCGF, TSF/TMF	Mice: 30000–35000 Humans: 30000–35000	T_H cells Some T_{CTL}	T_H & T_{CTL} B-cells NK cells	Growth factor
IL-3	Mast cells Growth factors	Mice: 28,000 and 32,000 Humans: 30,000–50,000	T-cells	Stem cells Mast cells	Growth and differentiation factors
IL-4	BCGF-1, BSF BCGF	Mice: 13,000–20,000 Humans: 13,000–14,000	T-cells	B-cells T-cells Mast cells	Growth, enhances Ia expression on B-cells
IL-5	BCGF II BCDFI TRF	Mice: oligomer 45,000	T-cells	B-cells Thymocytes	Proliferation and differentiation
IFN-α	Type I IFN pH 2 insensitive	16,000–22,000	leukocytes	NK cells	Induces antiviral state activation of T_{CTL} and NK cells
IFN-β	Type I IFN (ph 2 insensitive)	30,000	fibroblasts	T_{CTL} virus-infected cells	Enhanced Class I expression
IFN-γ	Type II IFN (ph 2 sensitive) Immune IFN	40,000 (dimer)	T-cells	Above plus B-cells and macrophages	Above plus enhanced Ia expression, stimulates IL-1, IL-2, and Ig productio
Afferent-suppressing cytokines					
SIRS	Soluble immune response substance	48,000–67,000	Probably made by T_S cells and activated macrophages	B-cells	Inhibits proliferation and Ab production
T_SF	Id$^+$, I-J$^+$ factors	Variable	T_S cells (see text)	B- & T-cells	Inhibits induction (tolerance) and proliferation

Table 8.3 (*Continued*)

Name	Alternative name	M.W. (daltons)	Source	Target	Function
			Efferent cytokines		
MIF	Migration inhibition factor	15,000–70,000	T_H cells Fibroblasts	Macrophages	Inhibits macrophage migration from inflammatory area by inducing polymerization of tubulin
MAF	Macrophage activation factor (may be IFN-γ)	10,000–70,000	T-cells	Macrophages	Activates macrophages to kill tumors and certain bacteria
TNF		Dimer, trimers	Macrophages	Many, including tumor cells (see text)	Antitumor factor, induces fever, elevates serum lipid levels, and causes cachexia (wasting disease)
	Cachetin Necrosin	17,000 (monomer)			

hydrophobic segment is the fourth region. The fifth region is exposed into the cytoplasm. Each of the three surface segments is composed of 100 amino acids and contains disulfhydral bonds spaced 60 amino acids apart such that each folds into a β-pleat. The external portion of the polypeptide coded by its Class I gene is noncovalently associated with the second polypeptide, a 12,000-dalton molecule called β_2-*microglobulin.* In mice, β_2-microglobulin is coded for by a gene on chromosome 2. Thus, two proteins coded for by genes on different chromosomes come together to produce the histocompatibility proteins.

Regions I in mice and Dr in humans code for immune response (I_r or Ia) molecules. A simplified diagram of this region is shown in Figure 8.2. This region codes for Class I molecules that consist of α and β peptides of molecular weights of 32,000 and 28,000 daltons, respectively. The region is divided into several sections. The A region contains three genes. Two of these, the A_A and A_B genes, code for an IA molecule. In the B region the gene E_A produces an IE molecule. IA and IE, collectively referred to as *Ia molecules,* are present on the surfaces of B-cells, macrophages, and related APC. Class II molecules are involved in MHC-restricted macrophage–T-cell and T-cell–B cell interactions that will be discussed later.

The S region of the MHC gene complex codes for some of the components of the complement cascade such as C4, C2, and Factor B.

Genes coding for immunoglobulins, the TCR, Class I and II antigens, and other

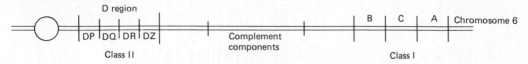

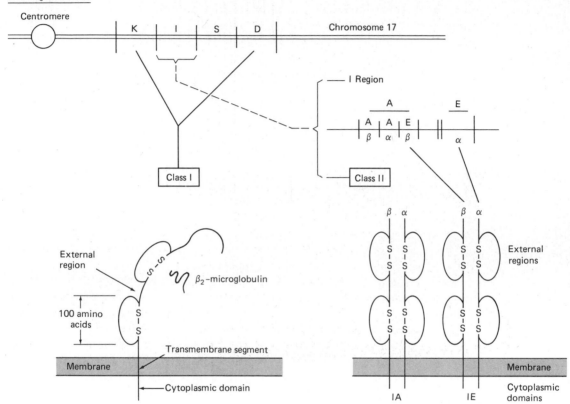

Figure 8.2 The major histocompatibility complexes of mice and humans are similar in function although the terminology used to describe them differs. In mice the system is called the major histocompatibility complex (MHC); in humans it is called the human leukocyte antigen (HLA) complex. It is becoming common, however, for the system in humans also to be referred to as the major histocompatibility complex. Genes located in the K and D regions in mice and the A, B, and C regions in humans code for proteins present on almost every nucleated cell of the body. These are the class I proteins. Regions I in mice and Dr in humans code for the class II molecules, which regulate the immune response. The products of the class II genes are present on the antigen-presenting cells.

immunologically important molecules appear to have evolved from a common primordial gene and are members of the immunoglobulin (Ig) superfamily of proteins.

CLONAL SELECTION THEORY AND RECEPTORS FOR ANTIGEN

The hallmark of the inducible immune system is specificity. For example, if an individual becomes infected with mumps virus, an immune response specific for mumps virus develops. However, the individual remains susceptible to other viruses (for example, measles), thus demonstrating specificity for the virus to which the response occurred. Upon reexposure to mumps virus, the immune system "remembers," and a rapid, enhanced immune response ensues, eliminating the virus before clinical symptoms develop. The rapid secondary response is often called an *anamnestic* or *immunologic memory response.*

One of the early questions that puzzled immunologists was how immunological specificity was achieved. It was assumed that lymphocytes possessed receptors for antigens, but the nature and distribution of antigen receptors was unclear. Linus Pauling, in the early 1950s, suggested that immunoglobulins are pliable molecules that can acquire a specific shape by "folding around" antigens. That is, an antigen would interact with the receptors on B-cells and "instruct" them to secrete immunoglobulins with shapes complementary to the antigen. This is called the *instructional theory of antibody production.* When scientists learned that antibody specificity is a result of the primary structure of antibody molecules, the instructional theory could no longer explain specificity.

Sir MacFarlane Burnet, in the late 1950s, advanced the theory that numerous individual clones of lymphocytes exist, each of which possesses a receptor for one or a few structurally related antigens. Upon primary exposure to an invasive pathogen, those lymphocytes with complementary receptors would bind the pathogen, become activated, undergo cell division, and differentiate into functionally reactive cells. Thus, the antigen or pathogen would "select" appropriate cells and induce clonal expansion. This concept is called the *clonal selection theory,* and many subsequent studies have substantiated it (Chapter 5). When one is reexposed to a pathogen (secondary exposure), the number of antigen-responsive cells is already large as a result of the first exposure and a large, rapid, secondary response results. The selective activation of lymphocytes with receptors complementary to the antigen is the basis for achieving specificity in inducible immunity.

Once the validity of the clonal selection theory had been established, the next problem was the determination of the biochemical nature of the receptor for antigen on B-cells and T-cells. Indeed, at least a portion of the molecule had to vary from receptor to receptor to account for antigen specificity. The antigen receptor on B-cells is an immunoglobulin (IgM or IgD). A hydrophobic amino acid sequence at the carboxyl end of the conserved portion of the heavy chains anchors the monomeric surface IgM into the B-cell membrane. The immunoglobulin receptors bind free antigens to the B-cells.

The antigen receptor on T-cells is similar in structure in a general way to an Fab fragment of immunoglobulin. It is composed of two chains (α and β) that have an M.W. of 40,000–50,000 daltons each. Each chain possesses a variable (V) region of 100 amino acids and a constant (C) region of 100 to 110 amino acids. Both chains combine to form a β-pleated molecule with the combined V regions exposed on the outer surface to form an antigen binding site. Both chains are anchored in the T-cell membrane by a hydrophobic transmembrane segment and both have a small portion extending into the cell cytoplasm. The TCR is associated with three or four integral membrane proteins of 20,000 to 25,000 daltons each. The receptor and the membrane proteins together are called the T_i/T_3 *complex* (see Chapter 11, Figure 11.4). Unlike the immunoglobulin receptor on B-cells, the TCR cannot bind free antigen. It can only bind to small segments of antigen complexed to Class I or II glycoproteins exposed on the cell surface. Thus, the TCR must bind both antigen and ''self'' simultaneously. It remains to be established whether the receptor actually binds a portion of the processed antigen plus a portion of self or instead binds a new shape created by a combination of the two (a neoantigen). Since Class I or II histocompatibility antigens must be associated with the antigen for recognition by the T-cell to occur, the interaction of TCR and antigen is thus said to be *MHC restricted.*

There is a population of T-cells that contain a receptor composed of γ/Δ chains (instead of α/β). These T-cells generally do not circulate in the lymphatic system but reside within the thymus. Although they are probably involved in the killing of abnormal cells, the nature of their antigen specificity and exact functions remain to be determined.

Upon exposure to a pathogen, only lymphocytes with receptors complementary to the molecular configuration of the pathogen become activated. Experiments indicate that about 1 in 2000 B-cells and 1 in 2000 T-cells may respond when an individual is injected with an antigen that has only one type of antigenic determinant; for example, polymerized flagellin. With pathogens, the number of antigenic molecules is large and, therefore, the number of responding cells would be considerably greater.

Immunologists believe that an individual can respond to between 10^6 and 10^7 different antigens. Accordingly, there would have to be at least from 10^6 to 10^7 B- and T-cells, each with different antigen receptors. Since there are various B- and T-cell subsets (that is, T_H, T_S, and so on), each subset of functional lymphocytes would require this level of receptor diversity for an animal to be immunocompetent. Originally, geneticists believed that a separate gene was required to code for each unique receptor. If true, this would require more than 10 percent of an organism's DNA to be used to code for lymphocyte antigen receptors. We know that this is not true, but rather that a series of ''mini-genes,'' or movable DNA segments, recombine to generate antibodies and TCR diversity. This topic is discussed in Chapter 7.

THE IMMUNE SYSTEM

A diagram of the major components of the immune system is shown in Figure 8.3a. Organs that provide mature lymphocytes—that is, the bone marrow in mammals, the bursa in chickens, and the thymus—are termed *primary lymphoid organs.*

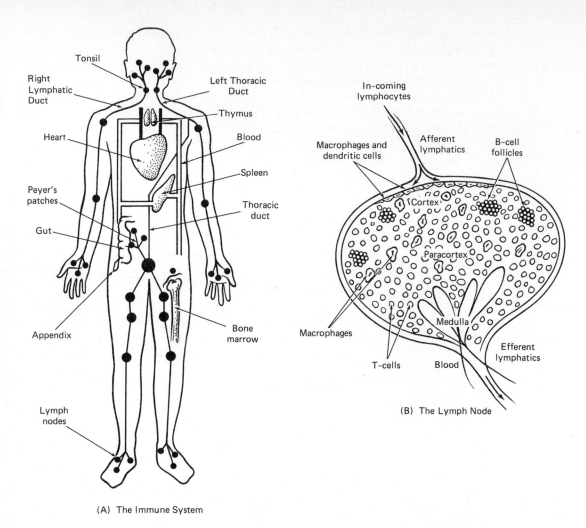

Tonsil
Right Lymphatic Duct
Left Thoracic Duct
Thymus
Heart
Blood
Spleen
Peyer's patches
Thoracic duct
Gut
Appendix
Bone marrow
Lymph nodes
In-coming lymphocytes
Macrophages and dendritic cells
Afferent lymphatics
B-cell follicles
Cortex
Paracortex
Macrophages
Medulla
Efferent lymphatics
T-cells
Blood

(A) The Immune System

(B) The Lymph Node

Figure 8.3 The anatomy of the immune system: (a) The major components of the immune system of humans. The system consists of lymph nodes connected by lymph ducts; the Peyer's patches, which are masses of lymphocytes in the gut wall; the thymus; and the spleen. The other major component of the system, the bone marrow, which exists in bones throughout the body, is indicated by the drawing of a section of a femur. (b) The lymph node has a complex anatomy. Afferent lymph ducts bring lymph-containing antigens into the lymph nodes. In the cortical region of the node there are numerous macrophages and dendritic cells. Contact of antigen with these antigen-presenting cells initiates the immune response. As a result, B-cell colonies (germinal centers) containing many plasma cells develop, and antibody is produced and released. The antibody leaves the node by the efferent lymphatic ducts that empty into the blood system. Lymphocytes also leave the node by the efferent duct to colonize other parts of the body.

Those that receive and maintain functional lymphocytes are called *secondary lymphoid organs.* Secondary lymphoid organs include lymph nodes, the spleen, Peyers patches (lymph nodes along the gut, also referred to as gut associated lymphoid tissue, or GALT), appendix, tonsils, and adenoids. Lymph nodes develop throughout the body and are most highly concentrated in areas where pathogens are most likely to enter the body. They are especially concentrated in areas in the head around the eyes, mouth, and nose, and in the gut and limbs. The lymph nodes and spleen are connected by lymphatic channels (Figure 8.3*a*). The spleen, thymus, and bone marrow are connected to the rest of the immune system by the blood.

Lymphocytes within the immune system are not fixed within tissues but constantly migrate throughout the body during their lifetime in search of foreign material in a process called *lymphocyte trafficking.* Lymphocytes present in lymph nodes may leave them via the efferent lymphatics, circulate in lymphatic vessels and lodge in other lymph nodes, or enter the blood via one of the two major lymphatic ducts (Figure 8.3*a*). In the blood, lymphocytes circulate through the spleen and peripheral circulation; then they ultimately enter venules from which they migrate back into the lymphatic system. Both T- and B-cells recirculate by this route.

Within the secondary lymphoid organs, lymphocytes are found in distinct areas such that they will be able to mount a maximal immune response. The architecture of a typical lymph node is shown in Figure 8.3*b*. A similar though more complex arrangement exists in the spleen. If an antigen enters the tissues, it will probably make its way into the lymphatics and enter the lymph nodes. If the antigen is in the blood, it will be "filtered-out" in the spleen. Within these organs, macrophages and other APC are strategically positioned so that they can capture foreign material by phagocytosis. Under the layer of macrophages are found T-cells and a few macrophages. This area is called the *paracortical region.* Within the paracortex are found discrete regions, called *follicles,* that contain B-cells. Upon infection, which of course causes antigenic stimulation, B-cells divide within the follicle; the follicular region increases in diameter and may merge with an adjoining follicle. Regions containing rapidly dividing B-cells are called *germinal centers.* During an infection, lymph nodes enlarge as a result of both B- and T-cell proliferation. One sign of a localized immune response is an enlarged lymph node. Activated B- and T-cells will leave the lymph nodes and spleen, and disperse throughout the body.

DEVELOPMENT OF THE IMMUNE SYSTEM

Embryonic Development of Lymphoid Organs and Tissues

The basic pattern of the immune system found in the adult animal is developed during embryogenesis. During the formation of the lymphoid organs, cells of endodermal and mesodermal origin form a loose matrix of connective tissue that becomes filled with developing lymphocytes. The cells in the matrix of the thymus and bone marrow not only provide structure for the organ but also provide factors required for lymphocyte and stem cell differentiation. We will first look briefly at the formation of the organs and then at the development of the cells within them.

All components of the human immune system begin formation during the first three months *in utero.* After about six weeks of development, the thymus, spleen, and bone marrow begin to form. In the formation of the thymus, endodermal tissue from the bronchial gill clefts grows inward, and two lobes of tissue are found on either side of the throat. These lobes migrate into the thoracic cavity, coalesce, and form a recognizable thymus by week 10. The development of the thymus is completed when the matrix of endodermal origin becomes filled with developing lymphocytes of mesodermal origin that migrate from the yolk sac and bone marrow (described later). In bone marrow and spleen formation, mesodermal cells form a loose connective tissue network that becomes populated with developing lymphoid and stem cells.

The last portions of the immune system to form are the lymphatic channels (the lymphatic duct system) and lymph nodes. In humans, six lymphatic sacs of mesodermal tissue form. As the fetus develops, these elongate into channels. At about three months masses of mesodermal cells form beside the channels, a connective tissue capsule forms around them, and they become vascularized. The newly developed lymph nodes sink into the channels and become populated with lymphocytes from the thymus and spleen. Lymph node development is completed within a short period after parturition.

During embryonic development, cells that give rise to lymphocytes can be identified in the yolk sac and are called *pluripotential hematopoietic stem cells.* The yolk sac is of endodermal origin (an outpocketing of the gut), but cells of mesodermal origin are thought to migrate there and develop into stem cells. In mammals, stem cells migrate from the yolk sac into the developing thymus (of endodermal origin) and the fetal liver (mesodermal), and then from the fetal liver into the bone marrow. Following differentiation and development, lymphocytes leave the thymus as T-cells and the bone marrow as immature B-cells that migrate into the spleen. From the spleen, lymphocytes migrate to the developing lymph nodes and the blood. Immature pre–T-cells also emigrate from the bone marrow to the thymus, where they complete development. Self-renewing stem cells can be found in the bone marrow of humans in the spleen and in the bone marrow of mice throughout the life of the animal.

Differentiation of Pluripotential Hematopoietic Stem Cells

Cells involved in both the constitutive and inducible immune systems, and all the cells present in blood, develop from a common stem cell, the pluripotential hematopoietic stem cell (Figure 8.4). This stem cell, under the influence of the soluble cytokine interleukin-3 and other factors, undergoes a complex sequence of differentiation steps during embryogenesis and throughout the life of adult animals. The exact sequence of events is uncertain, but it is known that totipotent stem cells first differentiate into progenitor cells that are committed to develop into a specific cell type; that is, they develop surface receptors for cytokines that provide

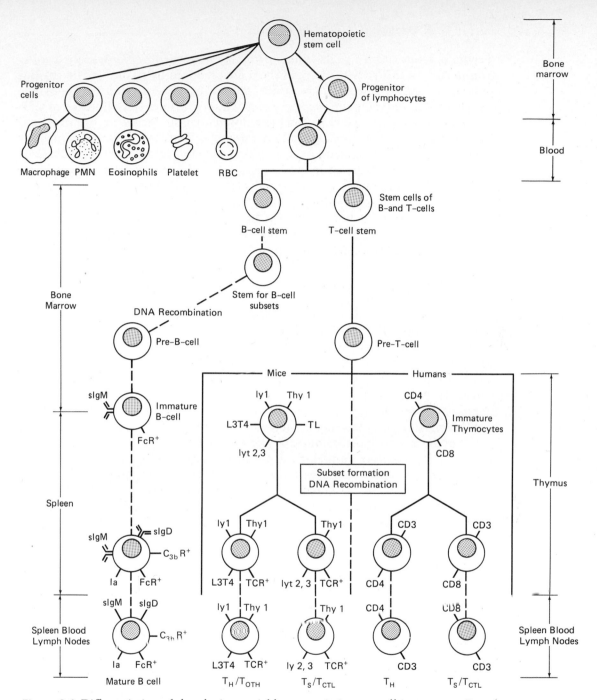

Figure 8.4 Differentiation of the pluripotential hematopoietic stem cell into mature B- and T-cells: The basic developmental steps of human and rodent B-cells are similar. It is known that murine B-cells develop into cells of various subsets; subsets in humans are still undefined. During development in the thymus, human and murine thymocytes undergo subset formation. Ag-responsive T-cells are designed as TCR$^+$ in mice and CD3$^+$ in humans.

specific differentiation signals. These cytokines are called *hematopoietic colony stimulating factors (CSF)*. Many of them are produced by tissues of the thymus and bone marrow. Accordingly, these tissues have been referred to as the *hematopoietic-inducing microenvironment tissues*. Under the influence of CSF, progenitor cells are induced to complete differentiation. Known progenitor cells include granulocyte-macrophage–colony forming cells (GM–CFC) that ultimately develop into macrophages and neutrophils; eosinophil–colony forming cells (EO–CFC) that become mature eosinophils; megakaryocyte–colony forming cells (MC–CFC) that become megakaryocytes and platelets; and bursa-forming unit–erythrocytes (BU–E) that produce erythrocytes.

The progenitor for lymphocytes is less clear, but it also develops from the pluripotential stem cell. It is currently thought that the lymphoid progenitor differentiates into secondary progenitors for B-cells and T-cells. Then, tertiary progenitors for various B- and T-cell subsets are formed. Finally, generation of antigen specificity takes place, resulting in production of lymphocyte populations with various specific antigen receptors (Figure 8.4).

In developing B-cells in the bone marrow, DNA coding for V, D, and J mini-gene segments of the heavy chains and VJ genes of the light chains rearrange to produce a functional V-domain (Chapter 7). A similar series of V, D, and J recombinational events takes place in T-cells (thymocytes) in the thymus. This rearrangement of DNA takes place during embryogenesis and throughout the life of the animal. It occurs in the absence of antigen and is referred to as *antigen-independent lymphocyte differentiation*.

During antigen-independent lymphocyte differentiation, mini-gene rearrangement produces an almost infinite array of B- and T-cell receptors. It is likely that some of these receptors would bind to molecules or tissues normally present in the body. This, of course, would be undesirable as then the immune system would respond to and attempt to remove or destroy normal components of the host. (This actually happens in certain autoimmune diseases.) However, the immune system has the ability to distinguish self from nonself molecules by a mechanism termed *self-recognition*, or *tolerance*. Unfortunately, it is still unclear how tolerance is achieved, but some current ideas are incorporated in this chapter. It is important to remember that stem cells constantly replenish the supply of lymphocytes throughout the life of the animal and that these lymphocytes recognize an infinite number of foreign, but not self, antigens.

Antigen-independent Differentiation of B- and T-Cells

The earliest B-cell one can identify in mice and humans is found in the bone marrow and is called a *pre–B-cell*. It is a large cell, 10 μm in diameter, and has the IgM heavy chain within its cytoplasm (Figure 8.4), thus demonstrating that heavy chain gene rearrangement has already occurred. As this cell matures, monomeric IgM appears on its surface. The cell is called an *immature, virgin,* or *unprimed B-cell.* Immature B-cells are affected by the presence of antigens. In the presence of antigen in high concentration (that is, self-antigens or large amounts of antigen exogenously supplied), any immature B-cell that responds to that antigen is either deleted or has its surface receptors for the antigen permanently internalized, making the cell nonreactive. Much remains to be learned about B-cell tolerance.

About this time or slightly later, the immature B-cell leaves the bone marrow and finishes its development in the spleen. In completing its development into a mature B-cell, the cell synthesizes and inserts the following receptor molecules onto its surface: an IgD molecule that possesses the same antigen-binding specificity as the IgM, an Fc receptor for the IgG, a receptor for C_{3b}, and a number of lymphocyte (ly) alloantigens, including lyb3 and lyb5 in mice and numerous CD surface markers in humans. In addition, both Class I and II MHC molecules are inserted into the surface membranes of B-cells by the time they are mature. Mature B-cells can be found in B-cell follicles of the spleen and lymph nodes, and circulating in the blood.

In adult animals, pre–T-cells begin development in the bone narrow and migrate through the blood to the cortex of the thymus, where they develop from immature to mature thymocytes. Thymocyte differentiation is an important step in the development of the immune system. In the thymus, V, D, and J DNA segments rearrange within the nucleus of thymocytes to produce the genes coding for the TCR. The DNA must be rearranged before it is expressed to produce a TCR. Thus T-cells obtain antigenic specificity within the thymus. Upon maturation thymocytes also express a receptor for IL-2, which serves as a growth factor inducing their clonal expansion.

Within the thymus, thymocytes differentiate into mature T-cells. However, only 1 percent of developing thymocytes leave the thymus; the remainder die within it. It appears that only those thymocytes reactive to nonself-antigens are allowed to mature (clonal deletion). Self-reactive T-cell clones either are not allowed to mature or are in some way made nonfunctional under normal circumstances.

As pre–T-cells develop into mature lymphocytes, a series of markers appears on their surfaces. In mice, pre–T-cells have low levels of thy 1 and ly 1 on their surfaces as they leave the bone marrow, but within the thymus they become immature thymocytes with high levels of thy 1 and ly 1. They also express at this time a differentiation marker called *TL (thymus leukemia antigen)* and develop high levels of both lyt 2,3 and L3T4. At about this stage, the T-cell antigen receptor appears on the cell surface and thymocytes mature into functionally distinct subsets; for example, in mice L3T4$^+$, ly 1$^+$(T_H), or lyt 2,3$^+$(T_{CTL} or T_S). Functionally mature T-cells are found in the medulla of the thymus, from which they rapidly migrate to all parts of the lymphoid system through the blood. A similar series of steps occurs during T-cell development in humans (Figure 8.4).

Following antigen-independent differentiation, mature lymphocytes remain in the resting stage (G_0) of the life cycle. They circulate through the body in search of foreign antigens or "abnormal" self-antigens. If a lymphocyte "meets" an antigen complementary to its receptor, it undergoes proliferation and differentiation. Cellular interactions and factors that influence antigen-dependent activation and differentiation of B- and T-cells will be described next. If a lymphocyte does not encounter an appropriate antigen, it will die (and thus be removed from the lymphocyte pool) at the end of its normal life span.

Activation of the Immune System by Antigen

To a large extent, the rate, length, and nature of the immune response that follows entry of a pathogen or other antigen-bearing object is regulated by the amount, site of entry, and biochemical composition of the antigen itself. Thus, in a sense one cannot describe *the* immune response, since it differs with each situation. Figure 8.5 diagrams some of the events that might take place following the introduction of antigen. It is unlikely that all of the events would be induced by a single infectious agent.

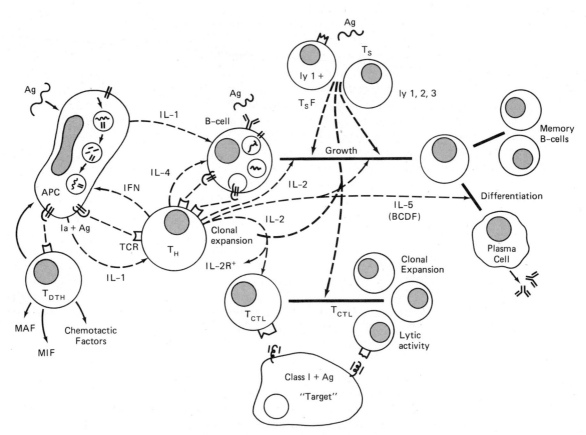

Figure 8.5 Possible sequences of events during an immune response following introduction of antigen: The antigen-presenting cell (APC) ingests antigen, processes it, and presents it to the T_H cells. These cells then undergo clonal expansion. They interact with B-cells, which also ingest, process, and present antigen, and with T_{CTL} cells. As a result of these interactions, in part mediated by cytokines (e.g., IL-1, IL-2, etc.), clonal expansion of these cells takes place with the production of antibody, T-cytolytic effector cells, and memory cells.

Macrophages: Antigen Processing and IL-1 Production

Generally, if an antigen is introduced into the skin or muscle, it will by phagocytized by macrophages in lymph nodes; if the antigen is introduced into the circulation, it will be phagocytized in the spleen. Within the macrophage, the contents of the endocytic vesicles become acidified. This change in pH leads to the activation of cathepsinlike proteases and fragmentation of the antigen. Within the endocytic vesicle, some of the fragments become associated with Class II (Ia) molecules, whereas other fragments are completely degraded in the lysosomal vesicles. Endosomal vesicles return the antigenic segment complexed to Class II molecules to the cell surface. It is also possible that the antigen is fragmented in the macrophage and is returned to the cell surface, where the fragments combine with Ia. As a result, a combination of the antigen segment bound to an Ia molecule is expressed on the macrophage surface. These processes are known as *antigen processing* and *antigen presentation*, respectively. In order for a protein fragment to be expressed, it must be of an appropriate size (thought to be 11–20 amino acids long) and of the correct charge and hydrophobicity to bind to Ia molecules. Segments of antigens that can make a successful interaction with Class I and II MHC molecules are generally termed *T-cell epitopes* because they provide induction signals for T-cells.

Antigen-presenting macrophages make direct contact with those T-cells of the T_H and T_{DTH} subclasses that bear complementary receptors. This interaction stimulates T-cell activation. It also stimulates macrophages to produce and secrete the monokine (IL-1). This monokine was originally termed *lymphocyte activation factor (LAF)* and is an important growth regulator (Table 8.3). IL-1 production is induced not only by contact with T-cells but also by phagocytosis of a wide variety of agents (for example, latex, muramyl dipeptide [a component of Complete Freunds Adjuvant], various endotoxins, and Ag–Ab complexes).

IL-1 is a 15,000-dalton protein that affects the growth of cells of various types. For example, IL-1 increases the number of IL-2 receptors on T-cells (thus enhancing T-cell clonal expansion); enhances Ia expression on B-cells; promotes the growth of fibroblasts; induces liver hepatocytes to synthesize and release acute phase proteins, including C-reactive protein; acts on chondrocytes and osteoclasts for bone resorption; forms a chemotactic gradient for neutrophils; and serves as an endogenous pyrogen, which produces fever. Thus, IL-1 plays an important role both in the inducible immune system and in inflammatory reactions

T-cell–Macrophage Interaction

As noted earlier, regulatory T_H cells cannot respond to antigens directly. Because of this, if purified T_H cells are incubated with antigens, they do not become activated. They only respond upon contact with antigens expressed in association with Ia on macrophages, B-cells, or other APC. Thus, direct macrophage–T-cell contact is required for T-cell activation. Since the APC expresses multiple copies of T-cell epitopes on its surface, the interaction of the APC and T_H cell results in cross linking of the TCRs (T_i/T_3 complex). This creates a transmembrane signal that activates certain biochemical pathways. One initial pathway that is activated is thought to cause the hydrolysis of intramembranous phosphatidylinosital bi-phosphate to inosital triphosphate and diacylglyerol. Both inosital triphosphate and diacylglyerol act as secondary intracellular messengers and elicit a series of physiologic responses.

One of the earliest proteins induced following the activation of T_H cells by contact with antigen or APCs is a 32,000-dalton glycoprotein, IL-2. It is a growth factor for T-cells. At the same time, activated T_H cells synthesize and express on their surfaces a receptor for IL-2; that is, they become IL-2 receptor positive. The binding of IL-2 to the IL-2 receptor induces clonal expansion. As long as antigen is present on APC, activated T_H cells synthesize IL-2 and the IL-2 receptor, and the binding of IL-2 to the IL-2 receptor serves as a signal for continued expansion of the T-cell clone. However, since the receptor–IL-2 complex is continually internalized by endocytosis, once antigen is cleared the T_H cells stop synthesizing the receptor. Then they are no longer susceptible to the growth factor activity of IL-2, and clonal expansion ceases. T_H cells have thus developed an antigen-controlled autocrine system for regulating their clonal expansion.

In the presence of processed antigen, T_H cells not only undergo cell division but also interact directly with B-cells and secrete a variety of regulatory lymphokines. Some of these lymphokines, which are considered next, enhance the immune response (Table 8.3), whereas others shut the system off.

B-Cell Activation and Antibody Production

Upon encountering an antigen, B-cells become activated (that is, acquire sensitivity to induction signals), proliferate, and develop into "memory cells" or differentiated plasma cells. A B-cell must receive a number of induction signals to differentiate into an antibody-producing plasma cell. Not all of the steps are clear, and they may differ between mice and humans.

At least in mice, there are two subpopulations of B-cells that differ in their need for induction signals. B-cells that possess the lyb5$^+$ receptor can produce antibodies without direct contact with T-cells, whereas B-cells of the lyb5$^-$ phenotype cannot. The former cells respond to a group of antigens called *T-independent antigens:* For example, *Pneumococcal polysaccharide* Type III (SIII) can induce antibody-producing lyb5$^+$ cells in the absence of T-cells, whereas it cannot induce antibody production by lyb5$^-$ cells in the absence of T_H cells. To cause lyb5$^+$ cells to produce antibody, the antigen must bind to the Ig receptors on B-cells. Cross linking of the receptors then induces a transmembrane signal initiating intracellular events similar to those described for T_H cells. As a result the cell becomes activated, begins proliferation, then differentiation, and finally secretes antibody. IL-1 is important in inducing clonal expansion of the lyb5$^+$ cells.

In lyb5$^-$ cells antigen is thought to bind on B-cells, but cross linking of the Ig receptors either does not occur or is insufficient to induce activation. The antigen receptor complex and nearby Ia molecules are internalized into endosomal vesicles, and antigen processing takes place that is similar to that by macrophages. Then a combination of the peptide fragments, bound to Ia, appears on the cell surface of the activated B-cell. IL-1 helps the system to develop by enhancing Ia expression. Next, T_H cells with receptors complementary to the antigen Ia complex make contact with the B-cells, cross link the molecules, and provide the induction signal for proliferation, differentiation, and antibody secretion.

Activated T-cells secrete a variety of lymphokines that serve as B-cell growth factors that promote clonal expansion and B-cell differentiation, and that convert dividing B-cells into plasma cells. A variety of factors has been shown to have growth factor activity, including B-cell stimulating factor, IL-1, IL-2, and IFN-γ. B-cell stimulating factor (called *IL-4*) has been shown to be important in the activation of antigen-primed B-cells. The signal for stimulating dividing B-cells to become differentiated plasma cells was originally termed *T-cell replacing factor* or *B-cell differentiation factor-1* (Table 8.3), is currently called *IL-5*.

As long as antigen is present (for example, as long as an infectious disease persists), B-cell proliferation will continue. Some of the newly produced B-cells will differentiate into plasma cells. These cells have a life span of about five days. During that time they secrete about 2000 antibody molecules per minute per cell. Plasma cells are produced as long as they are needed. The B-cells that do not become plasma cells become "memory" cells. Some 40 to 200 memory cells are generated from a single activated B-cell. Thus, upon secondary exposure to antigen, an increased number of antigen-reactive cells is available to respond.

Induction of Cytotoxic T-Cells

Cytotoxic T-cells possess the lyt 2,3$^+$ phenotype in mice and the CD8$^+$ phenotype in humans. T_{CTL} cells mount the primary cell-mediated response against virus-infected host cells; aberrant self (tumor) cells; some protozoa, fungi, and worms; and cells in foreign tissue and grafts. As their name implies, they lyse their respective "target" cells in an antigen-specific manner. Like T_H cells, T_{CTL} cells do not respond to free antigens. The receptor of T_{CTL} only reacts with foreign (probably processed) antigens that are bound to Class I molecules. The interaction between T_{CTL} and antigen is thus restricted by Class I determinants; however, very rarely some cells may be Class II restricted. A good example of T_{CTL} restriction can be seen in their interaction with virus-infected cells (for example, influenza). It is well known that when a virus infects a cell, it uses the metabolic processes of the host to produce its own proteins. Some viral proteins may be "sorted out" by the host cell and packaged into endosomal vesicles. Here the viral antigens are processed into segments that bind to the Class I molecules found in endosomes. The process is similar to antigen processing by APC. The viral antigen–Class I complexes are inserted into the membrane on the cell surface in the course of the normal endosomal cycle. In a sense, this "blows the cover" of the intracellular virus. T_{CTL}, present in the spleen, blood, and lymph nodes, traffic throughout the body, and those with appropriate receptors may bind to the virus-infected cells. The interaction activates the T_{CTL}, causing clonal expansion and cytolytic activity. These activated T_{CTL} only kill homologous virus-infected host cells; they do not kill uninfected host cells or cells from other individuals infected with the same virus. They also will not kill APC displaying the same virus fragments in association with Class II MHC.

Not all T_{CTL} killing, however, is MHC restricted. That is, T_{CTL} can kill foreign (allogeneic) cells; for example, cells in a foreign skin or organ graft (see Chapter 11).

Upon exposure to antigen presented by an antigen-presenting cell, T_{CTL} may become activated, undergo clonal expansion, and differentiate into effector cells. It was once believed that T_H cells were required for T_{CTL} activation. Recently it has been reported that T_H cells are not always required. In general, however, the presence of T_H cells amplifies the production of T_{CTL}. Upon antigen activation, the T_{CTL} becomes IL-2R$^+$. The release of large amounts of IL-2 by T_H cells greatly increases T_{CTL} clonal expansion. Other soluble mediators produced by T_H cells, for example, IFN-γ, also enhance T_{CTL} activity.

The killing of the target cell by T_{CTL} requires direct contact with the cell. There is no evidence that T_{CTL} release toxic substances; only cells with which contact is made, not other cells nearby, are killed. Once the antigen is eliminated, the T_{CTL} cell reverts to IL-2$^-$ type and clonal expansion ceases.

Activation of T_{DTH} Cells

Like T_H cells, T_{DTH} cells recognize processed antigen complexed to Ia that is expressed on the surfaces of macrophages and other APC. Upon activation, T_{DTH} cells undergo IL-2–mediated clonal expansion. T_{DTH} cells secrete a variety of lymphokines that activate macrophages and form a chemotactic gradient that guides neutrophils and other granulocytic cells to the site. The end result is an inflammatory reaction, usually leading to the elimination of the foreign material. If the foreign material cannot be eliminated because it is not degradable (for example, asbestos) or because it resists killing (for example, the tubercule bacillus) the inflammatory reaction persists and becomes chronic.

Because the delayed type hypersensitivity reaction is mediated by cells that must migrate to the site, it generally takes longer for the reaction to become clinically recognizable than is the case for reactions mediated by antibodies. This is why the response is called a *delayed type hypersensitivity reaction,* and the T-cells that mediate it *T-delayed type hypersensitivity cells* (Chapter 10). The antibody-mediated reactions, in contrast, are called *immediate hypersensitivity reactions* because they occur within minutes of exposure to antigen. Examples of T_{DTH} cell-mediated responses are the tuberculin reaction (diagnostic for *Mycobacterium tuberculosis* infection) and the reaction to poison ivy and poison oak.

Regulation of the Immune Response by Cytokines

It should be clear from the discussion so far that the immune response is regulated not only by antigen and by cell-to-cell contact (for example, macrophage–T-cell interaction) but also by soluble factors called *cytokines.* A list of the most important of these factors is given in Table 8.3. Cytokines are biologically active at concentrations from 10^{-10} to 10^{-15}M and usually mediate their effects over a short range (that is, they usually only affect nearby cells). This is because they only act on cells that have appropriate receptors, and these are often in the same areas as the secreting cells. Because cytokines are produced in such small amounts, they are difficult to isolate. They were originally named for their biologic activity; for example, LAF (lymphocyte activation factor). However, as a single factor may have multiple activities, a single compound often ended up with several names. A standard nomenclature has been devised for naming cytokines. The name for LAF in this system is IL-1. The current names and some of the common synonyms for the better-characterized cytokines are included in Table 8.3.

Cytokines that regulate the immune system are called *afferent,* or *inductive,* cytokines. They may either enhance or suppress the immune response. The roles of many of the enhancing afferent cytokines have already been discussed. The two major classes are the interleukins (IL) and the interferons (IFN). In general, the interleukins stimulate the activation, growth, and proliferation of a variety of types of cells. They are from 15,000 to 35,000 daltons in the monomeric form but are often found as oligomers. Most are glycoproteins. Some have roles in stem cell differentiation (IL-3) and some affect antigen-dependent B- and T-cell differentiation (IL-1, IL-2, IL-4, IL-5).

The interferons function both as afferent-inducing and -suppressing cytokines. They also have effector functions. There are at least 16 proteins that demonstrate antiviral activity and therefore are considered interferons. The three major groups of interferons are interferon alpha (IFN-α), produced by macrophages and other white blood cells; interferon beta (IFN-β), produced primarily by fibroblasts; and immune, or gamma, interferon (IFN-γ), produced by T_H cells. IFN-α and IFN-β retain biologic activity after exposure to solutions at pH 2, a characteristic of type I interferons, whereas IFN-γ does not (type II). All three interferons have a variety of functions in common. At low concentrations they activate T_{CTL}, induce expression of Class I MHC determinants, and activate natural killer cells. In addition, IFN-γ also induces Class II (Ia) expression, stimulates IL-1 and IL-2 production, and increases antibody production.

When present in high concentrations, the interferons react differently than when present in low concentrations. At high concentrations interferons suppress cell division, thus preventing further clonal expansion. In general, the interferons tend to be produced later in infections than are the interleukins. Thus, the presence of low concentrations of interferons during the early phases of the infection stimulates the immune response and induces production of effector cells; but when higher concentrations are present later in the infection, they inhibit the immune response and stop effector cell production. The production of large amounts of interferons early in the infection would not be advantageous as this would prematurely halt clonal expansion and the immune response.

A variety of factors in addition to the interleukins and interferons also turn off or suppress the immune response (Table 8.3). Many of these have not been well studied. The best-defined are ones that suppress antibody production. The relatively well-studied T-suppressor factor ($T_S F$), for example, may be important in maintaining tolerance.

Effector Cytokines

In addition to regulating the immune system, some cytokines have direct effector functions. As stated previously, the interferons produce an antiviral response within the host that directly affects the growth and infectivity of viral pathogens.

Macrophage migration inhibition factor (MIF) prevents macrophages from migrating out of an area of inflammation. Macrophage migration inhibition factor appears to mediate its effect by inducing the polymerization of tubulin. Macrophage activating factor activates macrophages so that they become able to kill tumors and some intracellular bacteria and protozoa that they were not able to kill before activation. IFN-γ demonstrates macrophage activation factorlike activity when present at low concentrations and macrophage inhibition factorlike activity at high concentrations. An effector cytokine that has generated considerable interest is tumor necrosis factor, or cachetin. As the name implies, it exhibits antitumor activity both *in vitro* and *in vivo.* Tumor necrosis factor also causes a variety of pathologic effects. It is present in high levels in animals with cachexia, which is a wasting disease. It is thought that it may be partially responsible for the extreme weight loss observed in terminal cancer patients. The factor suppresses lipoprotein lipase activity, resulting in increased lipid levels in the serum, instead of in tissues. Thus, the factor may be a double-edged sword in tumor biology, both suppressing tumor growth and damaging the host. Tumor necrosis factor induces fever both directly by affecting the hypothalamus and indirectly by inducing IL-1 production. Thus this single molecule mediates a variety of important effects and may be considered both an afferent and an effector monokine.

T-Suppressor Cells

It is well know that if a mouse is first given a subimmunogenic dose of certain antigens—for example, *Pneumococcal polysaccharide* III—it will fail to produce antibodies when subsequently injected with an immunogenic dose of the material. The unresponsiveness (suppression) can be transferred to another mouse by transfer of T-cells. This clearly demonstrates the presence and function of T-suppressor (T_S) cells. However, of all of the T-cell subsets, T_S cells are the most controversial. It is unclear how many different subsets there are, although it is agreed that there are subsets of T_S cells. How T_S cells interact, and the biochemical nature and mode of action of the $T_S F$ they produce are areas of active study.

There are at least two, and perhaps three, subsets of T_S cells required for the induction of suppression. The first cell of the set to become activated is an inducer of T_S cells. It induces the $T_S 1$ cell. It has the $ly1^+,2,3^-$ phenotype in mice, and is CD4 in humans. In mice it can be distinguished from the normal T_H cells in that it has an additional surface marker, I-J, and unlike all other T-cells, it can bind free antigen. Upon activation by antigen, the $ly1^+,2,3,^+$ $T_S 1$ cell becomes activated and releases a soluble mediator. This factor then activates a second T_S cell subset, $T_S 2$. In some systems, this is a $ly1^+,2,3,^+$ T_S effector cell (CD8 in humans). In other systems, it appears that an intermediate ($ly2^+$, I-J$^+$) T_S cell is required. Ultimately, the T_S effector cell, either directly or through the release of another factor, can suppress the activation and clonal expansion of T-cells. They may also suppress B-cell proliferation and block the differentiation of B-cells into plasma cells. T_S cell activation occurs both during embryogenesis and throughout the life of the animal. It is a factor in preventing the development of autoreactive T- and B-cell clones (that is, it induces tolerance). T_S cells are also important in regulating an immune response once it has been initiated.

SUMMARY

The maintenance of health and recovery from infectious disease are mediated by both the constitutive (noninducible, or innate) and the inducible (adaptive, or acquired) immune systems. Inducible immunity is achieved by lymphocytes of various subsets, each with different immunological roles. Every lymphocyte in the body has a receptor expressed on its surface that allows it to interact with only one epitope (or several structurally related ones). Following introduction of a pathogen, those lymphocytes with receptors complementary to the antigens of the pathogen will be stimulated to respond. This requirement ensures specificity. Once activated, a lymphocyte undergoes a complex series of changes, including activation, growth, proliferation (clonal expansion), and differentiation. These changes require a sequence of induction signals provided either by direct contact with other lymphocytes and monocytes, or indirectly through cytokines. Bursal cell (B-cell) activation leads to the production of antibody that binds with the epitope on the pathogen that induced its production. As a result, the pathogen is usually destroyed by complement-mediated lysis or by Fc/C_3b receptor-mediated phagocytosis. Thymic helper (T_H) cells interact with antigen displayed in association with Class II Ia determinants on APC. The antigen-specific activation induces T_H cells to undergo clonal expansion and to release a variety of immunoregulatory lymphokines. Lymphokines provide positive or negative induction signals to cells in the appropriate state of differentiation, including signals aiding antigen-primed B-cells to produce antibodies, signals to T_{CTL} cells inducing them to differentiate into cytolytic cells, and signals to macrophages inducing them to become activated. T_{CTL} cells directly eliminate certain viral and microbial pathogens by destroying their host cells and may destroy tumors and foreign grafts. The introduction of various pathogens may activate T_{DTH} cells to orchestrate an inflammatory reaction or may stimulate T_S cells to prevent or suppress a response. Once the pathogen has been eliminated, immunoresponsive cells either die, as do plasma cells, or return to a resting state, as do memory cells. Many lymphocytes are available in increased numbers after contact with a parasite, however, and are thus available to combat a subsequent encounter with the pathogen. This fact accounts for the hallmark characteristic of the inducible immune system, immunologic memory.

SUGGESTIONS FOR FURTHER READING

J. A. Bellanti. *Immunology: Basic Processes*, 2nd edition. W.B. Saunders Company, Philadelphia, 1985.

D. D. Davies and H. Metzger. "Structural basis of antibody function." Ann. Rev. Immunol. *1:*87, 1983.

H. N. Eisen. *Immunology: An introduction to Molecular and Cellular Principles of the Immune Responses*, 2nd edition. Harper & Row, 1980.

H. H. Fudenberg, J. R. L. Pink, A. C. Wang, and G. B. Ferrara. The Genetics of Immunoglobulin Molecules. In *Basic Immunogenetics*, 3rd edition. Oxford University Press, London, 1984.

P. J. Gearhart. "Generation of immunoglobulin variable gene diversity." Immunol. Today *3:*107, 1982.

T. Honjo. "Immunoglobulin genes." Ann. Rev. Immunol. *1:*499, 1983.

D. Male, B. Champion, and A. Cooke. *Advanced Immunology.* Gower Medical Publishing Company, London, 1987.

A. Nissonoff. *Introduction to Molecular Immunology,* 2nd edition. Sinauer Associates, Sunderland, Massachusetts, 1985.

I. Roitt. *Essential Immunology,* 6th edition. Blackwell Scientific Publications, Oxford, England, 1988.

S. Sell. *Basic Immunology: Immune Mechanisms in Health and Disease.* Elsevier, New York, 1987.

R. Wall and M. Kuehl. "Biosynthesis and regulation of immunoglobulins." Ann. Rev. Immunol. *1:*393, 1983.

Antibody-mediated

Antibod
The wor
The
The two
the latte
high affi
of antibc
on macr
The
there is r
act of bii
where it
surround
an endoc
nism ana
attachme
After
merge wi
usually a
gen-indep
following
following
The
efficiency
constituti
C3b is de
receptors
about by
with a ra
Antib
microbes.
composed
cell walls
choic acid
extensivel
binding fi
ocytosis b
of anti–M
bacteria. A
been well
pneumocc

Chapter 9

Specific Host Resistance

The Effector Mechanisms

Na
An
Cy
The
F
SUGGESTION

INTRODUCTIO

Spec
para
pers
in th
8). T
rapi
path

were
gens
anism
of th
syste
N
or po
many
speci
can b
a mi
medi
magn
oped

I
are re
proto

E
follov
tion
mune
agent

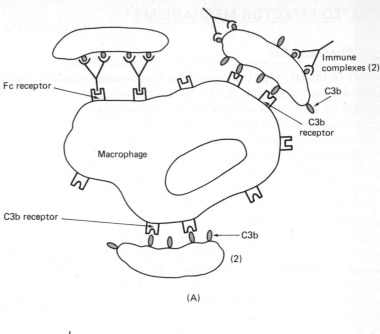

(A)

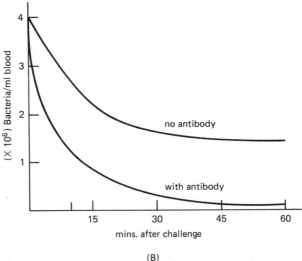

(B)

Figure 9.1 Phagocytosis of bacteria opsonized by IgG or by bound C3b: (a) Fc receptors can mediate both attachment and ingestion of antibody-coated particles. Multiple interactions can occur since many IgG molecules per bacterium trigger attachment to several of the many (up to 100,000) Fc receptors on a macrophage. Internalization occurs by endocytosis. C3b receptors mediate attachment of bacteria to macrophages, and their ingestion if the phagocytic cell is activated. Immune complexes (1) may initiate C3b deposition on parasites by the classical pathway or C3b deposition may occur in the absence of antibody by the alternate pathway (2). (b) Avirulent pneumococci are rapidly cleared from the circulations of rabbits after injection. Virulent pneumococci on the other hand resist phagocytosis. The presence of antibody causes virulent microorganisms to be cleared as are avirulent microorganisms. (Adapted with permission of Macmillan Publishing Co. from *Introduction to Immunology* by John W. Kimball. Copyright 1985.)

capsule. In its absence the microbes are not phagocytized and reproduce unimpeded by the host. As a result the host may die of a severe pneumonia.

Inactivation of Toxins by Antibody

Microbial toxins are of two types, exotoxins and endotoxins. They differ in chemical nature, and the host deals with them in distinct ways. Exotoxins are proteins secreted by only a few of the many bacterial pathogens, but they may be extremely potent virulence factors for the microbes that secrete them. Some exotoxins produce disease when they are ingested with food or water. In such cases there may be no microbial infection or growth in the poisoned individual. Botulism and staphylococcal food poisoning are examples of this. The production of food poisoning in the absence of infection is clearly of no use to the microbe. It is possible that such toxins perform functions important to the microbe that are still unknown and that it is only chance that makes them toxic.

The roles of many exotoxins in the pathogenesis of disease are clear. The toxins secreted by the clostridia causing gas gangrene, for example, kill the host's tissue and digest it, thus making food available for the infecting organism. Many toxins secreted by streptococci and staphylococci kill or impair the functions of leukocytes, preventing phagocytosis of the microbes. Coagulase causes deposition of fibrin on the staphylococci that produce it, providing an antigenic disguise for the microbe. Regardless of the function of the toxin in the microbe's ecology, its inactivation is important to the host.

Exotoxins are very immunogenic. Inactivation is a result of the binding of antibody to sites on the molecule that are responsible for the toxic effects. In many cases antibody can block intoxication if it is available before the toxin binds to its target but cannot reverse damage already done. This is the case with tetanus antitoxin. It must be given prophylactically and is of little use for treatment. If antitoxin is given, it is given just after injury, before infection can develop. It then prevents intoxication. Prophylactic immunization with toxoid, which is a detoxified but still immunogenic toxin, permits a rapid secondary antibody response by the host after infection and provides an antibody that neutralizes the toxin that is secreted, thus blocking intoxication.

The toxin antibody complexes formed are removed by the macrophages of the reticuloendothelial system (Figure 9.2). In the absence of antitoxin, the phagocytic cells are very susceptible to the action of toxins.

Antibodies that can be formed in response to immunization with a toxoid are important in resistance to diseases caused by a variety of exotoxin-producing microbes. Some examples of such diseases are gas gangrene caused by *Clostridium perfringens*, diphtheria caused by *Corynebacterium diphtheriae*, tetanus caused by *Clostridium tetani*, and botulism caused by *Clostridium botulinum*.

The endotoxins are lipopolysaccharides. They are a part of the cell walls of Gram-negative enterobacteria. They are not secreted, but are released when the bacteria die and disintegrate. Endotoxin does induce antibody production, but the antibodies do not neutralize the endotoxin. Endotoxin of enterobacteria is an efficient activator of complement through the alternative complement pathway. It

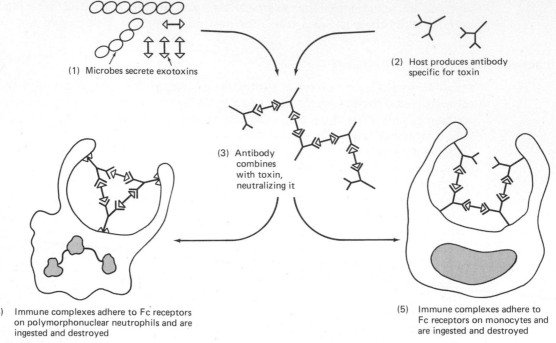

(1) Microbes secrete exotoxins

(2) Host produces antibody specific for toxin

(3) Antibody combines with toxin, neutralizing it

(4) Immune complexes adhere to Fc receptors on polymorphonuclear neutrophils and are ingested and destroyed

(5) Immune complexes adhere to Fc receptors on monocytes and are ingested and destroyed

Figure 9.2 Microbial exotoxins (1) are rendered innocuous by neutralization by specific IgG type antitoxins (2). After combination with antibody, the immune complexes (3) are ingested and degraded by phagocytic cells of the polymorphonuclear (4) and monocytic types (5).

is primarily the complement system that protects the host from the effects of endotoxin. When complement is activated, it induces phagocytosis of the endotoxin through C3b receptors. The phagocytes reduce the ingested endotoxin to nontoxic fragments.

Prevention by Antibody of Attachment of Microbes to Host Cells

Antibodies of the IgG, IgM, and secretory IgA classes that are directed toward appropriate surface components of an intracellular parasite such as a virus can prevent attachment to, and thus infection of, the host cell. The IgG antiviral antibody in the blood, for example, is responsible for the lifelong immunity to infection of neurological cells by polio virus that develops following immunization.

Secretory IgA antibody to the capsules or fimbriae of bacteria that use these structures to adhere to mucosa can inhibit their colonization of mucosal areas. Antibody to capsules and fimbriae inhibits colonization of the trachea and lungs by pseudomonads, for example. Antibody to some intracellular protozoan parasites can prevent their attachment and entry into their host cells. The attachment of antibody by itself does not kill the parasite. To some degree antibody-mediated inhibition of attachment to the red blood cell of the protozoan that causes malaria contributes to antimalarial immunity.

Bacteriolysis

Antibody alone does not bring about lysis of parasites; when antibody binds to the surfaces of parasites, however, the immune complexes that are formed activate complement. It is the products released by the activated complement that may lyse the parasites. Antibodies of the IgM and IgG classes activate complement. Gram-negative bacilli are particularly susceptible to complement-mediated lysis. Secretory or dimeric IgA that is secreted onto mucosal surfaces protects these surfaces from colonization by microbes in part by blocking microbial attachment as noted earlier but also by functioning when aggregated by activation of complement.

Protection by complement-mediated bacteriolysis probably occurs *in vivo*. Complement components generated early in the reaction also provide potent opsonins that cause microbes to undergo phagocytosis. Since the various antibody and complement systems induce several responses, it is rather artificial to attempt to discuss their effects separately.

Agglutination

Although agglutination of parasites by antibody does not kill them, the agglutinated pathogens are adversely affected. Agglutination results in a decrease in the number of infectious units available for dissemination. The agglutinated microorganisms are also much easier to ingest by phagocytic cells than are the single cells. Clumps of parasites are readily filtered from the blood by phagocytes in the spleen. Antibodies to the flagella of motile bacteria can prevent their movement and thus inhibit their spread.

Agglutinating antibodies to *Mycoplasma* may inhibit their growth. This may be because the antibodies block receptors for nutrients. In general, however, antibody-mediated agglutination alone is not a major impediment for microbial growth.

Table 9.1 summarizes the major antimicrobial actions of specific antibodies.

Table 9.1   LIST OF THE ANTIMICROBIAL ACTIONS OF ANTIBODIES

1. Opsonization for phagocytosis
2. Complement activation, enhancing phagocytosis and inducing lysis
3. Prevention of attachment to host cells
4. Prevention of penetration of host cells
5. Neutralization of toxins
6. Inhibition of motility of parasites
7. Agglutination of parasites
8. Inhibition of microbial growth and metabolism

COMPLEMENT-MEDIATED EFFECTOR MECHANISMS

Introduction

As noted in Chapter 4, there are two pathways for activation of the complement system, the classical and the alternative (Figure 9.3). The term *classical* is used because this pathway was discovered prior to the alternative pathway. The reactions in both pathways activate the same effector mechanisms.

The complement components, designated by a capital C, are all serum proteins. They are each identified by a numbered suffix, C1, C2, and so on, that reflects the order in which they were originally identified rather than the order in which they

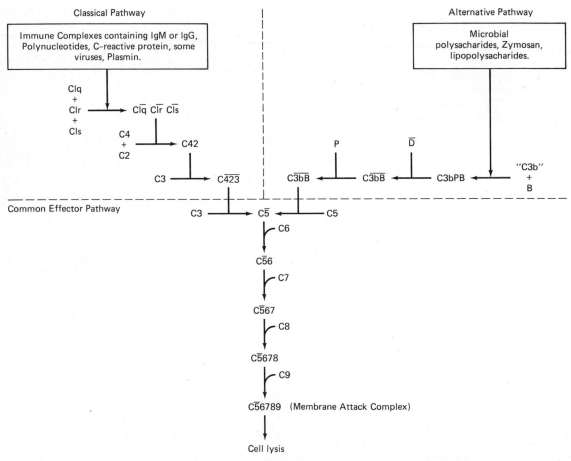

Figure 9.3 The reaction sequences of the complement components in the classical and alternative pathways. Activating substances for each pathway are shown in the boxes. The two pathways differ not only in the nature of the initiation step, but also in the subsequent amplification reactions leading to cleavage of C5. The pathways share the same effector mechanisms, including the membrane attack complex.

react. Fragments of the complement components produced during activation are designated by lower-case letters, for example, C3a and C3b. The complement components circulate in the blood in inactive form. During the activation process they may change in conformation, undergo proteolytic cleavage, or undergo aggregation. Any one of these mechanisms can generate a protein with an enzymatic site or a binding site not present on the inactive component. The sites that are generated enable each component to react with the next component in the cascade. As noted earlier, the effector mechanisms developed by complement activation are the same for complement activated by either of the two pathways. Biological activities are produced by components of C3 and by components C5 through C9.

The complement cascade involves factors B and D, as well as properdin (P), regardless of the method of activation. In the classical pathway these factors amplify the reaction after it is initiated. The significant difference between the two pathways is the nature of the substances that trigger them. In the classical pathway, complement is activated by immune complexes containing IgG or IgM, by C-reactive protein, and by some viruses (Figure 9.3). In contrast, alternative pathway activation occurs following contact with the polysaccharide-bearing surfaces of a variety of microorganisms and by lipopolysaccharide from some Gram-negative bacteria. Alternative pathway activation does not require the presence of antibody. It is thought that the alternative pathway evolved first since it provides an antimicrobial defense in the absence of a specific immune response.

Complement activation is controlled by three serum proteins. These inhibitors of the reaction will be described later, along with the reaction step they inhibit.

Antibody-dependent Activation of Complement: The Classical Complement Pathway

As previously noted, the classical pathway is triggered by immune complexes, among other things. Lysis of bacteria or other cells can occur when activation occurs on their surfaces. Although lysis of an infected host cell or of a parasitic microorganism is of obvious benefit to the host, other less obvious benefits occur as a result of complement activation. Some of the most important contributions to host defense that result from complement activation result from the biologic activities of the fragments cleaved from complement proteins during activation. Such biologically active fragments are generated at various points in the complement cascade. By convention, these fragments are designated by placing a bar above the symbol for the component, for example, $\overline{C1}$.

The first step in activation of complement by the classical pathway is binding of C1 to the Fc portions of antibody molecules in immune complexes. The C1 component must encounter at least two adjacent IgG molecules or one IgM molecule bound to antigen to initiate the cascade (Figure 9.4). C1 consists of subunits called *C1q, C1r,* and *C1s.* There is only one C1q subunit, but there are two each of C1r and C1s. There are globular "bulbs" at the ends of the stalks of C1q. These bind to receptors within the Fc region of the IgG or IgM molecule. The binding of C1q triggers an internal rearrangement in one of the C1r molecules to give an activated form ($\overline{C1r}$), which is an enzyme that cleaves a peptide bond within the

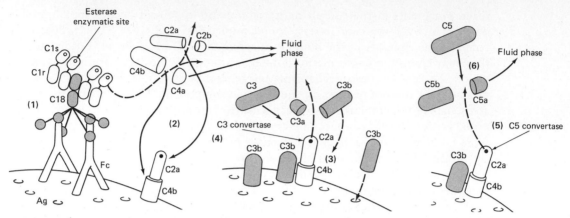

Figure 9.4 The initial reactions of the classical complement pathway occur on membranes or other surfaces or on immune complexes in solution. The first reaction is the recognition of IgG (or IgM) antibody bound to antigen by the C1q subunit (1). Self-activation by rearrangement and cleavage within C1 generates a C1s esterase that cleaves both C4 and C2 (2). The membrane-bound C4b2a (3) serves first as a C3 convertase (4) and then as a C5 convertase (5) following attachment of C3b to C4b C2a. The split complement components (6) in the "fluid phase" have potent inflammatory activities. (Reproduced from *The Biology of Immunologic Disease,* Sinauer Associates, Sunderland, MA, 1980, with the permission of the publishers.)

second C1r molecule. As a result, both C1r molecules acquire enzymatic capacity and cleave the C1s molecules to generate the activated form of C1s ($\overline{\text{C1s}}$), which is a serine esterase.

The second step in the cascade is cleavage of C4 and C2 by the serine esterase. Since the serine esterase ($\overline{\text{C1s}}$) is able to act on many C4 and C2 molecules, the small initial reaction is amplified. Each serine esterase may cleave approximately 200 C4 molecules into $\overline{\text{C4a}}$ and $\overline{\text{C4b}}$ fragments. The $\overline{\text{C4b}}$ fragment, which is the larger of the two fragments, binds to cell membranes of any cell near the activating immune complex (Figure 9.4). The C2 molecule is also cleaved by the serine esterase. Cleavage yields a large fragment ($\overline{\text{C2a}}$), which binds to the membrane-bound $\overline{\text{C4b}}$ to form a $\overline{\text{C4b2a}}$ complex. Cleavage also yields a small fragment, $\overline{\text{C2b}}$. The small fragments resulting from cleavage of C4 and C2, $\overline{\text{C4a}}$ and $\overline{\text{C2b}}$, diffuse from the area where they were produced. These soluble fragments are pharmacologically active and enhance the inflammatory reaction that develops at sites of immune complex formation.

The $\overline{\text{C4b2b2a}}$ complex affects C3 and is therefore called *C3 convertase.* The enzymatic site on each $\overline{\text{C2a}}$ fragment of the $\overline{\text{C4b2a}}$ complex may cleave as many as 100 C3 molecules. The fragments produced are called $\overline{\text{C3a}}$ and $\overline{\text{C3b}}$. The larger fragment, $\overline{\text{C3b}}$, binds to several sites. One site is the $\overline{\text{C4b2a}}$ complex. At this site it forms a $\overline{\text{C4b2a3b}}$ aggregate that now possesses a new enzymatic site specific for C5. Cleavage of C5 by this C5 convertase is the last enzymatic step in the pathway. Each molecule of C5 convertase may split from 50 to 100 C5 molecules. The small fragments resulting from complement activation, $\overline{\text{C3a}}$ and $\overline{\text{C5a}}$, diffuse away from their sites of production. The $\overline{C5a}$, at least, is chemotactic and attracts leukocytes.

The $\overline{C5b}$ fragment is hydrophobic and binds to the lipid bilayer of cells near its site of production. The $\overline{C5b}$ fragment on the membranes of cells serves as the initiation point for the assembly of the remaining complement components, C6 through C9, into a structure termed the *membrane attack complex.* The assembly of the complex occurs in several steps. The $\overline{C5b}$ fragments bind C6, C7, and C8. The $\overline{C5b678}$ complex brings about the polymerization of up to 16 C9 molecules. The polymerized C9 molecules form a cylindrical tubule that inserts into the cell membrane, making a hole. This transmembrane channel permits water to flow into, and ions to flow out of, the cell. As a consequence the cell swells and bursts. Nucleated cells often simply lose their cytoplasm through the pores rather than swelling and bursting (Figure 9.5).

The membrane attack complex usually enters the membranes of cells to which antibody is bound. A few of these complexes, however, may become detached from the antibody-coated cell on which they formed and be deposited on adjacent cells. This may result in loss of healthy host cells in the vicinity of immune complexes. When this occurs, it is referred to as a *bystander* effect of complement activation.

The Alternative Pathway of Complement Activation

Activation of complement by the alternative pathway requires the three serum proteins, Factors B and D, and Properdin (P), and a stabilizing microbial surface. The alternate route of complement activation is a mechanism for generating com-

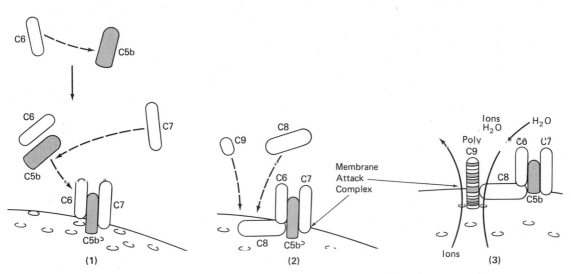

Figure 9.5 Outline or the assembly of the complement proteins into a membrane attack complex. The deposition of C5b at a site (1) as a trimolecular complex of C5b67 allows the binding of C8 and many C9 molecules to the site. The C9 molecules form a transmembrane tubule (2) that allows the free passage of water into the cell, and ions out of it, resulting in lysis (3). (Reproduced from *The Biology of Immunologic Disease*, Sinauer Associates, Sunderland, MA, 1980, with the permission of the publishers.)

plement components with inflammatory activity and for assembling the C5–C9 lytic complex in the absence of antibody.

Activation of complement by the alternative pathway begins in the plasma. Component C3 hydrolyses spontaneously to form a $\overline{C3b}$-like molecule. The $\overline{C3b}$-like molecule associates with Factor B to form a complex. This complex, which is unstable, must be deposited on a cell wall or membrane for further steps in the complement cascade to occur. The lipopolysaccharide of Gram-negative bacteria and the carbohydrates of yeast cell walls provide particularly suitable sites for deposition and stabilization of this complex. After deposition on the microbe, the Factor B in the complex undergoes a conformational change and cleaves additional C3 to form $\overline{C3a}$ and $\overline{C3b\text{-}B}$ (Figure 9.6a). The $\overline{C3b\text{-}B}$ complex is susceptible to the action of Factor D, which exists in the serum as an active enzyme. It cleaves $\overline{C3b\text{-}B}$ into $\overline{C3bBb}$ and $\overline{Ba}$. The $\overline{C3bBb}$ is a C3 convertase. When it is stabilized by the binding of Properdin (P) molecules, it cleaves many C3 molecules. The stabilized large complex of $\overline{C3b\text{-}Bb\text{-}C3b(n)\text{-}P(n)}$ eventually undergoes a conformational change to expose another enzymatic site on $\overline{Bb}$, which is a C5 convertase. The assembly of the C5–9 membrane attack complex then occurs.

On some cell membranes there is a "decay-accelerating factor." This factor rapidly dissociates the $\overline{Bb}$ from the membrane, preventing the complement cascade from developing further.

The generation of the effector mechanisms by both pathways is amplified by the components B, D, and P, which are involved in the initiation of the alternative pathway. Any $\overline{C3b}$ generated by the classical pathway may initiate the reactions of the alternative pathway (Figure 9.6b).

Biological Activities of Complement Components

Complement activation induces inflammation, produces membrane attack complexes, and facilitates phagocytosis of the parasite. The inflammatory events that occur result in the influx of large numbers of leukocytes into the site and thus increase the likelihood of ingestion of parasites that are present.

Various of the processes that occur at an inflammatory site are induced by complement components (Table 9.2). The inflamation-inducing complement components $\overline{C4a}$, $\overline{C3a}$, and $\overline{C5a}$ are called *anaphylatoxins.* Anaphylatoxins trigger the release of histamine from platelets, mast cells, or basophils. Histamine causes vasodilation, increases capillary permeability, and is a constrictor of bronchial smooth muscle. The changes that histamine causes in capillaries facilitate emigration of leukocytes from the blood into the inflamed site. They cause edema, which is the accumulation of plasma in the tissues. The plasma contains all kinds of serum proteins, including antibodies and complement. The complement fragment $\overline{C2b}$, which is not usually considered an anaphylatoxin, also increases vessel dilation.

Chemotactic factors are substances that attract leukocytes. Under their influence polymorphonuclear leukocytes and monocytes move into the inflamed site. They move along the concentration gradient of the factor toward the higher levels at the inflamed site. $\overline{C567}$ is weakly chemotactic; $\overline{C5a}$ is strongly chemotactic. It is at least 100 times more potent a chemotactic factor than is $\overline{C3a}$ or $\overline{C567}$.

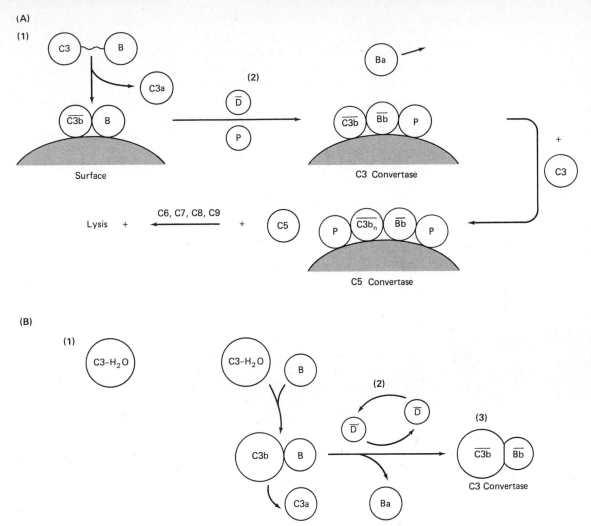

Figure 9.6 Outline of the alternative complement pathway reaction and the positive-feedback loop that amplifies both pathways. (A) The assembly of the C3 and C5 convertases occurs on a membrane or surface that protects C3 from decay (1). The Factors D, B, and P (2) contribute to this protection. The positive-feedback loop depends on a hydrolyzed molecule of C3 and a binding of factor B to it. (B) C3-H_2O (1) is "C3b-like" in function. It can bind Factor B and, in the presence of the enzyme, Factor D (2) and can generate many fluid-phase C3 convertase molecules (C3b-Bb) (3).

Immune adherence brings about attachment of leukocytes to parasites and other foreign antigens. The complement components responsible for immune adherence are $\overline{C4b}$ and $\overline{C3b}$. Immune adherence may be the first step in phagocytosis; $\overline{C4b}$ and $\overline{C3b}$, which mediate immune adherence, are potent opsonic substances.

Table 9.2   BIOLOGICAL ACTIVITIES OF COMPLEMENT
COMPONENTS

Component	Activity
$\overline{C2b}$ (fluid phase)	Kininlike, increased vasodilation
$\overline{C4a}$	Anaphylatoxin–histamine release
$\overline{C3a}$	Anaphylatoxin
$\overline{C5a}$	Anaphylatoxin–strong chemotactic factor
$\overline{C4b}$ (membrane)	Immune adherence, opsonization
$\overline{C3b}$ (membrane)	Immune adherence, opsonization
$\overline{C567}$	Weak chemotactic factor
$\overline{C9}$ (polymer)	Membrane disruption

Regulation of Complement Activity

Since the activation of complement generates potent products that may cause injury to host cells in the vicinity, the activation of the cascade must be regulated to prevent adverse reactions. The enzymatic step mediated by C1 is inhibited by a normal serum protein, C1-inhibitor, which binds C1s. A key step in both the classical and alternative pathways is the deposition of $\overline{C3b}$ on cells. Factor I in normal serum is a $\overline{C3b}$-inactivator that degrades $\overline{C3b}$ to C3bi unless it is bound to a surface. This reduces the likelihood of bystander damage during complement activation. Another normal serum protein, Factor H, enhances the inhibitory action of Factor I.

The various factors in the plasma that stimulate or inhibit complement activation are in exquisite balance. In the absence of parasites or other foreign antigens, complement activation is completely inhibited. Even in the presence of parasites and other foreign antigens, activation is controlled so that it occurs only in the immediate vicinity of the initiating factor. Such control is vital to prevent the occurrence of a chain reaction that would destroy the host as well as the parasite.

CELL-MEDIATED EFFECTOR MECHANISMS

Introduction

The distinctive characteristic of cell-mediated immunity is that it can be transferred from an immunized animal to a naive recipient by transfer of T-lymphocytes but not by transfer of serum. Cell-mediated immunity is a major factor in control of viruses, bacteria, and protozoa that grow in nonphagocytic as well as phagocytic cells. The control of intraphagocytic parasites is accomplished by activation of macrophages to a state characterized by a heightened ability to kill the parasites they ingest. The control of viruses and other parasites in nonphagocytic cells is by host cell lysis by cytolytic T-lymphocytes (T_{CTL}). Parasitic worms that dwell in tissues may also be killed by cell-mediated immune mechanisms.

The role of macrophage activation in resistance to parasites that develop inside macrophages was first shown by George Mackaness and his colleagues. In the early 1960s they clearly demonstrated that transfer of T-cells transferred immunity to *Listeria monocytogenes,* a parasite that grows inside of macrophages (Figure 9.7). The most surprising outcome of this study was the observation that with the transfer of resistance to *L. monocytogenes,* resistance to unrelated pathogens such as *Mycobacterium bovis* or *Salmonella typhimurium* also developed in the recipients of the lymphocytes. These individuals and others subsequently demonstrated that the relatively nonspecific resistance that developed to the parasites was a result of a T-helper cell-mediated enhancement of the macrophages' ability to kill the parasites they contained.

In general all of the effector responses of cell-mediated immunity require T-cells. This means that with the elimination of T-cells by any means, the cell-mediated protective response is eliminated. The only exception to the rule that T-cells are required for cell-mediated immunity are those portions of the immunity mediated by nonactivated macrophages and by natural killer lymphocytes, which appear not to be thymic lymphocytes but rather cells of a separate lineage.

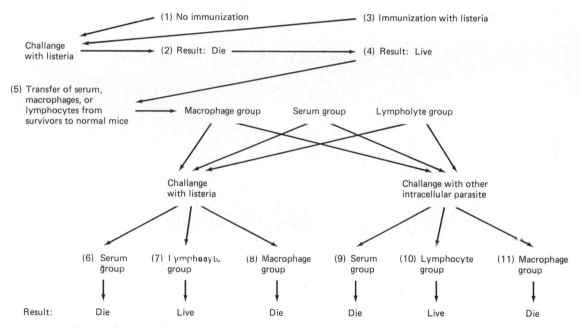

Figure 9.7 The mechanism of immunity to *Listeria monocytogenes* in mice. Unimmunized mice (1) die upon challenge with listeria (2). Mice adaptively immunized with *L. monocytogenes* (3) when challenged with listeria display heightened resistance (4). The nature of the immune effector mechanisms is revealed by the transfer experiments (5). Mice that receive immune lymphocytes (7, 10) but not immune serum or macrophages (6, 8, 9, 11) resist challenge with listeria and with unrelated intracellular parasites. Thus, the triggering of the immune response is antigen specific but the anti-microbial activity generated is nonspecific.

Delayed Type Hypersensitivity and Antimicrobial Activity

The skin reaction that develops following tuberculin injection is just a visible manifestation of events that may occur in any tissue where tubercule bacilli exist. The events that occur at the site of tuberculin injection in a tuberculin-sensitive individual are the same as those that occur in appropriately sensitized individuals when tissue-dwelling worms, intracellular protozoa, bacteria, or viruses release antigen at their sites of growth. The reaction is normally beneficial to the host and damages the parasite. If it becomes excessive, however, tissue damage also occurs.

For delayed type hypersensitivity to be induced by a parasite, sensitization of a distinct subpopulation of thymic lymphocytes termed *delayed type hypersensitivity lymphocytes* (T_{DTH}) must occur. Clonal expansion of the T_{DTH} cells reactive with the particular antigen follows sensitization. The T_{DTH} cells are only sensitized by antigen if it is presented on the surface of an antigen-presenting cell in association with a Class II Ia molecule (Figure 9.8). The T_{DTH} lymphocytes have most of the same membrane differentiation markers as thymic helper lymphocytes. The T_{DTH} cells in mice are Lyt-1+ and in humans are CD4+. For convenience, the cells are referred to as *T4+ helper cells* in mice and *CD4+ cells* in humans.

To induce a clonal expansion of T_{DTH} lymphocytes, macrophages are required

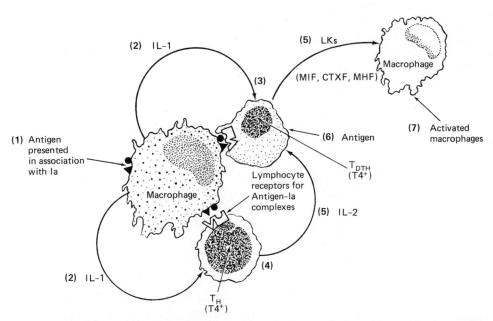

Figure 9.8 Mechanism of sensitization of T_{DTH} and T_H cells by antigen (1) presented in association with Class II MHC I-region products (Ia). The IL-1 (2) produced by the antigen-presenting cells drives the differentiation of the T_{DTH} (3) and T_H (4) cells (T4+). The T_{DTH} and T_H cells elaborate other lymphokines (5) upon reexposure to the sensitizing antigen (6); the lymphokines, among other functions, activate macrophages (7). (Reproduced from *Immunology III,* J.A. Bellanti, W.B. Saunders Co., Philadelphia, 1985, with permission of the publishers.)

not only for the presentation of antigen but also for the secretion of interleukin-1. Interleukin-1 has multiple biological activities. In addition to its effects on T_{DTH} lymphocytes, it is involved in inflammation. Exposure of T4+ lymphocytes to interleukin-1 brings about changes so that they respond to T-cell growth factor or interleukin-2.

Following sensitization either by infection or by injection of antigen, the clonal expansion that occurs provides enough of the appropriate T_{DTH} cells to mount a delayed hypersensitivity response at any site where there is antigen deposition.

The hallmark of the delayed type reaction is a massive infiltration of lymphocytes and macrophages into the site where the antigen occurs. Only 0.1 percent of the T-cells in a sensitized host respond *in vitro* to the antigen used to sensitize the host, and only 5 percent of the lymphocytes in a delayed type reaction in an animal sensitized by passive transfer are lymphocytes that were transferred. The sensitized T_{DTH} cells must therefore recruit a large number of unsensitized lymphocytes and macrophages to the site. This recruitment is accomplished by the elaboration of mediators of delayed type hypersensitivity by T_{DTH} cells in response to antigen.

The lymphocytes and macrophages that accumulate at the site of antigen deposition during the delayed hypersensitivity response in a sensitized animal produce an array of effector molecules. The mediators secreted by the lymphocytes are lymphokines and are named for their activities. More than 30 lymphokines associated with delayed hypersensitivity reactions have been described; however, only a few have been well characterized. Some of those lymphokines may cause several responses and thus may have received several different names.

Macrophage chemotactic factor is a lymphokine that *in vitro* attracts monocytes and other types of macrophages. *In vivo* the factor probably acts to attract phagocytes to the site where the T_{DTH} cell encounters the antigen. Another lymphokine, *migration inhibition factor,* greatly hinders the normally vigorous movement of macrophages over a glass surface and, presumably, *in vivo* prevents the macrophages from leaving the site of inflammation. The lymphokine called *mitogenic* or *blastogenic factor* acts on T4+ cells that are present to initiate cell division. This lymphokine has been purified and has been shown to be the molecule also called *interleukin-2* or *T-cell growth factor.* Interleukin-2 is a polypeptide hormone. The lymphokine called *macrophage activating factor* is probably really a mixture of several peptide hormones. They have the important function of activating macrophages to enhance their ability to kill intracellular protozoa, bacteria, and viruses. One of the most potent lymphokines of the macrophage activating factor complex is *gamma interferon.* This is a molecule that induces macrophages to become strongly parasiticidal and tumoricidal. The actions of several mediators are depicted in Figure 9.9.

Macrophage Activation and Tumoricidal and Microbicidal Activity

The activation of macrophages by T-cell products provides an effector mechanism for the inducible response. The activated macrophages are strongly antimicrobial and also have tumoricidal capabilities. The enhanced capacity of activated macro-

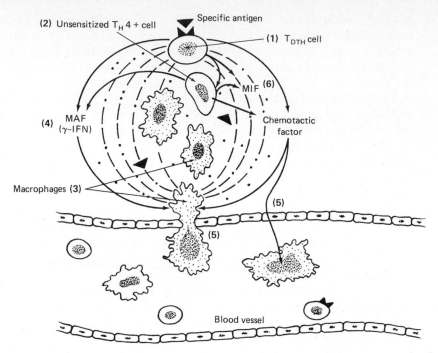

Figure 9.9 The sites of action of several lymphokines in the generation of a delayed type hypersensitivity reaction. The antigen-stimulated T_{DTH} cell (1) releases lymphokines that act on T_H4+ cells (2) and on macrophages (3), for example. The lymphokines bring about various changes in the cells upon which they act, involving activation (4) and migration (5) into and retention in the site (6).

phages to destroy not only the microbe inducing the activation but others as well is the basis of the use of the bacillis of Calmette-Guerin (BCG), an attenuated *Mycobacterium bovis*, as a therapeutic agent for treatment of solid tumors. The BCG is injected into the tumor mass. The monocytes that concentrate at the site differentiate into macrophages that upon activation may destroy the tumor cells as well as the mycobacteria that induced the activation.

The destruction of tumor cells by activated macrophages appears to be accomplished by a neutral protease with cytolytic activity that is secreted by the macrophage upon binding to the tumor cell. The activated macrophage may also secrete tumor necrosis factor-alpha (TNF-α), a tumoricidal monokine. The latter factor was discovered in serum of mice that were rejecting solid tumors following treatment with BCG and lipopolysaccharide. The activated macrophages bind to the tumor cell before releasing the cytolytic factors (Figure 9.10).

Macrophage activation at the site of a delayed type reaction can be analyzed into a series of events that take place over a few hours (Figure 9.10). The monocytes that enter the area can be considered to be potentially responsive macrophages. They pass through a stage in which they are considered to be "primed," and finally become fully activated. The signal driving the transition of the macrophages from responsive to primed is a gamma interferon. As noted earlier, gamma interferon,

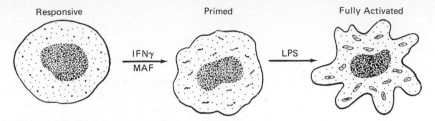

Figure 9.10 The sequence of events involved in the activation of macrophages. Responsive macrophages differentiate into primed macrophages that may be rapidly transformed into fully activated macrophages with tumoricidal abilities. The mediators shown are those best studied, but may not be the only ones.

which is produced by T_{DTH} lymphocytes, has some antiviral activity. Gamma interferon is probably the major active component in the presently available crude lymphokine preparations with macrophage-activating ability. It may not be the only component of the preparation that induces the primed state, however. A compound required for the rapid transition of a primed macrophage to a fully activated one *in vitro* is bacterial lipopolysaccharide. Only a few nanograms of lipopolysaccharide are required. The compound that induces full activation *in vivo* is still not known but is likely also to be lipopolysaccharide or some other component of the infecting microorganism itself. Lipopolysaccharide in high concentration can by itself trigger macrophage activation.

The fully differentiated macrophages are actively phagocytic but have only a poor capacity for antigen presentation to T-cells. Poor antigen presentation is probably a result of the efficient antigen degradation carried out by activated macrophages.

During macrophage activation arachidonic acid metabolism is enhanced. This results in greatly increased secretion of prostaglandins and leukotrienes, although by the same basic reactions as were described in Chapter 4. These products, as noted in Chapter 4, mediate inflammation. Activated macrophages have an increased capacity for oxidative metabolism. The metabolic burst of activated macrophages following phagocytosis is 20 to 50 times that of resting macrophages. The metabolic burst is carried out by an NADPH-dependent oxidase enzyme complex that resides in the macrophage's membrane (Figure 9.11). These enzymes generate a superoxide (O_2^-) ion that is rapidly dismutated to H_2O_2 and hydroxyl radicals. The generation of these reactive oxygen intermediates that have very potent antimicrobial activity was described in detail in Chapter 3. All of the effector mechanisms used by macrophages in the inducible immune response were developed as parts of the constitutive resistance system. The inducible response amplifies their effects, however.

Natural Killer Cells

Natural killer cells are a distinct class of lymphocytes that do not fit into either the T-cell or B-cell lineages. They have distinct surface differentiation markers and they lack surface Ig and T-cell markers. They possess large cytoplasmic

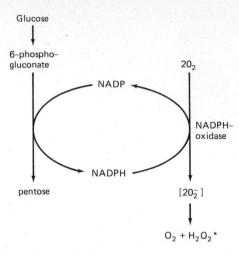

Figure 9.11 Some mechanisms used by phagocytes in production of the respiratory burst. Degradation of glucose is linked through the NADP-NADPH cycle of glucose metabolism to activation of oxygen. The various active oxygen products are antimicrobial because they are strong oxidizers. Two antimicrobial compounds yielded by these reactions are indicated by a star (*). The ones indicated in this diagram are superoxide (O_2) and hydrogen peroxide (H_2O_2). Others may also occur.

granules that resemble those of the granular leukocytes but are less numerous. Because of this attribute, another name given to natural killer cells is *large granular lymphocytes*, and they can be separated from other lymphocytes by their density.

Natural killer cells probably kill microbial pathogens without prior sensitization. Thus, natural killer cell activity may be a component of constitutive resistance; however, natural killer cells have receptors for the Fc portion of IgG and can therefore be mobilized as effector cells by antibody through the antibody-dependent cell cytotoxicity mechanism. In this latter respect they may be effectors for the inducible immune system.

Natural killer cells lyse a wide range of target cells with no apparent restriction by the major histocompatibility complex (MHC); in this they are distinct from cytotoxic T-lymphocytes. Natural killer cells become much more cytolytic if exposed to gamma interferon. Treatment with the lymphokine apparently causes them to differentiate into a more effectively lytic form (Figure 9.12*a*). The mechanism whereby natural killer cells cause cytolysis is not known, but appears to be different from that used by the T_{CTL}.

Natural killer cells have been shown to kill cells transformed by viruses; to aid in rejection of allografts; to contribute to resistance to some cancers, especially leukemias; and to contribute to resistance to infection by some fungi and protozoa. Following their discovery, it was proposed that they carry out immune surveillance against malignant disease. On the basis of recent information about them, however, it appears that their main function may be control of differentiation of cells of the lymphoid system, not host defense.

Antibody-dependent Cell Cytotoxicity

Antibody-dependent cell cytotoxicity is an effector mechanism that depends upon the joint activity of leukocytes of various types and antibody. One class of

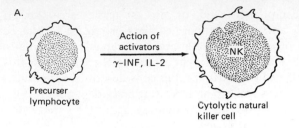

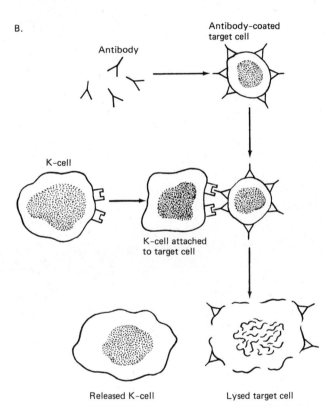

Figure 9.12 (A) Natural killer cells differentiate into strongly cytolytic cells through the effects of gamma interferon (γ IFN), which is released by thymic helper-lymphocytes following antigenic stimulation. (B) Antibody-dependent cell cytotoxicity (ADCC) is mediated in part by a class of lymphocytes called K-cells. The specificity of the reaction is dictated by IgG antibody. Other cells bearing receptors for the Fc portion of antibody also may serve as effector cells for ADCC. These include macrophages and eosinophils.

lymphocytes that participate in antibody-dependent cell cytotoxicity is called *killer lymphocytes,* or *K-cells.* They have some of the properties of immature T-cells. The antibody involved is of the IgG type (Figure 9.12*b*). To bring about cytolysis, the K-cells must be bound to the target cell by receptors on the Fc portion of the antibody coating the target cell. K-cells also have receptors for the

C3 component of complement and, in mice at least, carry the Thy-1 marker. They lack surface Ig and do not adhere to glass or engage in phagocytosis as do macrophages. Cells other than K-cells are also capable of mediating antibody-dependent killing, but to a lesser extent. Some of the cells with this capacity in addition to the K-cell and the natural killer cells described earlier are neutrophils, eosinophils, macrophages, and platelets. Antibody-dependent cell cytotoxicity may be an important part of the host defense against a variety of parasites, including worms, fungi, and protozoa.

Cytolytic T-Lymphocytes

Cytolytic T-cells are lymphocytes programmed to destroy target cells in an antigen-specific fashion. They have been extensively studied because they are the cells primarily responsible for graft rejection, which is described in Chapter 11. The T_{CTL}'s are capable of recognizing virus and other parasite-produced components that are present in the membranes of host cells in association with the MHC molecules (Figure 9.13). The recognition and destruction of host cells infected by viruses that are not lytic and of cells containing other intracellular parasites is the only way the host can eventually rid itself of such infections.

For cytotoxic lymphocytes to kill, contact is required. After contact is made the membrane of the cell bearing the parasite antigen is damaged, and the cell

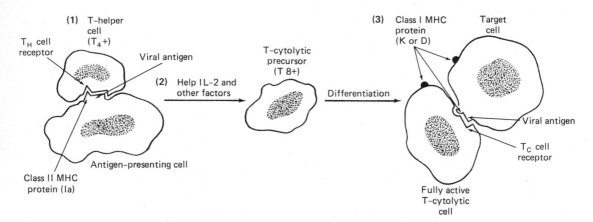

Figure 9.13 This figure outlines the cellular events bringing about the induction of cytolytic T-lymphocytes capable of reacting to parasite antigen in a host cell membrane. The helper lymphocyte (T_H) recognizes the antigen in the context of Class II (Ia) molecules on an antigen-presenting cell (1). The T-helper cell secretes lymphokines (2) that induce T-cytolytic precursors to differentiate into fully active cytolytic cells. The T_c cell lyses the target cell only in the context of Class I MHC molecules (3). Cytolysis of targets by cytolytic lymphocytes is further restricted to target cells with the same Class I MHC antigens as occur on the cytolytic lymphocyte. Antigens to be recognized by cytolytic lymphocytes must be associated with products of either the H-2 or H-2D region of the mouse MHC gene complex. A viral antigen is used as an example here.

swells and lyses. The cytotoxic lymphocyte is unharmed by the reaction and can destroy a number of infected cells.

The Biological Significance of Major Histocompatibility Complex Restriction of Cytolytic T-Lymphocytes

The single most important mechanism among the many mechanisms governing the sensitization and effector activities of T-cells is that which permits antigen recognition only if the antigens are presented as a complex in association with membrane proteins encoded by genes of the MHC complex.

Major histocompatibility restriction of antigen recognition by cells of the inducible immune response is a complicated mechanism that was not eliminated during evolution. It must therefore have utility. It cannot have arisen to prevent graft acceptance, but rather must have arisen as part of the mechanism required to prevent colonization of the host's tissues by parasites. As noted earlier, antigen-presenting cells display parasite components on their surfaces. It would not be in the interest of a host to use its cytolytic mechanisms to destroy these cells.

Self-recognition is also required to permit differentiation from nonself. If all members of a species were identical in self-components, some parasite could perhaps develop at least an outer coat similar to that of the host's self and thus escape detection in all members of the species. As each member of the species has distinct self markers, however, no parasite can develop a pattern to deceive all members of the species. The diversity of self types that exists in vertebrates is generated by a system of reassortment of genes during gamete formation and fertilization. This system precludes any parasite becoming self to all members of the vertebrate species. Self-recognition and MHC restriction are thus systems that permit parasite recognition in the face of unique individuality.

SUGGESTIONS FOR FURTHER READING

D. O. Adams and T. A. Hamilton. "The cell biology of macrophage activation." Ann. Rev. Immunol. *2*:283, 1984.

O. G. Bier, W. Dias da Silva, D. Gotze, and J. Mota. *Fundamentals of Immunology,* 2nd edition. Springer-Verlag, Berlin, 1986.

F. MacFarlane Burnet. *Cellular Immunology.* Cambridge University Press, London, 1969.

F. J. Dixon and D. W. Fisher. *The Biology of Immunological Diseases.* Sinauer Associates, Sunderland, Massachusetts, 1983. (From *Hospital Practice* feature articles.)

J. W. Kimball. *Introduction to Immunology,* 2nd edition. Macmillan, New York, 1986.

D. S. Nelson. *Macrophages and Immunity.* American Elsevier, New York, 1969.

G. Rook. Cell-mediated Immunity. In *Immunology.* I. Roitt, J. Brostoff, and D. K. Male, *eds.* Gower Medical Publishing, London, 1985.

R. H. Schwartz. "Immune response (Ir) genes of the murine major histocompatibility complex." Adv. in Immunology *38*:31, 1986.

S. Sell. *Immunology, Immunopathology and Immunity,* 4th edition. Elsevier, New York, 1987.

H. Smith and J. H. Pearce. *Microbial Pathogenicity in Man and Animals.* Cambridge University Press, London, 1972.

K. A. Smith. "Interleukin 2." Ann. Rev. Immunol. *2:*319, 1984.

K. A. Smith. "Interleukin 2: Inception, impact, and implications." Science *240:*1169, 1988.

S. T. Tonegawa. "The molecules of the immune system." Scientific American *253:*122, 1985.

Chapter 10

Immunologically Mediated Diseases and Allergic Reactions

CAROLINE C. WHITACRE

Department of Medical Microbiology and Immunology
College of Medicine
The Ohio State University

INTRODUCTION

The purpose of the immunological response is to protect the host. The beneficial effects we expect to see are, for example, eradication of an infectious agent or immunity following vaccination. In order to carry out such beneficial effects, a complex interaction of lymphocytes, macrophages, interleukins, antibodies, complement, and other biochemical factors is necessary: They are all regulated by an exquisite system of checks and balances. In some cases the regulation fails and inappropriate responses, as for example reaction to self-components, occur. In other cases the response is properly developed but the effector mechanisms produce effects so intense that the host's tissues as well as the parasite may be injured. In this chapter we will discuss some of these "inappropriate" responses, including the responses to self-antigens and excessive responses to environmental antigens.

As has been stated previously, the central role of the immune system is to discriminate between what is self and what is nonself. It is thought that the primary means by which the immune system recognizes foreign antigens is through comparison with self major histocompatibility complex (MHC) determinants. Therefore, the cell surface MHC class I and II molecules serve as a self "yardstick" against which foreign determinants can be measured. Obviously, then, a mechanism must exist by which an individual can recognize its own self-antigens. At the same time, mounting an immune response against those self-antigens would be most dangerous. Therefore, recognition of self-determinants and immunologic reactivity against self-determinants are two very different processes and should not be confused. Recognition of self-determinants is normal and occurs during the generation of nearly all immune responses, whereas immunologic reactivity against self-determinants can lead to autoimmune disease.

AUTOIMMUNE DISEASES

In the early 1900s Paul Ehrlich introduced the term *horror autotoxicus,* meaning that an individual would not form an immune response against self-constituents. A corollary to this concept was the recognition that if indeed immune responses of sufficient strength and duration are made to self-determinants, then the outcome would be harmful autoimmune disease. In the years since the introduction of the horror autotoxicus concept, abnormal autoimmune responses have been recognized to be the primary cause of, or a secondary contributor to, several human diseases.

How is it that autoimmune responses can be generated in the face of immunological tolerance that supposedly prevents us from forming immune responses against self-antigens? It is probable that immunological tolerance can be explained by three primary mechanisms: (1) the deletion of all self-reactive clones of lymphocytes, a process occurring very early in the life of an individual; (2) the preferential inactivation of helper T-cells specific for self-reactive immune responses; and (3) the activity of suppressor T-cells, one of whose jobs it is to control self-reactive immune responses. The emergence of autoimmune disease is postulated to be due to mutation of a non–self-reactive lymphocyte into a self-reactive one, the activation of previously tolerant helper T-cells, or the inhibition of suppressor T-cells.

Table 10.1 lists some of the more common autoimmune diseases and the self-antigen recognized by the immune system in each disease. There are at least two broad types of autoimmune diseases based on the location of lesions produced by the diseases. The first is the *organ-specific type* of autoimmune disease, in which disease involvement is limited to a single organ such as the thyroid, stomach, adrenal gland, or pancreas. An example of this type of disorder is Hashimoto's thyroiditis, where pathology is limited to the thyroid gland and the symptoms of the disease are the result of disturbances in thyroid function. In this disease antibodies directed against thyroglobulin, a major component of the thyroid follicular fluid, prevent production of thyroid hormone. The second is the non–organ-specific type of autoimmune disease, in which the manifestations of disease are much more widespread, often occurring in many organ systems. In these disorders, autoimmune responses are directed against antigens that are widely disseminated throughout the body, and lesions are often present in the skin, joints, kidney, and muscle. A classic example of a non–organ-specific autoimmune disease is systemic lupus erythematosus, referred to as SLE or lupus. SLE occurs most frequently in females (9:1 female:male), usually between the ages of 20 and 50 years. Symptoms include fever, extreme fatigue, weight loss, skin rashes, sensitivity to sunlight, central nervous system signs, and arthritis occurring in several joints. In these patients, autoantibodies are produced against DNA (both double-stranded and single-stranded), RNA, lymphocytes, red blood cells, and platelets. Complexes of these antibodies, with their specific antigen, are deposited in the skin, joints, muscle, and glomeruli of the kidney. It is the deposition of immune complexes in the kidney that is the most damaging and can result in life-threatening glomerulonephritis. Figure 10.1 shows a section of kidney with the immune complexes that have been deposited in the glomeruli visualized by immunofluorescence. The mechanism thought to be responsible for causing the pathology ob-

Table 10.1 AUTOIMMUNE DISEASES

Autoimmune disease	Self-antigen recognized
Organ-specific diseases	
Hashimoto's thyroiditis	Thyroglobulin
Pernicious anemia	Gastric parietal cells
Graves' disease	Thyroid-stimulating hormone receptor
Juvenile insulin-dependent diabetes	Pancreatic islet cells
Multiple sclerosis	Central nervous system myelin
Non–organ-specific diseases	
Systemic lupus erythematosus	dsDNA, ssDNA, platelets, red blood cells, lymphocytes, neuronal cells
Rheumatoid arthritis	Gamma globulin
Goodpasture's syndrome	Basement membrane

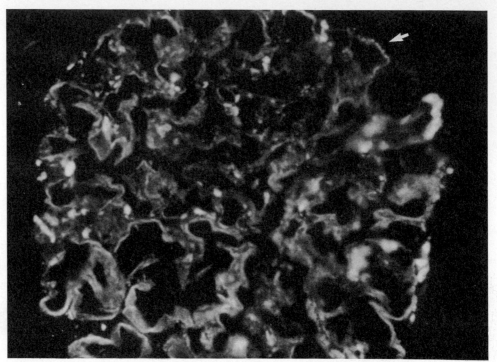

Figure 10.1 A micrograph of a section of kidney from an individual with lupus, demonstrating the presence of immunoglobulin in the glomerular capillary loops. The section was stained with fluorescent labeled antiglobulin. Arrow indicates an individual capillary loop, demonstrating granular immunofluorescence.

served in SLE and other immune complex diseases will be discussed in the section entitled "Type III Hypersensitivity."

Certainly, one of the most common of autoimmune diseases is rheumatoid arthritis, which afflicts a significant proportion of older persons. In fact, it is estimated that as many as 80 percent of the population of the United States will experience some form of rheumatic discomfort at some time in their lives. Clinically, rheumatoid arthritis is characterized by inflammation of the joints, with pain upon movement. Individuals with rheumatic arthritis have in their serum IgM or IgG autoantibodies that are reactive with the Fc portion of IgG; such autoantibodies are referred to as *rheumatoid factor.* These autoantibodies complexed with IgG are thought to deposit in the joints and blood vessels and to play a key role in the joint inflammation and vasculitis characteristic of this disease.

Although the vast majority of autoimmune diseases listed in Table 10.1 are thought to be due to humoral immunity and autoantibody formation, there are autoimmune diseases in which cellular immunity is the primary mediator. For example, multiple sclerosis (MS) is postulated to be due to a cellular immune response to the myelin in the central nervous system. In this disease, which is usually first observed in adults between 20 and 40 years of age and results in vision and motor abnormalities, there are accumulations of lymphocytes and macrophages surrounding the blood vessels of the central nervous system.

THE HYPERSENSITIVITIES

Among immunologists, the term *hypersensitivity* has come to mean any harmful immune reaction that causes tissue damage. Some examples of reactions considered to be hypersensitivities are allergy due to ragweed pollen, transfusion reactions following introduction of mismatched blood, the skin reaction following contact with poison ivy, and the often severe glomerulonephritis that occurs following introduction into an animal of antiserum prepared in another species of animal. In the 1950s, Coombs and Gell devised a scheme for classifying hypersensitivities based upon the immunological mechanism involved. Their scheme divided these reactions into four types, called types I, II, III, and IV. The first three types are antibody-mediated, and the fourth is due to the actions of T-lymphocytes and macrophages. Actually, the autoimmune diseases covered earlier in this chapter fall under the broad definition of hypersensitivity and can also be classified into Coombs and Gell's scheme. We will treat each type of hypersensitivity individually.

Type I Hypersensitivity

Type I hypersensitivity (Figure 10.1) is also known as *immediate hypersensitivity* because of the speed with which the immunologic reactions take place, occurring within minutes following antigen challenge. The most common type of immediate hypersensitivity reaction is seasonal rhinitis, or hay fever, which afflicts from 10 to 15 percent of the population of the United States. The symptoms of hay fever develop following exposure of the individual to ragweed or other pollens. These are found in their highest concentrations in the atmosphere of the northern hemisphere in the months of August, September, and October. After exposure to the environmental allergens, these individuals experience symptoms that include itchy and watery eyes, sneezing, runny nose, and photophobia. Other types of immediate hypersensitivity reactions less common than hay fever are bronchial asthma, an allergic dermatitis known as urticaria, and some food allergies.

In order for immediate hypersensitivity reactions to occur, an individual must first come in contact with an antigen and produce IgE antibody in response to that antigen. It is currently thought that genetic factors may play a role in determining whether a given individual will produce IgE or antibody of another class in response to antigen. For example, recent studies have shown that if both parents have allergies, then a child has a 75 percent chance of being allergic; if only one parent is allergic, then there is a 50 percent chance. However, 38 percent of allergic individuals have no parental history of allergy.

Once IgE antibody is formed in response to antigen, it becomes fixed to mast cells in the tissues and to basophils in the blood. These cells possess high affinity receptors specific for the Fc portion of IgE antibodies. The IgE antibodies are bound to mast cells and basophils by the Fc portion, leaving the antigen-binding portion (Fab) of the IgE exposed (Figure 10.2). The interaction of IgE with the mast cell surface is a relatively stable one, since mast cells have been shown to remain sensitized with IgE molecules for up to 12 weeks.

A variety of events take place on the mast cell. Upon reexposure to the sensitizing antigen, the IgE molecules on the mast cell surface become cross linked, thus activating the mast cell. Mast cell activation is accompanied by the release of intracellular granules that contain potent mediators of inflammation (Figure 10.2). It is these mediators that are responsible for the symptoms of rhinitis, asthma, and dermatitis associated with type I hypersensitivity.

Tissue mast cells are found in highest concentration in the skin and gastrointestinal tract. Their major function appears to be storage of granules that contain mediators important in inflammation and repair processes. There are at least two different types of mast cells in humans: the connective tissue mast cell that is located throughout the body, particularly around blood vessels, and the mucosal mast cell that is located predominantly in the mucosa of the gut and lung. Within the gastrointestinal tract, the type of mast cell may vary, a finding that may have implications for individuals with food allergies. For example, in the mouth, tongue, esophagus, and proximal stomach, the connective tissue mast cells predominate; whereas in the distal stomach, duodenum, jejunum, ileum, and colon, mucosal mast cells are more plentiful. The two types of mast cells differ in appearance, content of granules, and T-cell dependence. The connective tissue mast cell is

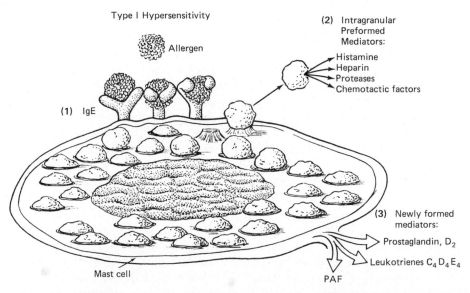

Figure 10.2 Reactions occurring in type I hypersensitivity. Allergen-reactive IgE binds to the mast cell surface by IgE-specific Fc receptors (1). When the allergen reacts with the cell-bound IgE, the mast cell degranulates releasing preformed mediators (2) and initiating the synthesis of arachidonic acid metabolites (3).

larger, contains many more granules, and has a higher histamine content than the mucosal mast cell (Figure 10.3). Moreover, the mucosal mast cell has been shown to proliferate following an influx of T-lymphocytes, suggesting an association between the two cell types. In spite of their differences, both the connective tissue mast cell and the mucosal mast cell bind IgE antibodies and degranulate following exposure to appropriate antigen, thus releasing potent mediators of inflammation. In addition to the mast cell, the blood basophil also binds IgE and participates in immediate hypersensitivity reactions. These cells comprise only about from 0.5 to 2 percent of circulating white cells and contain substantially fewer of the inflammatory mediators than do mast cells.

The biochemical events that occur following receptor cross linking and result in mast cell degranulation have recently received much attention. Once antigen bridges two IgE receptors and brings them into close apposition, several intracellular systems are activated. Among these systems is the adenylate cyclase pathway that serves to convert ATP to cyclic AMP and activates protein kinase A. In addition, other intracellular events take place such as the formation of inositol triphosphate and the activation of protein kinase C. The result of activation of these pathways is to increase the intracellular concentration of calcium, which

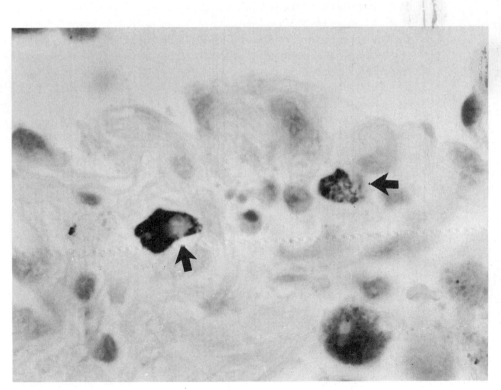

Figure 10.3 Photomicrograph of mucosal cells from the lung alveolar septa stained with methylene blue. Note the intensely staining granules within these mast cells. Arrows indicate mast cells in the tissue. (Oil immersion view.)

directly and indirectly causes the formation of membrane fusogens. These cause fusion of the membranes surrounding the mast cell granules with the plasma membrane of the cell, resulting in the spillage of the granule contents into the extracellular environment. In addition, metabolism of the phospholipids contained in the plasma membrane of the mast cell results in the generation of the inflammatory mediators outlined next.

The mediators released from mast cells can be divided into those substances that are preformed and packaged into granules and those that are membrane-derived lipids. The first group includes histamine, proteases, heparin, eosinophil chemotactic factor, and neutrophil chemotactic factor. These substances are present in mast cell granules and are released immediately upon degranulation. The various types of mast cell mediators have a variety of biological effects (Table 10.2). For example, histamine, which is the major preformed mediator present in the human mast cell, causes such effects as contraction of the smooth muscle in the bronchioles, vascular dilation with increases in vascular permeability, and increases in nasal secretion. Such effects are usually evident within one to two minutes after exposure of an allergic individual to the inciting antigen. Proteases such as tryptase and chymase may increase vascular permeability by digesting the blood vessel basement membrane. Heparin, also a preformed constituent of mast cell granules, may complex with the proteases within the granule and may decrease their deleterious effects once the granules are released into the extracellular space. Finally, factors chemotactic for eosinophils and neutrophils have been shown to be present in the granules and to account for the influx of cells of these types into areas of mast cell degranulation.

The second class of mediators released by mast cells as a result of allergic

Table 10.2   MEDIATORS OF IMMEDIATE HYPERSENSITIVITY REACTIONS

Mediator	Biological effects
Preformed mediators (present in granules of mast cells and basophils)	
Histamine	Vasopermeability, bronchoconstriction
Heparin	Complex with proteases, anticoagulant
Tryptase	Digestion of basement membranes
Chymase	Digestion of basement membranes
Eosinophil chemotactic factor (ECF)	Influx of eosinophils
Neutrophil chemotactic factor (NCF)	Influx of eosinophils
Membrane-derived mediators (formed *de novo* after cell activation)	
Prostaglandin D_2	Vasopermeability, bronchoconstriction
Leukotrienes C_4, D_4, E_4	Vasopermeability, bronchoconstriction
Platelet activating factor (PAF)	Vasopermeability, bronchoconstriction, chemotaxis, platelet aggregation

Source: Modified from W. E. Serafin and K. F. Austen, "Mediators of Immediate Hypersensitivity Reactions," *New England Journal of Medicine* 317:30–34, 1987.

exposure are the newly formed mediators, which are produced by metabolism of phospholipids within the mast cell. During IgE-mediated reactions, mast cell and basophil membrane phospholipids are phosphorylated; these phosphorylated lipids activate the enzymes phospholipase A_2 and C. As a consequence, there is formation of arachidonic acid. Arachidonic acid is then available to be further metabolized by enzymes of one of two enzymatic pathways: the cyclooxygenase pathway that produces the prostaglandins or the 5-lipoxygenase pathway that produces the leukotrienes. During allergic reactions, prostaglandin D_2 induces vasodilation, increases in vascular permeability, and bronchoconstriction. The leukotrienes C_4, D_4, and E_4, previously referred to collectively as the slow-reactive substance of anaphylaxis, mediate bronchoconstriction, vasopermeability, and mucus secretion. Another derivative of phospholipid, platelet activating factor (PAF), brings about aggregation of platelets, causing microthrombi; it also causes severe bronchoconstriction, increases in permeability, and chemotaxis of neutrophils. Whereas mast cells have been shown to produce prostaglandin D_2, the leukotrienes, and PAF, basophils apparently synthesize only the leukotrienes (see Chapter 4).

Allergies to certain foods, dust, or animal dander can be controlled by avoidance of the allergen. However, ubiquitous allergens such as ragweed, grasses, or certain tree pollens are difficult to avoid. In these instances immunotherapy by the injection of increasing doses of allergen has proven successful in some cases. Although the explanation for the observed clinical improvement is unknown, it is thought that IgG antibody may be produced in response to systemic injection of allergen, which may block the allergen-IgE reaction. Furthermore, immunotherapy may also lead to an increase in suppressor T-cell activity, causing a decrease in IgE production.

Therapy for allergy has also been based on attempts to inhibit the release of inflammatory mediators from mast cells. Cromolyn sodium, which was introduced relatively recently, has a beneficial effect on patients with allergic disorders and is thought to act by stabilizing lysosomal membranes, thus inhibiting degranulation. Another therapy is based on drugs that interfere with the actions of the inflammatory mediators. For example, antihistamines are administered to interfere with the reaction of histamine with histamine receptors on shock organs. Likewise, diethylcarbamazine interferes with the action of the leukotrienes. Corticosteroids have frequently been administered to persons with allergies, and it is now known that in the presence of corticosteroids mast cells fail to reaccumulate histamine following degranulation.

Type II Hypersensitivity

Type II hypersensitivity is often referred to as *cytotoxic hypersensitivity* because in these reactions IgG or IgM antibody directed against cell surface components causes damage to, or lysis of, the affected cell. Complement can participate in these reactions by effecting cell lysis or through opsonization of the antibody-coated cell. Some examples of cytotoxic hypersensitivity are transfusion reactions, in which the transfusion of incompatible blood results in antibody and complement-mediated destruction of the transfused cells, and autoimmune hemolytic anemia, in which antibodies effect lysis of erythrocytes. In some autoimmune hemolytic anemias, the antibodies are directed against erythrocyte components, whereas in others they are produced in response to drugs and result when the antibody binds to the drug or drug metabolites that are adsorbed onto the erythrocyte surface.

The critical event in any of the type II cytotoxic reactions is the binding of IgG or IgM antibody to cell surface antigens (Figure 10.4). What happens after that initiating event depends upon the class or subclass of the antibody bound and the nature of the target cell involved. If the antibody is IgM, IgG1, IgG2, or IgG3, then the Clq component of complement is bound and activated. This initiates complement activation by the classical complement pathway and terminates with the formation of the $\overline{C5b6789}$ membrane attack complex and subsequent lysis of the affected cell (see Chapter 9). The membrane of the cell on which antibody is bound may also become coated with the $\overline{C3b}$ component of complement. This complement split product serves as an opsonin and facilitates uptake of the entire cell-antibody-$\overline{C3b}$ complex by phagocytic cells.

There are also complement-independent means by which antibody can cause cell damage. For example, an antibody-coated cell can interact with a killer cell: The killer cell binds to the antibody-coated cell by its receptor for the Fc portion of IgG. Binding in this fashion can lead to destruction of the target cell by the killer cell through antibody-dependent–cell-mediated cytotoxicity.

A classic type II cytotoxic hypersensitivity disease is erythroblastosis fetalis, also known as hemolytic disease of the newborn. In this condition the mother becomes sensitized to the blood group antigens on the fetus's erythrocytes, which eventually leads to antibody-mediated destruction of the fetal erythrocytes. Rhesus D (RhD) is the most commonly involved blood group antigen in hemolytic disease of the newborn. The antibodies responsible for erythroblastosis fetalis arise when an Rh− mother carries an Rh+ fetus (Figure 10.5). During the birth of the baby, fetal erythrocytes are released into the maternal circulation and stimulate the

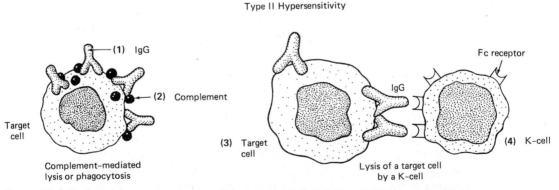

Type II Hypersensitivity

Figure 10.4 Reactions occurring in type II hypersensitivity. IgG or IgM (1) antibodies are directed against cell surface constituents. Complement binding (2) results in lysis or phagocytosis of the target cell. Alternatively, an antibody-coated target cell (3) can be lysed by a K cell (4) which bears Fc receptors.

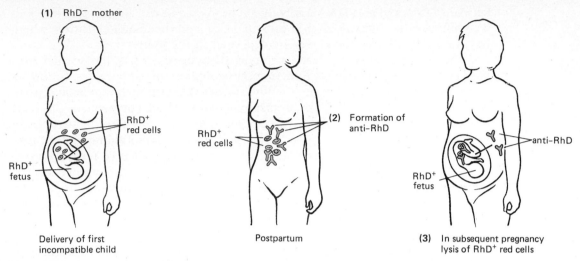

Figure 10.5 Immunologic events occurring in erythroblastosis fetalis. An RhD $^-$ mother carrying an RhD $^+$ fetus is exposed to fetal red blood cells carrying the RhD antigen during delivery of the baby (1). During the postpartum period, the mother forms antibodies directed against the RhD antigen (2). In subsequent pregnancies where the fetus is RhD+, maternal antibodies (containing anti-RhD antibodies) cross the placenta and can cause red cell destruction (3). Erythroblastosis fetalis can be prevented by giving the mother an injection of antibody directed against the RhD antigen upon birth of the fetus, thus eliminating the fetal cells from the maternal circulation before antibody can be formed.

mother's immune system to produce IgG antibodies directed against the RhD antigen. During subsequent pregnancies involving an Rh+ fetus, anti-RhD antibodies cross the placenta and cause red cell destruction.

The first Rh+ child born to an Rh− mother is usually unaffected, but subsequent children are at considerable risk from erythroblastosis fetalis. The mother is repeatedly immunized with each delivery, and her antibody to RhD increases with each pregnancy if no preventative measures are taken. This condition can now be prevented by immunologic means. If the Rh− mother receives an injection of anti-RhD antibodies at the time of the delivery of the first Rh+ child, sensitization of the mother to RhD antigens is prevented. This form of immunoprophylaxis has proven to be quite successful in preventing erythroblastosis fetalis.

Type III Hypersensitivity

Type III hypersensitivity is also known as *immune complex hypersensitivity* since the tissue damage results from deposition of immune complexes in the tissue. Complement participates in the tissue damage that occurs in these reactions through the anaphylactic properties of the split products of complement, $\overline{C3a}$ and $\overline{C5a}$. Some examples of immune complex–mediated diseases have already been discussed earlier in this chapter, namely, SLE, in which immune complexes formed between DNA and anti-DNA antibody are deposited in the glomeruli of the kidneys and at other sites where they cause damage, and rheumatoid arthritis, where IgG–anti-IgG immune complexes are deposited in the joints.

The sequence of events leading to type III hypersensitivity starts when antibody combines with antigen to form immune complexes of various sizes. Following complex formation, complement is bound and activated through the classical pathway. This results in the release of anaphylatoxins. These complement products induce basophils to degranulate, releasing histamine, thereby causing increases in vascular permeability. In addition, $\overline{C5a}$ also attracts polymorphonuclear neutrophils. These cells bind to the immune complexes through their Fc and C3b receptors and phagocytize the immune complexes. In the process of phagocytosis, the neutrophils release some of their intragranular enzymes, causing local tissue damage. This entire process may take place within blood vessel walls or along the glomerular basement membrane in the kidney (Figure 10.6).

The formation of immune complexes is a normal consequence of any immune response, but these complexes are only sometimes associated with disease. Normally immune complexes are removed from the circulation by cells of the reticuloendothelial system, that is, by macrophages located primarily in the liver, spleen, and lungs. There is some evidence that individuals who develop type III hypersensitivity have a defect in the system of macrophage clearance of immune complexes.

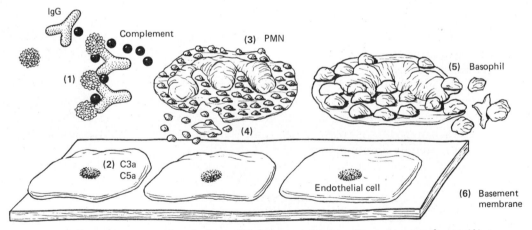

Figure 10.6 Reactions occurring in type III hypersensitivity. Immune complexes (1), formed when antigen and antibody combine, deposit on tissues (2), where they fix complement resulting in the release of the complement split products C3a and C5a. The C5a is chemotactic for neutrophils (3), which attempt to phagocytose the complexes, resulting in release of their intragranular enzymes that cause tissue damage (4). The complement products also cause basophil degranulation (5), resulting in release of vasoactive amines and an increase in vascular permeability. The net result of these effects is damage to the endothelial cells and underlying basement membrane (6), whether in the kidney, lung, or blood vessel walls.

There are other factors that also appear to play a role in immune complex–mediated tissue damage. First, the size of immune complexes in part determines their persistence in the blood. Large complexes are removed rapidly by the liver, but small complexes persist longer in the circulation. Second, the deposition of immune complexes in tissue appears to be triggered by an increase in local vascular permeability. For example, complement split products, as well as mediators released by mast cells, basophils, and platelets, participate in the release of vasoactive amines. When this release occurs within a blood vessel, these mediators cause retraction of endothelial cells, exposure of the underlying basement membrane, and increased blood flow and capillary permeability. The plasma containing the complexes passes into the tissues where they are deposited. Third, immune complex deposition is observed in certain locations within the body more often than in others. For example, sites of biological filtration such as the renal glomerulus or choroid plexus are particularly susceptible to immune complex–mediated damage. At these sites fluids in the blood pass through filtering membranes; the complexes are often retained on the filtering surfaces. Sites of high blood pressure and turbulence such as the glomerular capillaries are also susceptible to immune complex deposition; perhaps the turbulence brings the small complexes together and results in their aggregation and deposition.

Type IV Hypersensitivity

Type IV hypersensitivity is also known as *delayed hypersensitivity* since the obvious signs of these reactions are observed 24 hours or more after contact with antigen. In contrast to the first three types of hypersensitivity, which are antibody-mediated, type IV hypersensitivity reactions are mediated by T-lymphocytes and macrophages. The most commonly recognized form of delayed hypersensitivity is allergic contact dermatitis, best exemplified by the eczema that develops following exposure to poison ivy. More severe forms of delayed type hypersensitivity reactions have been observed in certain disease states such as leprosy or tuberculosis, where the antigen is persistent and cannot easily be eliminated by the macrophages.

The mechanisms responsible for delayed type hypersensitivity reactions are quite different from the antibody-mediated reactions discussed earlier (Figure 10.7). Thymic lymphocytes, sensitized by prior contact with the antigen, become activated upon reexposure to the allergen and release soluble mediators termed *lymphokines*. One of these lymphokines—macrophage activating factor, now known to be gamma interferon—is responsible for causing the differentiation of normal resting or responsive macrophages into activated macrophages. In this activated form, the macrophages are capable of enhanced phagocytosis and increased microbicidal activity. Another lymphokine released from activated T-lymphocytes is lymphocyte mitogenic factor, which acts to amplify the immune response by increasing the number of T-lymphocytes present in the vicinity. In this way, lymphocytes and activated macrophages recruited by lymphokines accumulate at the local reaction site.

Allergic contact dermatitis not only can follow exposure to poison ivy but can also occur following sensitization to certain soaps or to nickel, rubber, or any of

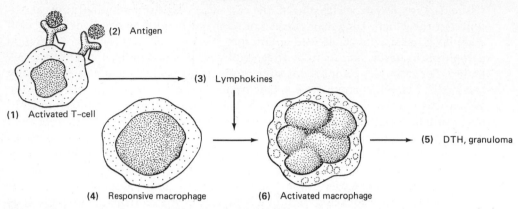

Figure 10.7 Reactions occurring in type IV hypersensitivity. Activated T-cells (1), upon reexposure to specific antigen (2), release lymphokines (3) such as gamma interferon. These lymphokines act on resting macrophages (4) causing them to become activated (6). Activated macrophages participate in cell-mediated reactions such as delayed hypersensitivity responses and granuloma formation (5).

many low molecular weight chemicals. The contact dermatitis that may develop following exposure to bath soap is a typical form of the condition (Figure 10.8). Upon gross examination, one observes fluid-filled vesicles in the epidermis; upon histologic examination, it is seen that both the epidermis and the dermis are infiltrated with lymphocytes and macrophages. The low molecular weight chemicals that cause contact dermatitis probably become immunogenic by complexing with skin proteins and forming a hapten-carrier conjugate of sufficient size to generate a T-cell–mediated immune response.

From a clinical standpoint, the most significant of the delayed type hypersensitivity reactions are the granulomatous reactions. It is often the case that following infection with certain bacteria such as *Mycobacterium tuberculosis, Mycobacterium leprae,* or worms such as Schistosoma, the host cannot adequately eliminate these agents and they persist within macrophages or in the tissues. The end result is that an intense area of inflammation is observed at the site of infection (Figure 10.9). This inflammatory response is characterized by a core of macrophages and epithelioid cells, the latter being the characteristic cell of a granuloma. Also contained within the granuloma core may be giant cells, visible as large cells with many nuclei at their outer edge. Epithelioid cells and giant cells are thought to be derived from macrophages and to represent terminal stages of differentiation. An area of actively proliferating lymphocytes is usually seen surrounding the core area of the granuloma. Thus in granulomatous hypersensitivity the pathology is, in large part, due to the inability of host macrophages to eliminate the infecting organism. Activated T-lymphocytes secrete lymphokines in the vicinity of the infection, serving to amplify the immunological reaction. With the help of these lymphokines, macrophages become activated and undergo terminal differentiation to epi-

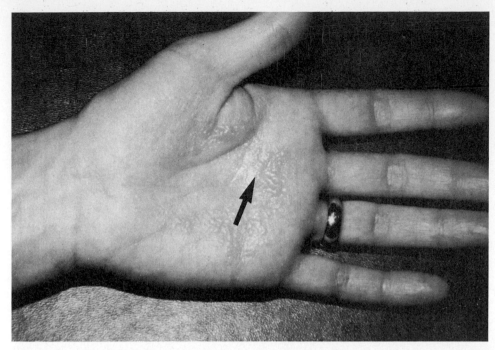

Figure 10.8 Photograph of a hand affected by allergic contact dermatitis (arrow) following exposure to bath soap. Low molecular weight chemicals contained in the soap bind to skin proteins, and the combination produces a hapten-carrier conjugate that is immunogenic. This reaction is T-cell–mediated and, histologically, both macrophages and lymphocytes are seen infiltrating the underlying tissue.

thelioid cells and giant cells. The end product of the interaction between the T-lymphocytes and macrophages is tissue death, called *necrosis* by pathologists.

SUMMARY

In this chapter we have discussed some of the ways in which the immune system can cause damage to the host. The immune system may react against self-antigens such as DNA in the case of lupus, or thyroid antigens in the case of thyroiditis. The end result may be systemic autoimmune disease in the former case, or organ-specific disease in the latter case. In addition to classification as systemic or organ specific, autoimmune diseases may be grouped using a broader classification based on the mechanism responsible for the immunopathology. Type I hypersensitivity, exemplified by hay fever, is due to the formation of excessive amounts of IgE antibodies specific for the allergen. These antibodies are capable of binding to the surfaces of mast cells and basophils. Following complexing with antigen, the mediators contained within cytoplasmic granules are released, causing tissue damage. Type II hypersensitivity, as illustrated by transfusion reactions, is caused by IgG

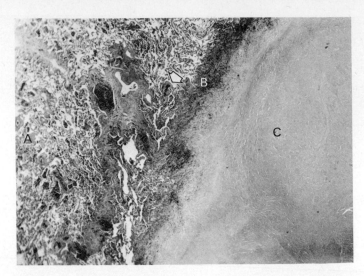

Figure 10.9 Photomicrograph of a tissue section containing a granulomatous reaction in the lung of an individual with tuberculosis. Note lung tissue (A), zone of inflammation with lymphocytes and macrophages (B), and remains of dead tissue (C). The lesion (C) is an example of caseous necrosis. Arrow indicates a multinucleate giant cell. (Low power view.)

or IgM antibody directed against a cell surface antigen. Binding of antibody to the cell is accompanied by fixation of complement and destruction of the cell to which the antibody is bound. Type III hypersensitivity, exemplified by systemic lupus erythematosus, is due to immune complex deposition in tissues. Fixation of complement by the immune complexes causes the release of complement split products, which are chemotactic for neutrophils and also cause basophil degranulation. The actions of the contents of neutrophil and basophil granules may damage host tissue. Type IV hypersensitivity, illustrated by leprosy, is caused by T-cell and macrophage activation in response to a skin-sensitizing compound or a persistent infection. Although these reactions may be classified into four discrete groups, it is important to remember that they may occur simultaneously in a given individual.

SUGGESTIONS FOR FURTHER READING

O. L. Frick. Immediate Hypersensitivity. In *Basic and Clinical Immunology*, D. P. Stites, J. D. Stobo, and J. V. Wells, *eds.* Appleton and Lange, Norwalk, Connecticut, 1987.

I. Roitt, J. Brostoff, and D. K. Male. *Immunology.* C. V. Mosby, New York, 1985.

W. E. Serafin and K. F. Austen. "Mediators of immediate hypersensitivity reactions." New England Journal of Medicine *317:*30, 1987.

A. N. Theofilopoulos. Autoimmunity. In *Basic and Clinical Immunology*, D. P. Stites, J. D. Stobo, and J. V. Wells, *eds.* Appleton and Lange, Norwalk, Connecticut, 1987.

in any particular case. In the absence of t
however, the destruction of grafted tissu

FORMS OF GRAFT REJECTION

The most practical definition of graft reje
cal manifestation, loss of graft function
progressive destruction of the graft. Curr
forms of graft rejection that can be disting
characteristics, and degree of susceptibilit
are hyperacute rejection, acute rejection

Hyperacute Rejection

This form of rejection occurs in graft reci
circulating in their blood prior to transpl
graft revascularization. Immunologically
deposition in the graft of antibody and co
tion of platelets in the capillary lumens, a
phonuclear leukocytes (Figure 11.1). As
and arterioles in the graft rapidly become b
graft stop blood flow to the graft. Tissue r
no known medical procedure that can s

Acute Rejection

Acute rejection occurs in graft recipien
lymphocytes. This form of rejection occu
implantation. Acute rejection is character
lymphocytes. First, small lymphocytes
walls. The lymphocytes pass through th
grafted tissue. With the passage of tim
diffuse. The infiltrating cells cause the pr
venules. Fluids accumulate in the tissue
grafted tissue is interrupted. With the fa
Acute rejection, unlike the other forms o
ate medical treatment.

Chronic Rejection

Chronic rejection occurs in graft recipien
acute rejection. Chronic rejection usuall
implantation. When chronic rejection oc
graft. Severe narrowing of the arteries i
intima thickens and the internal elastic l
remains intact. The narrowing of the art

The Host Response to Grafts and Transplantation Immunology

CHARLES G. OROSZ

Department of Surgery
College of Medicine
The Ohio State University

SPECIAL CONSIDERATIONS: RETRANSP
SPECIAL CONSIDERATIONS: TRANSPLA
SUMMARY
SUGGESTIONS FOR FURTHER READING

THE PHENOMENON OF REJECTION

Early attempts at tissue transplan
munologic responses that destroy tr
eliminate the possibility of tissue tra
recipients in the absence of tissue
practice of tissue transplantation is
difficult to explain the evolutionar
signed to prevent tissue exchange,
fact, graft rejection is caused by im
ployed to assure survival of the org
of foreign tissues is therefore the re
immunologic mechanisms, the func
nation of infectious agents.

In general, the vertebrate imn
efficient response to organisms inva
ganisms follows trauma to tissue or
be one of the initial factors alerting t
activates the bradykinin, clotting, f
initiates inflammation in the dam;
reproduction, then the immune s
contain the invader before it can bec
cannot know in advance the nature
the site of invasion, and thus it can
particular infectious agent but mus
the site of injury. This may explain
sites of tissue damage. Presumably,
localized inflammatory response b
croorganisms are encountered, the
response wanes. However, if micro
mechanisms are triggered that dir
sponse that is particularly effectiv
instead of a parasite at the site of
the same. An immune response is
.tion of the foreign tissue is accom
and considerable infiltration of th
immune effector mechanisms opera
these mechanisms are actually the

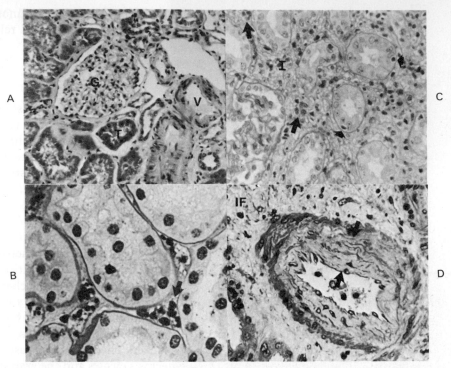

Figure 11.1 (A) Photomicrograph of a normal kidney. Glomerulus (G), tubule (T), vessel (V). (Hematoxylin and Eosin, original magnification 40×.) (B) Renal allograft undergoing hyperacute rejection. The peritubular capillaries are filled with neutrophils (arrows). (Periodic acid schiff, original magnification 160×.) (C) Renal allograft undergoing acute cellular rejection. The interstitium (I) is expanded by edema and a mononuclear cell infiltrate (arrows). Mononuclear cells focally invade the tubules (arrowheads). (Periodic acid schiff, original magnification 100×.) (D) Renal allograft undergoing chronic rejection. An artery shows fibrointimal hyperplasia (arrows) and there is interstitial fibrosis (IF). (Gomori's trichrome, original magnification 100×.)

and complement, and from formation of platelet and fibrin aggregates on the vessel walls. These deposits become covered with endothelium and are incorporated into the intima. The arterial narrowing causes reduction in blood flow, resulting in ischemia and progressive fibrosis. Currently, there are no satisfactory methods available to control chronic rejection.

MECHANISMS OF REJECTION

Acute rejection is the most studied and best understood of the three forms of rejection. This is probably because acute rejection is the most frequently encountered impediment to successful transplantation and because it is amenable to immunosuppressive therapy.

If hyperacute rejection does not occur first, immunocompetent vertebrate animals that receive a graft from another genetically distinct member of the same species (*allograft*) or from a member of a different species (*xenograft*) will invariably mount an acute graft-rejection response. Such an animal will, however, retain a graft from one part of itself to another (*autograft*) or a graft from a genetically identical individual (*isograft,* or *homograft*) for an indefinite period.

There is considerable evidence that acute allograft rejection is carried out primarily by T-lymphocytes. Mice that are made deficient in T-lymphocytes by neonatal thymectomy and the so-called nude mice that are genetically incapable of making T-lymphocytes fail to reject allografts. In contrast, a deficiency in B-lymphocytes does not interfere with allograft rejection. Chickens that have been neonatally bursectomized, making them deficient in B-lymphocytes, retain the ability to reject allografts. This does not mean that B-cells and antibodies are not involved in acute rejection. Rather, their involvement is not essential.

It has been shown that T-lymphocytes obtained by thoracic duct cannulation of dogs bearing allografts but not autografts have the ability to destroy cells derived from the donors of their grafts. This destruction is rapid, efficient, and specific for the graft. Unrelated or third-party cells from individuals not the graft donor are not destroyed by these lymphocytes. The cells that mediate this destruction are the cytolytic T-lymphocytes. Since these lymphocytes destroy graft cells *in vitro,* it has been hypothesized that they also destroy grafts *in vivo.* There is no doubt that cytolytic T-lymphocytes are present in grafts undergoing rejection, as they are easily recovered from graft sites. It is not clear, however, how they cause graft rejection. The behavior of cytotoxic lymphocytes has been extensively studied by *in vitro* techniques, primarily in mixed lymphocyte cultures.

MIXED LYMPHOCYTE CULTURES

When lymphocytes from two different individuals are mixed in tissue culture and antigen-presenting cells are present, lymphocyte stimulation and proliferation usually occurs in five to seven days. Proliferation can be detected either by counting cells or by analysis of incorporation of tritiated thymidine (Figure 11.2). Tritiated thymidine is a radioactive DNA precursor that is incorporated into DNA by dividing cells. In the mixed lymphocyte culture, the lymphocytes of the two populations recognize each other as nonself, or foreign, by recognition of the proteins on the cell surface called *histocompatibility antigens.* Contact with foreign histocompatibility molecules and antigen-presenting cells initiates the processes that cause the lymphocytes to proliferate.

To study the behavior of a single lymphocyte population in mixed culture, the second, or stimulating, lymphocyte population is either irradiated or treated with a DNA binding agent such as the drug Mitomycin C, which destroys its ability to proliferate without interfering with its ability to display histocompatibility molecules. The mixed lymphocyte culture is used to characterize the histocompatibility

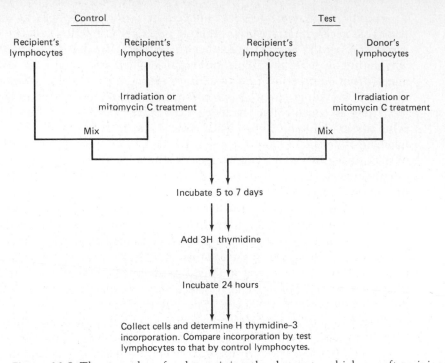

Figure 11.2 The procedure for determining the degree to which a graft recipient will be activated by alloantigens in a donors' lymphocytes. The donors' lymphocytes are treated by irradiation or with mitomycin C to prevent them from dividing. This treatment does not affect their ability to stimulate cell division of the recipient's lymphocytes. After mixing, the culture is incubated for five to seven days, then tritiated (^{3}H) thymidine is added; after 24 hours additional incubation, the degree of incorporation of label is determined. A compatible control using the recipient's lymphocytes is also run. A stimulation index (incorporation by test system divided by incorporation in control) indicates degree of compatibility.

molecules that stimulate lymphocytes and to study the behavior of lymphocytes following contact with alloantigens.

Cytolytic T-lymphocytes are generated in mixed lymphocyte cultures. Like the graft-reactive lymphocytes from the thoracic ducts of grafted animals, the cytotoxic lymphocytes that develop in mixed lymphocyte cultures can only lyse cells that display the alloantigens present on the stimulator cells. These cytotoxic lymphocytes are thus alloantigen specific.

It requires from five to seven days for cytotoxic lymphocytes to develop in mixed lymphocyte cultures. The presence of cytotoxic lymphocytes is assessed by determining the ability of the lymphocytes to lyse cells that have been radiolabeled with chromium 51 (Figure 11.3). The cells that may be destroyed are called *target cells.* Chromium 51 binds to proteins of the target cell cytoplasm. If the cell is lysed, the labeled cytoplasm leaks out. The amount of radioactivity released from the target cells is an index of the amount of lysis that occurred in the target cell

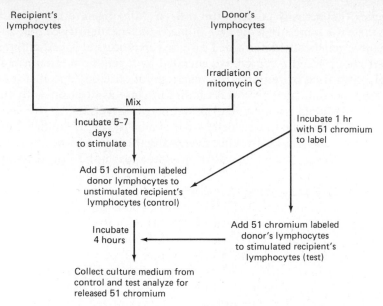

Figure 11.3 The degree to which cytolytic lymphocytes are generated in a mixed lymphocyte culture can be determined by the chromium-51 release assay. The donor's lymphocytes are labeled with ^{51}Cr, a label which binds to the proteins in the cytoplasm and is released along with the cytoplasm during cell lysis. The donor's lymphocytes are mixed with the recipient's lymphocytes and the cultures are incubated for five to seven days to permit generation of cytotoxic lymphocytes. Then fresh ^{51}Cr labeled donor's lymphocytes are added to the culture. After four hours the amount of radioactivity in the culture medium is measured. A cytotoxicity index is constructed by dividing the amount of radioactivity released in the test system by the amount released by labeled donor lymphocytes mixed with unstimulated recipients' lymphocytes. The larger the value of the index, the greater the incompatibility; an index of one indicates complete compatibility.

population. This method of detecting target cell destruction by cytotoxic lymphocytes is called the *chromium 51 release assay.*

THE T-CELL RECEPTOR

The specificity of a cytotoxic lymphocyte is determined by its antigen receptors. When a lymphocyte population is cultured with foreign cells, only a fraction of the lymphocytes in the population develop cytolytic activity; specifically, those lymphocytes with antigen receptors that can interact with the histocompatibility antigens on the foreign cells. The other lymphocytes are not stimulated and do not become lytic cells.

On all T-lymphocytes, the T-cell receptor is a complex protein aggregate. Part of the receptor complex is a 90,000-dalton combination of two linked but dissimilar proteins, collectively called *Ti.* The Ti is thought to be the part of the receptor complex that actually binds to the antigen. All antigen receptors on a given T-cell recognize the same antigenic determinant, and the identity of that antigenic determinant is genetically determined early in the process of T-cell differentiation. The repertoire of T-cell receptors is generated by a genetic mechanism similar to the mechanism used to generate the repertoire of antibody specificities.

The Ti component is always found in close association with three invariant 21,000–26,000-dalton membrane proteins, collectively called the *T3 complex* (Figure 11.4). T3 was first identified by use of a family of antibodies that reacted with determinants on the T3 proteins. Eventually the term *CD,* or *cluster of differentiation,* was used to categorize cell surface proteins, and T3 proteins became known as *CD3 proteins.*

The CD3 protein complex is displayed by maturing T-lymphocytes, but not by B-cells or macrophages. The T3 molecule (CD3) is thought to be the T-cell surface component that transmits activation signals from the T-cell receptor (Ti) through the T-cell membrane. There are many different additional proteins that are frequently associated with the T-cell receptor. Two of these, CD4 and CD8, are thought to help stabilize interactions between alloantigens and the T-cell receptor complex. The exact details of how all of these proteins cooperate to recognize specific antigenic determinants and of how antigen recognition is transmitted through the T-cell and translated into altered T-cell behavior are currently subjects of intensive investigation.

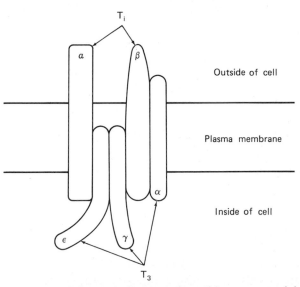

Figure 11.4 Schematic diagram of possible structure of the T-cell receptor (T_i/T_3 complex). The receptor consists of a number of molecules, some completely (α, β, δ,) and some partially (ϵ, δ) penetrating the cell membrane. The T_i part of the receptor is composed of the α and β proteins, and the T_3 of the δ and ϵ ones. When an antigen reacts with this receptor complex, the T_3 (CD3) proteins transmit a signal through the plasma membrane that initiates clonal expansion and differentiation of cytolytic T-cell precursors.

THE LYTIC MECHANISM USED BY CYTOTOXIC LYMPHOCYTES

The actual destruction of target cells by cytotoxic lymphocytes is a complex event that occurs in several stages. In general, active cytotoxic lymphocytes bind weakly and randomly to most cells. If they fail to encounter appropriate alloantigens, they dissociate without inflicting damage. However, if they encounter appropriate alloantigens, binding by their T-cell receptors is intensified in a process that requires metabolic energy and magnesium, and the bound cell is destroyed. Receptor-mediated binding initiates changes in the cytotoxic lymphocytes. These include reorganization of microtubules and reorientation of the Golgi apparatus and cellular granules. After reorganization the cytotoxic lymphocyte delivers the "lethal hit" to the targeted cell. This is a calcium-dependent and temperature-dependent process. During this killing process, granules are secreted onto the surface of the target cell. After granule secretion, the cytotoxic lymphocyte dissociates from the target cell and moves away, presumably in search of other target cells. The secreted granules remain in close proximity to the target cell, and one of the granule components, perforin, polymerizes on the target cell surface. The polymerized perforin enters the cell membrane and forms pores. The pores disrupt membrane integrity and cause lysis. Death results not only from loss of membrane integrity, but also from disintegration of the target cell nucleus, possibly due to enzymes that digest nuclear elements. A given cytotoxic lymphocyte can bind several target cells at one time, but target cell lysis occurs sequentially. Each lytic event requires intracellular reorientation of the cytotoxic lymphocyte.

ACTIVATION OF CYTOTOXIC LYMPHOCYTES

The generation of cytotoxic lymphocytes in mixed lymphocyte cultures and, presumably, *in vivo* is a complex process. Large numbers of inactive cytotoxic lymphocytes are normally present in the peripheral blood and lymphoid organs of healthy individuals. When a precursor lymphocyte encounters a relevant antigenic structure, it undergoes the first phase of lymphocyte activation. This is characterized by expression on the cell surface of new receptors for the lymphokines that trigger lymphocyte proliferation and differentiation. If these lymphokines are not present, activation does not occur. However, if these growth and differentiation factors are available, the partially activated lymphocyte differentiates, acquiring full cytolytic capability, and also begins to proliferate. By that mechanism, specific clones, selected by antigen, are activated and expanded; clones not reactive with the available antigen remain inactive.

The lymphokines inducing maturation and proliferation are produced by helper T-lymphocytes. Helper T-lymphocytes, like T-cytolytic lymphocytes, are also genetically committed to recognition of specific antigenic structures. They respond to contact with antigens by secreting the lymphokines that promote the activation and differentiation of other lymphocytes, and in this way helper T-lymphocytes orchestrate and regulate the immune responses that occur.

The activation of helper lymphocytes requires the participation of macrophages, which assist the activation process in two ways: First, macrophages present alloantigens in an appropriate manner to the helper lymphocytes (Figure 11.5). The alloantigens can be presented either directly by the foreign macrophages, or indirectly by self macrophages that have acquired the foreign alloantigens. Second, macrophages produce soluble proteins, called *monokines,* that are required for efficient helper lymphocyte function. One such monokine is called *interleukin-1* and facilitates helper lymphocyte proliferation.

Most T-lymphocyte behavior is regulated by sequential exposure to two signals. The first signal is contact of antigen-specific surface receptors with appropriate antigen. This triggers the display of the surface receptors for lymphokines and

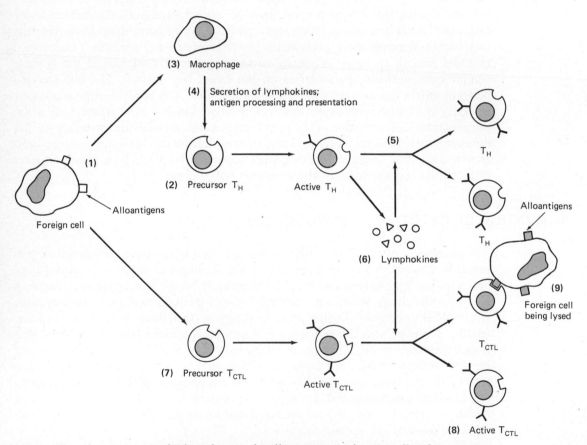

Figure 11.5 The activation of T-lymphocytes by alloantigens on foreign cells is by processes similar to activation by other antigens. The alloantigens (1) on the foreign cell are processed and presented to helper T-lymphocytes (T_H) (2) by macrophages (3) and the macrophages are induced to secrete lymphokines (4). These processes cause helper T-lymphocyte clones (CD44) of appropriate types to expand (5) and provide help (6) to appropriate precursor lytic (T_c) (7) lymphocytes (CD84). These lytic lymphocytes become activated and reproduce, yielding large numbers of active cytolytic lymphocytes (8) capable of lysing any foreign cells (9) bearing the alloantigen that induced the process.

monokines (collectively called *cytokines*). The second signal is contact of the T-cell with cytokines that bind to the newly displayed receptors. One such cytokine is called *interleukin-2*. This second contact triggers T-lymphocyte differentiation and proliferation. Only after the two signals have been received is the lymphocyte fully activated. This regulatory system assures that only the lymphocyte clones reactive with antigens present at the site become activated. This system also eliminates the necessity for a regulatory mechanism to actively suppress the activation of inappropriate T-lymphocyte clones.

LYMPHOKINES

As mentioned previously, helper T-lymphocytes produce a variety of lymphokines. The progeny of a single helper lymphocyte can produce a variety of lymphokines that collectively influence macrophages, B-lymphocytes, other T-lymphocytes, and lymphoid cell progenitors. Helper lymphocytes produce migration inhibition factor, which interferes with macrophage motility; gamma interferon, which causes macrophage activation; B-cell differentiation factor, which causes the shift from IgM to IgG production; B-cell growth factor, which causes B-cell proliferation; interleukin-2, which causes T-lymphocyte proliferation; and colony stimulating factor, which causes lymphoid differentiation from stem cell progenitors. This list of lymphokines is far from inclusive.

The ability to produce lymphokines is common to most types of T-lymphocytes, not just helper lymphocytes. The primary function of T-lymphocytes, in fact, may be to produce lymphokines and thus regulate and coordinate the behavior of the cells involved in immune responses. The lymphokines are the hormones of the immune system. As such, they operate like other peptide hormones, affecting many cell types that display the appropriate receptors. The reaction induced by a lymphokine is determined by the developmental stage of the receptive cell and by the type of cell on which it is acting.

HISTOCOMPATIBILITY ANTIGENS

Histocompatibility antigens differ in degree of antigenicity as defined by the period of time required for completion of the rejection of the graft bearing the antigen. There are strong histocompatibility antigens that cause vigorous rejection responses that take only 7 to 10 days to complete. There are also weaker histocompatibility antigens that cause milder rejection responses that take 20 or more days to complete. The strong histocompatibility antigens are all genetically encoded in the same chromosomal region, which is called the *major histocompatibility complex*, or *MHC* (Figure 11.6). In the human, the MHC encodes the so-called HLA (human leukocyte associated) antigens; in the mouse it encodes a similar set of antigens, called *H-2 antigens*. In both species, the weaker histocompatibility antigens are encoded at at least 40 different chromosomal sites and are collectively called *minor histocompatibility antigens*.

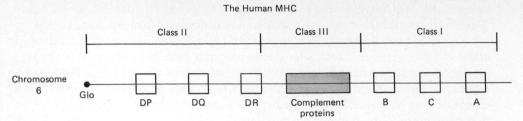

Figure 11.6 Strong human histocompatibility genes of the major histocompatibility complex (MHC) that are responsible for vigorous rejection responses are encoded on chromosome 6. At the gene loci (eg) DP, DQ, DR, B, C, and A, many alleles are available that are reassorted during sexual reproduction yielding many unique and therefore histoincompatible individuals. These genes, of course, have important functions in the immunological response quite apart from their role in tissue rejection. These are described in Chapter 8.

The cell surface proteins that bear the histocompatibility antigens are produced from genetic information by mechanisms used routinely by cells for protein production. These proteins have hydrophobic tail regions, which anchor them in the cell membrane. They also have glycosylated, hydrophilic regions that extend outward from the cell. This orients the protein for interaction with soluble extracellular proteins or with membrane proteins on other cells.

Major histocompatibility-encoded proteins are rapidly shed. As a result, histocompatibility proteins are not only present on cell surfaces but also in fluids surrounding cells. There is constant repopulation of the cell surface with histocompatibility proteins. The density of histocompatibility proteins on the cell surface can vary considerably. Density varies with the stage of cellular activation or differentiation, and is under the control of lymphokines. Macrophages and cells of the vascular endothelium increase their display of MHC-encoded proteins after contact with the lymphokine, gamma interferon. The increased display of histocompatibility proteins by these cells enhances their ability to participate in immune responses.

One striking characteristic of the MHC-encoded proteins is their high degree of polymorphism. Each of these proteins has as many as 20 or more different forms (or alleles) encoded at the same chromosomal site in different individuals. As each member of the species has genetic information for no more than two of these alleles, all other alleles at that site are foreign to that individual (Figure 11.7). The chance distribution of alleles determines the histocompatibility display of an individual.

There are several major regions in the MHC, each encoding a different type, or class, of protein. The Class I molecules are glycoprotein monomers with a molecular weight of approximately 44,000 daltons. Class I proteins have intracellular, intramembrane, and extracellular domains, and are always found complexed with an 11,000-dalton extracellular protein called *beta-2 microglobulin.* The role of beta-2 microglobulin may be to assist intracellular transport and subsequent cell surface display of Class I MHC proteins. Class I molecules are encoded in the

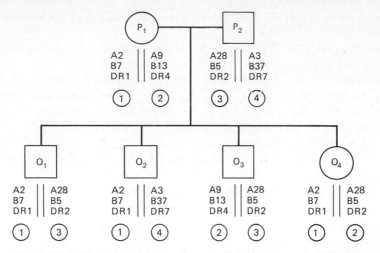

Figure 11.7 The reassortment of some of the histocompatibility genes. Each parent (P_1, P_2) has unique alleles at the various sites. The offspring (O_1, O_2, O_3 and O_4) have different combinations of the genes than their parents, a result of segregation of chromosomes during gamete formation and occasionally a recombination event during fertilization.

human MHC at three separate loci. Thus, cells from a given individual can display up to six different Class I proteins (two alleles at each locus) (Table 11.1). Three of these proteins (one allele for each locus) are contributed to individuals by each of their parents.

The Class II molecules are heterodimers composed of two noncovalently linked polypeptides; one is a 29,000-dalton glycoprotein, the other, a 34,000-dalton glycoprotein. Both polypeptides have intracellular, intramembrane, and extracellular domains. Neither polypeptide is found in association with beta-2 microglobulin. Class II molecules are encoded in the human MHC at three different loci (Table 11.1). Hence cells from a given individual can display up to six different Class II

Table 11.1   MHC-ENCODED PROTEINS

	Class I	Class II
Molecular weight	44,000 daltons	29,000 daltons
		34,000 daltons
Nature	β-2 microglobulin	Unknown
Human chromosonal loci	HLA-A	HLA-DR
	HLA-B	HLA-DP
	HLA-C	HLA-DQ
Function	Target structure for CTL and alloantibody	Induction of lymphokine secretion
Distribution	Most nucleated cells	Highly selective distribution

proteins. Again, three of these proteins are contributed by each of an individual's parents.

The Class III MHC-encoded proteins are complement components and will not be discussed further in this chapter (see Chapter 9).

All vertebrates studied to date possess an MHC. In the mouse, the MHC is found on the H-2 region of the seventeenth chromosome, and separate Class I proteins are encoded at the H-2K, H-2D, and H-2L loci. Additional Class II proteins are encoded at the H-2IA and H-2IE loci. In the human, the MHC is found on the HLA region of the sixth chromosome; separate Class I proteins are encoded at the HLA-A, HLA-B, and HLA-C loci. Additional Class II antigens are encoded at the HLA-DR, HLA-DP, and HLA-DQ loci.

Selected amino acid configurations on Class I MHC proteins serve as the primary target structures for alloantibody and for cytotoxic lymphocytes. Class I alloantigens are the primary antigenic stimuli for induction of cytotoxic lymphocytes. Class II alloantigens are efficient inducers of lymphokine production by helper lymphocytes. The observations leading to these conclusions were made on lymphocytes in mixed lymphocyte cultures. It is not clear whether this is how the system functions *in vivo*.

It is clear from experimental and clinical evidence that both *in vivo* and *in vitro* immune responses are strongest when there are incompatibilities in both Class I and Class II alloantigens. Allograft-rejection times are long, and mixed lymphocytic culture responses are suboptimal if the only incompatibilities are in one or the other of the major alloantigens. Long graft-rejection times and weak mixed lymphocytic culture responses also occur if the only incompatibility is in the minor histocompatibility antigens. Most minor histocompatibility antigens will not induce proliferation in primary mixed lymphocyte culture. Cells responding to minor histocompatibility antigens can only be detected in mixed lymphocyte cultures if the lymphocytes have been previously exposed to the same antigens *in vivo*. In general, the immune responses caused by minor histocompatibility antigens are thought to be analogous to, but weaker than, those caused by major histocompatibility antigens. Nonetheless, in the absence of immunosuppression, even the weaker histocompatibility antigens can eventually induce allograft rejection.

IMMUNOLOGIC MECHANISMS OF ALLOGRAFT REJECTION

A large number of immunologic events occur in mixed lymphocyte cultures: There is T-cell proliferation, reflecting the activation and clonal expansion of alloreactive helper and cytolytic T-cells. There is accumulation of lymphokines in the culture supernatant, and there is development of alloantigen-specific cytolytic activity. The immunologic events that occur in culture are thought to occur *in vivo* at a graft site and to be responsible for allograft rejection. This belief is currently the subject of considerable debate. The *in vitro* studies have focused almost exclusively on the behavior of T-lymphocytes; allograft rejection *in vivo*, however, is an extremely complex event that, although dependent on T-lymphocytes, is not exclusively a T-cell phenomenon. There is evidence that virtually every major immune effector mechanism participates in graft rejection. Antibody specific for the histocompatibility antigens accumulates in a graft. Antibody can mediate destruction by activating the complement cascade and by focusing the mechanism of antibody-dependent cellular cytotoxicity. A large fraction of the cells that infiltrate allografts are macrophages, and activated macrophages are mediators of antibody-dependent cellular cytotoxicity. Some lymphokines, such as lymphotoxin, can directly cause nonspecific tissue destruction. Tumor necrosis factor from activated macrophages also destroys cells. During rejection, the graft is thus subject to a variety of destructive mechanisms, all regulated by the products of activated T-lymphocytes.

CLINICAL STRATEGIES FOR AVOIDANCE OF GRAFT REJECTION

Treatments designed to prevent rejection of grafts must take into account the fact that rejection can occur by at least three dissimilar mechanisms. Hyperacute rejection mediated by antibodies is partially controlled by plasma pheresis, a process that selectively removes antibodies. To avoid hyperacute rejection, potential graft recipients are tested; those who have antibodies reactive with the graft are not transplanted. There are two primary strategies used to avoid acute allograft rejection: these are tissue matching and selective immunosuppression. Chronic rejection, a long-term effect of graft-reactive antibodies that presumably develops after transplantation, is untreatable.

Tissue Matching

Candidates for transplants are routinely screened for the presence of graft-reactive antibodies. These antibodies can develop after an earlier transplantation, after blood transfusion, or as a result of pregnancy. Serum samples from transplant candidates are tested for their ability to mediate complement-dependent lysis of lymphocytes obtained from the blood of the tissue donor. This test is the T-cell cross-match. Transplant candidates with no detectable donor-reactive antibodies have little risk of hyperacute rejection.

Hyperacute rejection can also occur when the graft donor and the recipient are of different ABO blood groups; ABO blood group antigens are important histocompatibility antigens as blood group antigens are present on vascular endothelium as well as on erythrocytes. Because of this, a primary criterion for transplantation is ABO blood group compatibility between a transplant candidate and the tissue donor.

To avoid acute rejection, attempts are made to match the histocompatibility proteins of the graft candidate with those of the tissue donor. Graft recipients also are immunosuppressed. In tissue matching, primary attention is given to the major histocompatibility proteins. Little effort is expended on attempts to match minor histocompatibility antigens. This is because there are so many of them that matching is virtually impossible, because immune responses to minor histocompatibility antigens are relatively weak, and because reactions to them are easily controlled by immunosuppression.

"Tissue typing" is the procedure used to determine the major histocompatibility antigens of donor and recipient. In this procedure, blood lymphocytes from the donor and the recipient are tested to determine if they can be lysed by antibodies and complement. A panel of antibodies, each antibody of which reacts with known HLA antigens, is used in this test. The antibodies are usually obtained from the sera of multiparous women. These sera contain high titers of complement-fixing antibodies specific for the major histocompatibility antigens of their children. The specificities of the antibodies in the sera are determined before it is used as a "typing serum." Antibodies are readily available to identify the proteins encoded by the HLA-A, HLA-B, HLA-C, and HLA-DR regions of the MHC, but antibodies that identify proteins encoded by the HLA-DP or HLA-DQ regions are rare. These latter proteins are usually identified by their ability to induce lymphocyte proliferation in mixed lymphocyte culture, a test that takes too long to be of practical use.

It is most often not possible to find a donor–recipient combination that is completely matched for all MHC-encoded antigens. Some matches are more important than others. For example, matching of HLA-DR is more important than matching of HLA-B, which is more important than matching of HLA-A, which is more important than matching of HLA-C.

Immunosuppression

Long-term graft survival in transplant recipients is largely a result of increased sophistication in the use of immunosuppressive agents. Without immunosuppression few, if any, allografts would survive, since it is virtually impossible to find a completely histocompatible donor–recipient combination; identical twins are the only exception. The importance of immunosuppression in graft acceptance is made apparent by the fact that with treatment with immunosuppressive drugs such as Cyclosporine, it is possible to perform successful transplants without regard for HLA matching.

A wide variety of immunosuppressive drugs and treatments have been evaluated in clinical transplantation studies. Many procedures, such as high-energy irradiation, which destroys all dividing cells, or thoracic duct drainage, which removes graft-reactive T-cells, are either too destructive or too complicated to be practical. Many drugs, such as cyclophosphamide, are similar to irradiation in that the negative effects of the treatment exceed the benefits. These treatments are often so immunosuppressive that they leave the patient susceptible to infection. Immunosuppressive drugs that improve graft acceptance with minimal undesirable side effects are azathioprine, prednisone, antilymphocyte globulin, and Cyclosporine.

Azathioprine is an analog of 6-mercaptopurine. It can be given orally. This drug competes for enzymes necessary for production of nucleic acids, and thus impairs synthesis of DNA and RNA. For this reason, rapidly dividing cells are most sensitive to azathioprine. Presumably, this drug is immunosuppressive because it interferes with the synthesis of lymphokines and with expansion of lymphocyte clones. Undesirable side effects of this drug include leukopenia, anemia, bone marrow depression, and hair loss.

Corticosteroids such as prednisone have wide-ranging physiologic effects, including immunosuppression. Prednisone or, more properly, its active metabolite, prednisolone, interferes both with lymphokine production by helper T-lymphocytes and with lymphocyte accumulation at a graft site. Prednisone is capable of reversing ongoing graft rejection. Undesirable side effects include avascular necrosis of bone, peptic ulceration, impairment of wound healing, and cataract formation.

Antilymphocyte globulin is a purified preparation of antibodies raised to lymphocytes. These antibodies interfere with immune responses by causing lymphocytes to be destroyed by complement-mediated lysis or by phagocytes of the reticuloendothelial system. These antibodies may also cause capping and shedding of surface proteins from lymphocytes, preventing antigen recognition. Since they are foreign proteins, patients eventually become sensitized to these antibodies and generate neutralizing antibodies, making therapy with antilymphocyte globulin or monoclonal antibodies ineffective.

Cyclosporine is a fungal metabolite. It has a relatively selective effect on helper T-lymphocytes. Cyclosporine blocks lymphokine production by helper T-lymphocytes. Cyclosporine thus interferes with all lymphokine-dependent immunologic mechanisms associated with allograft rejection. The disadvantage of Cyclosporine is that it does not stop immune responses once they have begun. Cyclosporine also has a number of undesirable side effects, including toxic effects on the kidneys and liver.

The various immunosuppressants operate by different mechanisms. In fact, therapy by combinations of these drugs is effective in controlling graft rejection.

Acceptance of allografts is facilitated by donor-specific blood transfusions. This procedure is only practical when tissues from a living donor are to be transplanted. Three transfusions of 200 cc of donor blood are given to the transplant candidate at biweekly intervals prior to transplantation. These transfusions can cause sensitization of the transplant candidate to histocompatibility antigens of the donor. The incidence of sensitization can be reduced by treating the transplant candidate with azathioprine during the three-week period when the transfusions are being given. When the transfusion process is complete, the lymphocytes of the transplant candidate are tested for reaction with the lymphocytes of the donor. If no reaction occurs, the candidate is transplanted with the donor tissue.

The effect of this procedure is to minimize the immune reactivity of the recipient to the donor's alloantigens. Reduced donor-reactivity makes immunosuppression easier and posttransplant clinical complications less frequent and more manageable. The reasons why this procedure works are unclear. It has been suggested that the transfusions stimulate production of a population of suppressive T-cells that, in turn, dampen immune responses to donor alloantigens after transplantation. It has also been suggested that the transfusions stimulate the production of antibodies that recognize the alloantigen binding structures on alloantibodies and on T-lymphocytes. These antiidiotypic antibodies would be circulating by the time of transplantation and would interfere with the ability of the immune system to respond to the alloantigens of the graft.

SPECIAL CONSIDERATIONS: RETRANSPLANTS

The immunologic events associated with retransplantation are not the same as events associated with primary transplantation. The most obvious difference is the accelerated rate and increased intensity with which graft rejection proceeds, even with immunosuppressant treatments that are highly effective against primary rejection. Lymphocytes from unsuccessfully transplanted individuals will proliferate and generate cytolytic activity in culture much more rapidly than naive lymphocytes. This second set response, like all secondary immunologic responses, is the result of the presence of large numbers of graft-reactive lymphocytes available to the immune system upon secondary contact with the alloantigens. The minor histocompatibility antigens, which are numerous but appear to contribute relatively little to primary acute rejection responses following the stimulation of the first encounter, may also make a significant contribution to the immune response to the secondary transplant.

The various immunosuppressive drugs are less effective at interfering with rejection of second transplants, perhaps due to their great intensity and rapid development. The net effect is that retransplants are rejected more often and more rapidly than primary transplants.

SPECIAL CONSIDERATIONS: TRANSPLANTATION OF SPECIFIC TISSUES

Most of the information available on allograft rejection is derived from studies of the most commonly transplanted organ, the kidney. Other organs and tissues behave differently.

Some tissues, such as corneas, are poorly vascularized and have little contact with the immune system; also, there are few technical complications with corneal transplants. For these reasons, corneal transplants are highly successful.

The most serious impediment to liver transplantation is the technical complexity of the surgical procedure, rather than control of subsequent rejection. Indeed, livers are not easily rejected. The large liver mass may overwhelm or absorb the immune responses directed at it. Nonetheless, liver transplant recipients must be immunosuppressed if rejection is to be avoided.

Transplantation of the pancreas has not been particularly successful. The major impediment to transplantation of the pancreas is the surgical procedure. For anatomic reasons, the pancreas must be transplanted with a segment of the donor gut. Infection of the immunosuppressed transplant recipient with microorganisms of the gut occurs frequently.

Heart transplantation is complicated by several factors. Hearts must be obtained from donors who are brain dead but whose hearts are still living. In addition, the organ must be rapidly transferred from donor to recipient. Heart transplant candidates are usually in poor health and it is unusually difficult to diagnose rejection before it becomes uncontrollable. The relative technical ease of the surgery and the efficiency of the immunosuppressive strategies now available have made cardiac transplantation a widely accepted procedure, however.

Skin transplantation is one of the least successful tissue transplant procedures. The reasons for this are unclear. The graft procedure is not technically demanding, and autografts are usually retained. The failure of foreign skin grafts to be accepted may result from the existence of an usually potent, skin-specific immune response or a unique system of histocompatibility antigens. The need for rapid vascularization of skin and the effect of immunosuppressants on the process of vascularization may also limit skin graft survival.

Bone marrow transplantation, which has enormous clinical potential, is still under development and has been increasingly successful. Bone marrow transplantation is most successful when the donor and recipient are completely histocompatible. Bone marrow transplantation is an immunologically unique procedure and has a variety of correspondingly unique complications. For this technically simple transplant procedure, bone marrow is aspirated by needle from the pelvis or sternum of the graft donor and transfused into a recipient who has been made immunodeficient by lethal irradiation or chemical preconditioning. Complications arise when immunocompetent lymphoid cells in the donor bone marrow recognize the foreign histocompatibility antigens of the immunocompromised recipient and initiate a rejection response, resulting in a potentially fatal attack on the host by the graft. Bone marrow recipients are also often severely immunocompromised and are thus susceptible to opportunistic pathogens.

SUMMARY

When a foreign tissue or organ is transplanted into a histoin compatible recipient, a number of immunologic events occur. There are inflammatory responses in the tissues damaged by the surgical procedure, and there is damage caused by the handling of the graft. The inflammatory response causes the damaged tissues to be infiltrated by a variety of inflammatory cells, including macrophages and T-lymphocytes.

At the same time, foreign cells and proteins escape from the transplanted tissues and are trapped by the lymph nodes along the lymph ducts draining the area. In the lymph nodes, T-cells respond to the foreign histocompatibility antigens and expand into populations of graft-reactive T-lymphocytes. These graft-reactive lymphocytes, which can secrete lymphokines and mediate cytolysis, leave the lymph nodes and travel through the blood to the graft site, where they enhance the local inflammatory response and participate in tissue destruction.

The activated T-lymphocytes that accumulate at the graft site participate in graft destruction by lysing graft cells. They, and other graft-reactive T-lymphocytes, secrete lymphokines that potentiate immunologic events at the graft site. Some lymphokines increase graft antigenicity by increasing the expression of MHC-encoded proteins. Other lymphokines directly kill graft tissues. Still others mobilize and orchestrate the graft-reactive immune responses of antibodies and macrophages.

There are a variety of ways for immunosuppressants to interfere with graft rejection. Many immunosuppressants destroy dividing cells, preventing the formation of clones of lymphocytes capable of rejecting the graft. Other immunosuppressants interfere with the basic signaling systems used by lymphocytes to potentiate immune responses at a graft site. In addition to these effects, some immunosuppressants interfere with the mechanisms by which lymphocytes are accumulated at the graft site. If immunosuppressants are used effectively, most primary acute allograft rejection can be avoided. However, there is a need for new immunosuppressive strategies that are effective against chronic graft rejection and against acute graft rejection in retransplanted patients. In general, much has been learned about the phenomenon of graft rejection, and therapeutic strategies have been developed to control it to some degree. Nevertheless, there is still much to be learned about the immunology of transplantation.

SUGGESTIONS FOR FURTHER READING

R. Calne. The Development of Immunosuppression in Organ Transplantation. In *Progress in Transplantation, Vol. 1*, P. Morris and N. Tilney, *eds.* Churchill Livingstone, New York, 1984.

C. Dinarello and J. Mier. "Lymphokines." New England Journal of Medicine *315:*940, 1987.

R. Flavell, H. Allen, L. Burkly, D. Sherman, G. Waneck, and G. Widera. "Molecular biology of the H-2 histocompatibility complex." Science *233:*437, 1986.

P. Halloran, A. Wadgmar, and P. Autenreid. "The regulation of expression of major histocompatibility complex products." Transplant. *41:*413, 1986.

P. Henkart. "Mechanism of lymphocyte-mediated cytotoxicity." Ann. Rev. Immunol. *3:*31, 1985.

C. Kirkpatrick. "Transplantation immunology." Journal of the American Medical Association, *258:*2993, 1987.

D. Mason. "Effector mechanisms of allograft rejection." Ann. Rev. Immunol. *4:*119, 1986.

M. Mickey. HLA Effects. In *Clinical Transplants 1987*, P. Terasaki, *ed.* UCLA Tissue Typing Laboratory, Los Angeles, 1987.

D. Steinmuller. "Tissue specific and tissue restricted histocompatibility antigens." Immunol. Today *5:*234, 1984.

N. Tilney, J. Kupiec-Weglinski, C. Heidecke, P. Leary, and T. Strom. "Mechanisms of rejection and prolongation of vascularized organ allografts." Immunol. Rev. *77:*185, 1983.

A. Weiss, J. Imboden, K. Hardy, B. Manger, C. Terhorst, and J. Stobo. "The role of the T3/antigen receptor complex in T Cell activation." Ann. Rev. Immunol. *4:*593, 1986.

Chapter 12

Pathogenicity and Virulence

LOLA WINTER

Department of Microbiology, Immunology and Parasitology
New York State College of Veterinary Medicine
Cornell University

INTRODUCTION

Any microorganism that is able to infect a host and produce disease is a pathogen. Microorganisms vary in their ability to produce disease. Some organisms, such as *Vibrio cholerae*, the agent of cholera, or *Yersinia pestis*, the cause of plague, are able to produce disease in normal, healthy hosts. These bacteria are thus overt pathogens and must be distinguished from those organisms that function as opportunists and produce disease only when a break in the host's normal defense mechanisms enables them to become established. Included in this latter group of opportunists are members of the normal flora, such as *Escherichia coli, Staphylococcus aureus*, and certain fungi, such as *Candida albicans*, as well as some free-living bacteria, such as *Pseudomonas aeruginosa* and *Legionella pneumophila*.

Whether disease ensues as a result of a host's encounter with a pathogen is dependent both upon the condition of the host and the particular characteristics of the microorganism. Those characteristics that contribute to the ability of a microorganism to produce disease are referred to as *virulence factors*. Most bacterial pathogens have many such factors and, although some have been identified, it is still not known in all cases precisely how each factor functions in the production of disease. It is known, for example, that enterotoxigenic *E. coli* adhere to the lining of the small intestine and produce a potent enterotoxin that is absorbed by the intestinal epithelial cells. This toxin produces an increase in the concentration of intracellular cAMP, which results in an increase in secretion of electrolytes into the intestinal lumen and an outpouring of water; the end result is diarrhea. Both the enterotoxin and the ability to adhere are coded for by plasmids carried by the bacterial cell. If the bacterium is cured only of the adherence plasmid, it cannot produce disease, even though enterotoxin is still produced. Unable to adhere, this organism can no longer maintain itself in the intestinal tract. The small amount of enterotoxin produced in transit may be insufficient to do harm or may be inactivated by intestinal secretions. If cured only of the plasmid coding for enterotoxin, the *E. coli* adheres but, again, no diarrhea results because the toxin is not produced. The pathogenesis of this particular disease syndrome is thus very well understood. By contrast, *S. aureus* produces many virulence factors and causes many different disease syndromes, but as yet there is a very incomplete understanding of how each factor functions in pathogenicity. Our understanding of virulence factors of other pathogens ranges between these two extremes. This chapter will present information about virulence factors, grouping them by mode of action and nature.

FACTORS MEDIATING ADHESION

Adhesins

Infections are initiated on the surfaces of the mucous membranes or through breaks in the skin. Most infections actually begin on the mucous membranes of the respiratory, gastrointestinal, or urogenital tracts. In these environments, the potential pathogen must first adhere to the host cell. Adherence prevents the microorganism from being flushed away in mucus secretions and renders it less susceptible to the effects of enzymes and secretory IgA. If disease is to result from the effects of a toxin, such as that of enterotoxigenic *E. coli,* close adherence of the bacterium assures that the toxin will be delivered in high concentrations directly to the host cell. If the organism is invasive, as is *Salmonella typhi,* adherence must occur before penetration of host cells is possible.

The observation that some bacteria affect particular hosts and specifically attach only to certain cells within these hosts suggests that adherence is a selective process. There are indeed specific structural moieties that function in adherence. Morphologically distinct structures or, in some cases, single molecules on the surfaces of bacteria that enable the organisms to adhere to host cells are referred to as *adhesins.* These adhesins bind specifically, much like a key in a lock, to receptors on the host cell surface.

Structural adhesins of Gram-positive organisms are known as *fibrillae.* An example would be the hairy surface appendages composed of lipoteichoic acid and M protein that have been demonstrated and identified in several streptococcal species (Figure 12.1). Work done with group A streptococci has further identified the lipid moiety of this complex as the adhesive molecule. The structural adhesins

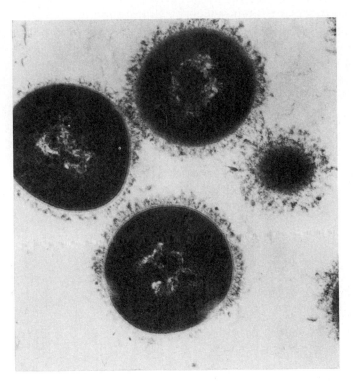

Figure 12.1 Electron micrograph of group G streptococci showing abundant surface fibrillae (magnification: 60,000×). (*Source:* A. L. Bisno, *Infection* and *Immunity 55:*753–757, 1987.)

of Gram-negative orgaisms are called *fimbriae.* They are tubular filaments, from 7.5 to 10 nm in diameter, and are made up of repeating protein subunits. Fimbriae have been identified in many different species, including *E. coli, P. aeruginosa, Bordetella pertussis, Neisseria gonorrhoeae, Neisseria meningitidis,* and *Hemophilus influenzae* (Figure 12.2). *Mycoplasma pneumoniae* attaches firmly to host cells of the respiratory epithelium via a surface protein located on a specialized terminal structure. Outer membrane proteins (*N. gonorrhoeae*), flagella (*Campylobacter jejuni*), lipopolysaccharide (*Shigella flexneri*), and the glycocalyx (*P. aeruginosa*) have also been identified as having roles in adherence.

There are thus many different factors that can function as bacterial adhesins. Moreover, it is now realized that many bacteria make use of not just one but several of these factors. In addition, some microorganisms such as *N. gonorrhoeae* have the genetic ability to alter the molecular composition of a particular adhesin and also to switch the type of adhesin expressed.

The expression of fimbriae is under the control of bacterial genes located either on the chromosome or on a plasmid. These genes can undergo "phase variations" that result in alterations in fimbrial states. The plasmids containing these genes can also be lost as well as acquired.

Most strains of *N. gonorrhoeae* can adhere both by fimbriae and by outer membrane proteins. Strain 9 of this species has been shown to express four different isogenic fimbrial variants simultaneously. Uropathogenic *E. coli,* which adhere to the epithelial cells of the urinary tract by means of P fimbriae, also have the ability

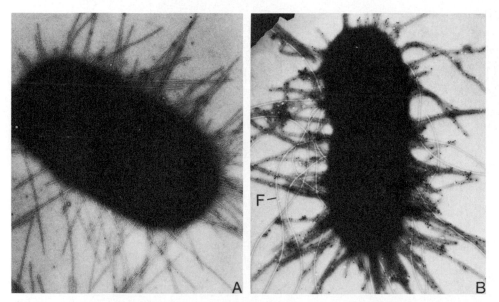

Figure 12.2 Electron micrograph of stained *Escherichia coli* showing (A) fimbriae and (B) fimbriae and flagella. Fimbriae are the structural adhesions of Gram-negative bacteria. Flagella (F) are the organs of motility of bacteria. (*Source:* S. Knutton *et al., Infection and Immunity 55:*86–92, 1987.)

to adhere by means of outer surface molecules. Multiple adhesin factors have also been demonstrated in other species, including *V. cholerae* and *C. jejuni.* Bacteria that are able to alter their adhesins may be better able to evade the defense mechanisms of the host.

The importance of adhesins as virulence factors has been demonstrated by comparing the virulence of mutants that have lost the ability to express an adhesin to that of the parent strain. Such comparisons, made with *E. coli, N. gonorrhoeae,* and *H. influenzae,* for example, have confirmed the role of adhesins in virulence. In addition, treatment with antibodies specific for the adhesin or treatment of the bacterial cell with enzymes to remove the adhesin prevent binding of the microorganism to the host cell, reducing the organism's infectivity.

Although it is generally held that adherence is a prerequisite for infection and the production of disease, there are some situations in which this characteristic is detrimental to the microorganism. Study of urinary tract infections with *Proteus* in rats revealed that, while the presence of fimbriae was required for establishment of infection in the urinary tract, these same fimbriae enhanced phagocytosis of the organism when it entered the bloodstream. Those organisms that can undergo phase variation to suppress adhesins therefore have a distinct survival advantage in systemic infections.

Adherence is a complex process involving specific components not only of the microbial cell but also of the host cell to which the adhesins bind. *In vitro* work with cell and organ cultures has helped to identify some of the receptors. This is done by treating cells with various enzymes or adhesin analogs and then testing for adherence. Thus, host receptors for *Streptococcus pyogenes* have been identified as glycoproteins, a sialoglycoprotein has been identified as the receptor for *M. pneumoniae,* and a glycolipid receptor binds *E. coli* through the colonizing factor antigens I and II (CFAI and CFAII).

Work with viruses has shown that many receptors that have an important role in normal biological functions of the host serve as viral receptors. There is evidence, for example, that a C3b receptor on phagocytes may serve as the receptor for the Epstein-Barr virus. The CD4 glycoprotein molecule present on T-lymphocytes is required for recognition of foreign antigens but has also been shown to be a receptor for the human immunodeficiency virus, the etiological agent of acquired immunodeficiency syndrome (AIDS). Recent work suggests that host cell receptors for acetylcholine may bind rabies virus.

The classical work with enterotoxigenic *E. coli* in swine has shown that host receptors are under genetic control. *E. coli* expressing the K88 antigen, a fimbrial protein, adhere to the intestinal epithelial cells of swine, whereas *E. coli* expressing K99 antigen adhere only to bovine cells. The observation that some swine were resistant to infection by *E. coli*–K88 suggested the possibility of breeding for resistance. The resistant swine were shown to lack the K88 receptor, which is coded for by an autosomal dominant gene. Among humans, *E. coli*–CFAI and –CFAII are the most frequent agents of urinary tract infections in females. Certain individuals are more susceptible than others to these infections, as is indicated by the recurrent nature of their infections. It has been suggested that these strains of *E. coli* bind more readily to the urogenital epithelial cells of susceptible women. It is known that CFAI and CFAII of *E. coli* bind to glycolipid receptors on the host cell; an increased concentration of these receptors may thus account for the higher incidence of infection in certain women.

In addition to naturally occurring receptors, new receptors may be expressed on host cells under certain conditions. For example, an increase of adherence of *S. aureus* to cells that are infected with influenza A virus has been demonstrated. Group B streptococci have also been shown to adhere preferentially to virus-infected cells. Some bacteria release enzymes that break down host tissue, thereby exposing new receptor sites that aid in their spread. *P. aeruginosa* produces a protease that breaks down host fibronectin, a high molecular weight glycoprotein present in the extracellular matrix and on the surfaces of many cells. This pseudomonad cannot adhere to fibronectin but can adhere to the cell surfaces exposed after its removal.

ANTIPHAGOCYTIC FACTORS

Adherence to a host cell is by no means the end of the microorganism's struggle to establish itself in the host. The potential pathogen must withstand attack by the phagocytic cells of the host: the polymorphonuclear leukocytes and the macrophages whose job it is to rid the body of invading organisms by ingesting and destroying them. There are several ways by which bacteria thwart this process.

Capsules

Many bacterial cells are surrounded by a gelatinous layer referred to as a *capsule*. Most capsules are polysaccharide in nature, but those of the genus *Bacillus* are composed of polypeptide. Capsules have been demonstrated by both direct and indirect staining techniques. Their presence has also been confirmed by chemical and antigenic analyses. Encapsulation is now known to play a very important role in microbial survival.

Extracellular parasites such as *Streptococcus pneumoniae* or *H. influenzae*, for example, can colonize the mucosal surfaces of the upper respiratory tract. Virulent strains, taking advantage of a compromised host, can invade the lower respiratory tract and other organ systems and produce severe disease. Such virulent strains have been shown to possess polysaccharide capsules that surround the bacterial cell and function to prevent phagocytosis.

That encapsulation does enhance virulence has clearly been shown in work with *S. pneumoniae* that demonstrated that unencapsulated, isogenic variants had little ability to cause disease. Further work with these bacteria suggests that not only the presence and the size of the capsule but also its composition determines virulence. Investigations with group B streptococci, major neonatal pathogens, have revealed that the sialic acid component of the capsule has a high affinity for proteins that inhibit the activation of complement by the alternate pathway. The K1 capsule of *E. coli* as well as the type B capsule of *N. meningitidis* are composed of homopolymers of sialic acid that function in an identical manner. Capsules also serve to block access of complement to the microbial cell wall, where surface components of both Gram-negative and Gram-positive bacteria are capable of activating complement in the absence of antibody. Although capsules do increase the surface charge of bacterial cells and thereby render them more repulsive to phagocytes, it is believed that the more important function of the capsule is to prevent the triggering of the alternate (antibody-independent) pathway of complement activation.

Encapsulation, however, does not always serve to benefit the invading microorganism. Although capsules may protect bacteria that are invading the blood stream, their presence on a cell may also block the function of adhesins and thereby hinder attachment to mucous membranes. It has been shown, for example, that the hyaluronic acid capsule of *S. pyogenes* hinders both the attachment of the phagocytes to the bacterial cells and also the adherence of the bacteria to the oral epithelial cells of the host. Encapsulation has also been shown to diminish the ability of *S. pneumoniae* to adhere to pharyngeal epithelial cells.

As was emphasized previously, the ability of an organism to modulate the expression of adhesins can influence its ability to survive in the host. The ability to shed or express capsules as situations change is also an important factor for microbial survival.

A glycocalyx, or exopolysaccharide slime layer, is characteristic of some bacteria when they are growing in colonies under certain environmental conditions. These structures are similar to capsules but have a less ordered morphology. The slime layer of *P. aeruginosa* has been identified as a glycolipoprotein, a separate entity from the lipopolysaccharide of the cell wall. The production of slime enables the bacterial cells to adhere to the host cells and to each other, resulting in the formation of adherent microcolonies. These slime-covered microcolonies are better able to withstand the effects of antibodies and complement than are microcolonies without a slime layer. If the microbes do not react with antibody and complement, they are less susceptible to phagocytosis than are microbes to which antibody and complement are bonded. Penetration of antibiotics is also reduced by microcolony formation; cells in the center of a colony may thus be protected from the antimicrobial effect of antibiotics. The observation that mucoid strains of *P. aeruginosa* are commonly isolated from hosts with abnormal microbial clearance systems but with a properly functioning immune system (for example, humans with cystic fibrosis), whereas nonmucoid strains are found in immune-compromised hosts (burn patients), has suggested that microcolony growth could be an adaptation to the environmental pressure of a functioning immune system.

Viridans streptococci, which are often found in vegetative cardiac lesions, are protected by dextran glycocalyces (Figure 12.3). This has been demonstrated by electron microscopy and offers a reasonable explanation for the poor clinical response of such patients to antibiotic therapy despite the fact that the infections are caused by antibiotic-sensitive strains of the microbe. Glycocalyces have also been demonstrated on *S. aureus.* Infections with this organism are a particular problem in patients with implanted prostheses and indwelling catheters. The K30 exopolysaccharide of *E. coli* also contributes to the formation of microcolonies and mediates adhesion of this microbe to the epithelial cells of the small intestine.

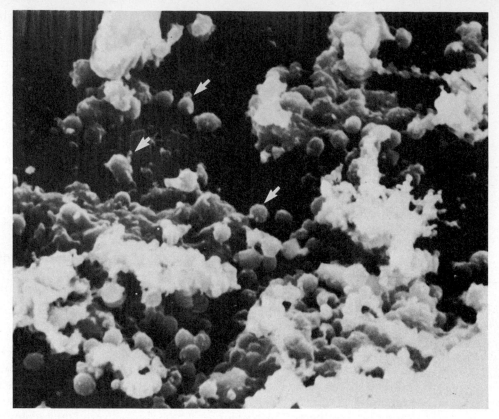

Figure 12.3 SEM showing staphylococci enveloped in their glycocalyx. These bacteria growing on the plastic surface of a cardiac pacemaker persisted in spite of aggressive antibiotic therapy. (*Source:* J. W. Costertonaud and J. J. Marrie, *Med. Micro.*, Vol. 3, C.S.F. Easmon, ed., Academic Press, London, 1983.)

M Protein

Reference has already been made to the lipoteichoic acid–M protein complex present on the surface of group A streptococci. It has been shown that whereas the lipoteichoic acid complex functions in adherence, the M protein functions to impede phagocytosis by binding fibrinogen to the bacterial cell wall and thus masking the microbial cell's receptors for complement. Antibodies against the M protein prevent the binding of fibrinogen and permit phagocytosis to take place.

Cytotoxin and Impairment of Chemotaxis

Bacteria make use of mechanisms other than capsule formation to prevent phagocytosis. Many organisms secrete exotoxins that either interfere with chemotaxis (the attraction of phagocytes to the site of the invading microbe) or kill the phagocyte.

P. aeruginosa secretes a protein that not only impairs chemotaxis but inhibits lysosomal fusion once phagocytosis has occurred. Several strains of this bacterium also produce a leukocidin, a protein that damages the cell membrane of white blood cells, resulting in leakage of essential nutrients and cell death. Exotoxin A, produced by most clinical isolates of *P. aeruginosa,* is similar in action to diphtheria toxin and is lethal to human macrophages.

The staphylococci, more commonly the virulent strains, produce several cytotoxins that act on a variety of cells. The staphylococcal hemolysins damage both erythrocytes and leukocytes, whereas the leukocidin is cytotoxic only for white blood cells. Although there is evidence that the hemolysin can function to impair both chemotaxis and subsequent lysosomal degranulation, the actual importance of these toxins in production of disease is not yet clearly defined. However, the production of the *E. coli* hemolysin, which is cytotoxic for leukocytes, correlates well with the virulence of the strain.

Group A streptococci produce two lysins, streptolysins S and O, which are cytotoxic for leukocytes, erythrocytes, and macrophages. These toxins cause damage to cell membranes, resulting in death of the cell.

SURVIVAL WITHIN THE PHAGOCYTE

In contrast to those organisms that have evolved means of preventing phagocytosis are those that have developed resistance to the killing mechanisms used by the phagocytes and as a consequence are able to survive and multiply within the phagocytes.

The ingestion of a microorganism by a phagocyte results in the formation of a phagosome. This event triggers the respiratory burst and the fusion of the phagosome with the lysosomes: the two microbicidal systems of the phagocyte. Any organism that has the ability to interfere with either of these two processes can therefore enhance its chances of intracellular survival.

Interference with the Oxidative Burst

Reactive oxygen radicals and other oxidizing agents resulting from the oxidative burst that occurs at the time of phagocytosis are contained within the phagosome. These substances, such as superoxide and hydrogen peroxide, are lethal to most bacteria. That the respiratory burst is important in the destruction of microorganisms intracellularly has been demonstrated both by observing the results of bacterial infections in persons lacking the ability to generate these substances and also by studying the bacteria that have evolved means of surviving within the phagosome.

Persons suffering from chronic granulomatous disease have an increased incidence of infection with staphylococci, aerobic Gram-negative rods, and fungi, all of which are catalase-positive. These individuals do not have a similarly high incidence of infection with catalase-negative organisms. The phagocytes of such patients have been found to have a poor ability to generate a respiratory burst; their phagosomes therefore are deficient in hydrogen peroxide and in products such as superoxide derived from hydrogen peroxide. If catalase is produced by the ingested microorganisms, the small amount of hydrogen peroxide produced is broken down and the already weak oxygen-mediated killing system fails.

L. pneumophila, the agent of Legionnaires' disease, is an opportunistic intracellular parasite that survives and multiplies within macrophages. There is evidence that these bacteria produce a toxin that inhibits the oxidative burst. Virulent strains of *Listeria monocytogenes* (an agent of infant meningitis) produce the enzyme superoxide dismutase, which neutralizes the oxygen radicals and contributes to the intracellular survival of bacteria. How virulent strains of *Salmonella typhi* suppress the oxidative burst is less clearly understood at the present time.

Prevention of Fusion and Degranulation

Work with the chlamydiae and *L. pneumophila* suggests that a component of the cell wall of these organisms can modify the phagosomal membrane and prevent fusion of the lysosomes with the phagosome. Chlamydiae that are killed by heating or treated with specific antibody are unable to prevent fusion, but envelopes of the chlamydial elementary bodies function as well as the viable chlamydiae in the prevention of fusion. Recent work has identified the adenylcyclase of *B. pertussis* as a potent inhibitor of degranulation. This enzyme is released from the bacterial cell and, when picked up by the phagocytic cell, stimulates an increase in cAMP, which inhibits degranulation. Work with mutants lacking the ability to produce this enzyme has demonstrated its importance in virulence. The production of adenine and guanosine monophosphate by virulent strains of *B. abortus* has also been shown to inhibit degranulation and to enhance the intracellular survival of these bacteria. Other parasites known to prevent phagolysosomal fusion include *Histoplasma capsulatum, Toxoplasma gondii,* influenza A virus, and *N. gonorrhoeae.*

Resistance to Lysosomal Enzymes

Some organisms that are unable to prevent fusion nevertheless can multiply within the phagolysosome because they are resistant to the effects of lysosomal enzymes. In the case of *Mycobacterium lepraemurium,* resistance is believed to be due to a capsular polysaccharide, whereas in *Salmonella typhimurium* the intact lipopolysaccharide is regarded as the resistance factor. The resistance of *Mycobacterium tuberculosis* has been attributed to a mycoside. Work with *Leishmania* has suggested that several factors may be involved: In addition to possessing a cell surface resistant to lysosomal enzymes, these organisms have been shown to release specific molecules that inhibit enzymatic activity. The alkaline environment resulting from the protease activity of the leishmanias can also contribute to a depression of activity of lysosomal enzymes because these enzymes require a low pH for proper function.

Escape from the Phagosome

Some microorganisms make use of yet another means of thwarting the phagocyte: They escape from the phagosome into the cytoplasm of the host cell before fusion occurs. The rickettsiae are believed to escape by an effect of phospholipase A on the phagosomal membrane, although it is not yet clear whether the enzyme is of microbial or host cell origin. Specific antibody to the parasite can prevent this effect and permit normal phagolysosomal fusion to occur. *Trypanosoma cruzi* has also been shown to escape from the phagosome. It actively penetrates the phagosome membrane.

SIDEROPHORES AND IRON ACQUISITION

Free ionic iron is present in the body fluids of animals, but only in very low concentrations. Most of the iron is either sequestered inside host cells, in association with functional molecules such as hemoglobin or myoglobin, or captured extracellularly by the glycoproteins lactoferrin and transferrin, which have a high iron-binding affinity. Lactoferrin is found primarily in mucosal secretions and milk, whereas transferrin is found mainly in blood and lymph. In response to a microbial infection, the host reduces the amount of iron bound to transferrin by transferring it to iron stores. Bacteria, however, require iron for their metabolism; the survival of the invading microorganism therefore depends upon its ability to scavenge iron from its environment.

Many bacteria produce *siderophores,* low molecular weight compounds that can acquire iron from the host's iron-binding proteins. This ability to scavenge iron has been demonstrated in many species and has been shown to enhance the virulence of invading bacteria.

Experiments have shown that virulence is greatly diminished in certain mutants that have lost the ability to obtain iron. Early work with *Y. pestis* showed that even 10^8 cells of a mutant that had lost the ability to acquire iron were not lethal for test animals, whereas as few as 100 cells of the parent strain killed the host.

Salmonella, E. coli, and *Klebsiella* produce *enterochelin,* an iron-chelating agent that can obtain iron from transferrin. This compound is only produced when iron concentrations are very low. It has been demonstrated that the virulence of an enterochelin-defective mutant of *S. typhi* can be increased 600-fold by the addition of enterochelin to a suspension of the organism prior to its injection into test animals. *Pyoverdin,* the siderophore of *P. aeruginosa,* has also been shown to stimulate the growth of this bacterium *in vivo.*

Some bacteria that apparently do not produce their own siderophores have specific surface receptors that enable them to make use of the chelators produced by other species. This has been observed in the campylobacters, shigellae, and some salmonellae. Pathogenic *Neisseria* are also able to obtain iron from iron-binding proteins, but the mechanism for this is not yet known.

Although most species of bacteria obtain iron from the host's glycoprotein storage molecules, there is evidence that some are able to acquire it from hemin. *Y. pestis* has already been mentioned. *E. coli* is another example: The hemolysin of *E. coli* lyses red blood cells, thus releasing heme that stimulates the growth of bacteria. Iron obtained by this method can permit development of fatal infections in individuals who have free blood in the abdominal cavity.

ENDOTOXIN

Patients suffering from Gram-negative septicemias show a variety of effects, including fever, hypoglycemia, intravascular coagulation, and shock. It has been known for many years that these signs are referable to the endotoxin common to all Gram-negative cells. Endotoxin has been identified as a component of the bacterial cell envelope and is composed of a complex of lipopolysaccharide with outer membrane proteins. The lipopolysaccharide is unique to Gram-negative bacteria. It is composed of three basic units: a lipid A molecule located in the hydrophobic zone of the outer membrane, an oligosaccharide core, and the O-polysaccharide side-chains that project from the cell surface. Results obtained with mutants defective in various phases of lipopolysaccharide synthesis as well as by chemical dissociation of the molecule have established that most of the toxic effects of endotoxins are due to the lipid A component of the lipopolysaccharide.

Most work to date on the characterization of lipopolysaccharide has been performed with *E. coli* and *Salmonella.* In these bacteria, O-polysaccharides are composed of repeating oligosaccharide units that differ in chemical composition among strains, thus accounting for the diversity of O serotypes. Virulent strains invariably possess O-polysaccharide. This holds true for bacteria of most other Gram-negative genera, but there are exceptions, such as *N. gonorrhoeae, Brucella ovis,* and *Brucella canis,* in which virulent strains lack O-polysaccharide.

The length and composition of the O-polysaccharide has been shown in some species to influence virulence. For example, in some *Salmonella* strains, the long O-polysaccharide chains projecting from the bacterial cell function as steric barriers to the bactericidal effects of complement. Complement is activated by lipopolysaccharide by the alternate pathway, and the macromolecular attack complex is deposited on the O-polysaccharide. The complex, however, is unable to insert into the lipid bilayer of the outer membrane of the *Salmonella* strains with the long O-polysaccharide chains and therefore cannot produce a lesion and allow access of other complement components to the cytoplasmic membrane. In a similar fashion, the long polysaccharide chains sterically hinder the attachment of antibodies, thereby blocking the activation of complement by the classical pathway. Some recent work suggests that certain sugars (2–6 dideoxyhexoses) in O-polysaccharides can prevent triggering of the alternate pathway of complement activation and that the presence of these sugars therefore constitutes an antiphagocytic mechanism.

Lipopolysaccharide also has a number of effects on neutrophil function. Endotoxin has been shown to bind via the lipid A moiety to the surface of neutrophils, resulting in increased adherence and aggregation of the cells. Exposure of neutrophils to lipopolysaccharide causes a decrease in chemotactic responsiveness as well as a decrease in the random migration of neutrophils. Finally, there is some indication that lipopolysaccharide can alter the metabolic and bactericidal properties of neutrophils.

ENZYMES AND EXOTOXINS

Enzymes

The presence of a microorganism in the host evokes an inflammatory response, resulting in a certain amount of tissue damage. In most cases this is limited, and a small price to pay for the elimination of a potentially harmful invader. Abnormalities in the host response can, of course, lead to more extensive tissue destruction, as can prolonged inflammation resulting from failure to eliminate the parasite. In addition, some bacteria have the ability to produce enzymes that can directly damage host tissue. The proteases of *P. aeruginosa* break down the fibrin and elastin connective tissue between cells, thus enabling the bacteria to spread more readily through the tissue and, at the same time, releasing nutrients that enhance bacterial growth. These same enzymes have been shown to inactivate complement and to cleave IgG.

Bacteria of several different species produce proteases that specifically cleave IgA, the immunoglobulin isotype most important in protection of mucosal surfaces. The enzymes act upon the hinge region of IgA, splitting the molecule into three fragments and thus separating the two Fab fragments, which combine with antigens, from the effector sites on the third (Fc) fragment. As a result of this cleavage, the function of the IgA molecule is greatly diminished. Such enzymes have been identified in *N. gonorrhoeae, N. meningitidis, H. influenzae, S. pneumoniae, Streptococcus sanguis,* and *Bacteroides* and are believed to contribute to the virulence of these organisms. However, these proteases have also been isolated from the nonpathogenic microbes constituting part of the normal flora.

Both virulent streptococci and staphylococci produce kinases that enhance the spread of the microbe by dissolving fibrin clots and inhibiting the clotting of plasma. Hyaluronidase, also associated with virulence in both streptococci and staphylococci, enhances dissemination of the infecting microorganism by breaking down the intercellular mucopolysaccharide hyaluronic acid that "cements" cells together. Virulent strains of staphylococci also produce coagulase, which causes the deposition of fibrin around the invading cocci and thus protects them from the phagocytes.

Collagenase produced by *Clostridium perfringens,* an agent of gas gangrene, produces breakdown of collagen in connective tissue. This results in the destruction of the muscle tissue and enhances the spread of the bacteria. This microbe also produces other powerful enzymes that contribute to its virulence.

Although most bacteria that cause disease produce enzymes that damage host tissue, it is not yet known how each functions in virulence.

Exotoxins

Exotoxins, which are proteins secreted by certain bacteria, are the most potent poisons known. It has recently been shown that most of these toxins are composed of two subunits: Fragment B, the carrier, binds to the host cell receptor and enables fragment A, the toxic or enzymatic unit, to enter the cell. The production of these highly specific toxins is under the control of genes carried on plasmids or by prophages. Exotoxins can be converted into toxoids, which are proteins that have lost their enzymatic activity but are still active antigenically. Treatment with formalin is a common way to convert a toxin to a toxoid. Toxoids are often used as immunogens for prophylactic immunization.

Exotoxin A, a single-chain polypeptide produced by most clinical strains of *P. aeruginosa*, catalyzes the transfer of adenine diphosphate dinucleotide from nicotinamide adenine dinucleotide to the ribosome binding elongation factor 2, resulting in inhibition of protein synthesis. This cytotoxin interferes with normal cellular immune functions. Efforts are now being made to use this toxin as an immunogen in persons at high risk of infection with these bacteria.

Corynebacterium diphtheriae produces a toxin that, although different in structure and cellular specificity, shares the same mechanism of action as exotoxin A of pseudomonas. Diphtheria was formerly a cause of very high morbidity and mortality among young children, but since the introduction of diphtheria toxoid as an immunizing agent (usually incorporated in the diphtheria–pertussis–tetanus, or DPT, vaccine) the incidence of this disease has been drastically reduced.

Shiga toxin, which is produced by strains of *S. typhimurium*, *Shigella*, *E. coli*, *V. cholerae*, and *Vibrio parahaemolyticus*, blocks ribosomal peptidyl elongation, resulting in the inhibition of protein synthesis.

The anaerobe *Clostridium botulinum* produces a potent neurotoxin that binds to specific receptors on presynaptic terminals of the peripheral nervous system and blocks the exocytosis of acetylcholine. This prevents the transmission of impulses from nerve to muscle and results in a flaccid paralysis that often leads to death.

Clostridium tetani, also an anaerobe, produces tetanus toxin, which binds to specific receptors in the central nervous system and blocks the normal postsynaptic inhibition of motor neurons by preventing the release of glycine. The resulting state of constant muscular contraction or spasm causes death.

Other exotoxins produced by bacteria involved in disease include the erythrogenic toxin of group A streptococci, which causes scarlet fever; the exfoliative toxin of some strains of *S. aureus*; the toxin of sudden toxic shock syndrome, also produced by *S. aureus*; the pertussis toxin of *B. pertussis*; and the edema-inducing toxin of *Bacillus anthracis*.

Those exotoxins that exert their activity in the gastrointestinal tract, producing symptoms such as nausea, vomiting, and diarrhea, are referred to as *enterotoxins*. Certain strains of *E. coli*, *S. aureus*, *Salmonella*, *Shigella*, *Vibrio*, and *C. perfringens* produce enterotoxins. Enterotoxin production may take place in contaminated food, as is the case with staphylococcal enterotoxin, or in the gastrointestinal tract, as occurs with *Salmonella* and the other bacteria. Although the mechanism of action varies, the end results are usually similar.

R-FACTORS

Although this discussion of virulence factors is by no means complete, it would be much less so if we did not discuss R-factors.

Plasmids are extrachromosomal DNA segments that carry genes for antibiotic resistance known as R-factors. They were first observed in the genus *Shigella* in 1959. These factors are readily transferrable by conjugation to bacterial cells of the same species as well as to cells of different species and even genera, and can confer resistance to many antibiotics.

Many bacteria of the normal flora carry these R-factors, but they present no problem until prolonged or improper use of antibiotics selectively enhances the survival of drug-resistant clones, making further therapy difficult.

SUGGESTIONS FOR FURTHER READING

C. S. F. Easmon, J. Jeljaszewicz, M. R. W. Brown, and P. A. Lambert, eds. *Role of the Envelope in the Survival of Bacteria in Infection: Medical Microbiology, Vol. 3.* Academic Press, London, 1983.

C. S. F. Easmon, J. Jeljaszewicz, M. R. W. Brown, and P. A. Lambert, eds. *Medical Microbiology, Vol. 4.* Academic Press, London, 1983.

C. A. Mims. *Pathogenesis of Infectious Disease.* Academic Press, London, 1982.

P. F. Sparling. "Bacterial virulence and pathogenesis: An overview." Review of Infectious Diseases 5(S4): 637, 1983.

The Bacteria

INTRODUCTION

Bacteria are microscopic organisms that may be considered to be more primitive life forms than plants, animals, and other eukaryotes; they certainly arose earlier than organisms of the latter groups. Bacteria are prokaryotes since they do not possess discrete nuclear membranes, chromosomes that condense during mitosis, or mitotic processes as found in the eukaryotes. The term *eubacteria* is used to separate most of the bacteria, including the pathogenic bacteria, from the cyanobacteria and Archaebacteria. The cyanobacteria are photosynthetic, "gliding" bacteria and are sometimes called *blue-green algae*. The Archaebacteria are unique organisms now considered to be distinct from other bacteria.

Not only do bacteria lack nuclear membranes, neither do these prokaryotes possess mitochondria, chloroplasts, or lysosomes as do eukaryotes. Thus, a bacterium is a morphologically simple single-cell organism surrounded by a cell envelope and a cell wall, and containing a single, coiled chromosome not bound by a nuclear membrane.

In this chapter, some of the essential features of bacteria will be described, followed by a description of a few of the common bacterial pathogens, arranged according to the organ or tissue in which the infection predominates.

MORPHOLOGY AND STRUCTURE OF BACTERIA

Shape and structure are useful properties that are widely used to aid in identification of bacteria. Many of the structural components and staining characteristics of bacteria correlate with their pathogenicity or virulence. A complete review of the attributes of bacteria can be found in any good introductory microbiology text.

Size and Shape

Bacteria can be stained, making them easily observable under the light microscope. Bacteria may be as small as $0.2\ \mu m$ in diameter, fairly close to the limit of resolution of the light microscope; as large as $2\ \mu m$ in diameter; or in the case of some rods, from 3 to $5\ \mu m$ long. More sophisticated techniques using phase contrast, dark field, or electron microscopy are needed to visualize many of the details of bacterial ultrastructure.

One rather simple means of classifying bacteria is based upon their size, shape, and grouping; all properties used for identification. By examination with the light microscope, it can be seen that bacteria usually occur as spheres (cocci), cylinders (bacilli), or corkscrews (spirochetes). Some, such as mycoplasms, have no cell walls and thus no fixed shape. If they are rod forms, they may occur as single cells, chains (streptobacilli), or pairs of cells (diplobacilli) (Figure 13.1). Some rods are curved or spiral shaped. Cocci occur as pairs (diplococci), chains (streptococci), or clusters (staphylococci). A few cocci divide in two planes, do not separate completely, and form tetrads; or they divide in three planes and form cubes (sarcinae). Spirochetes

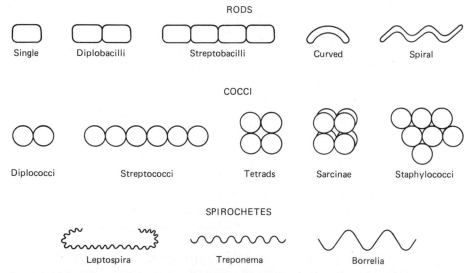

Figure 13.1 The shape and arrangement of bacteria. The three major shapes in which Eubacteria occur are illustrated. The names of genera or classes of bacteria often coincide with the name describing their shape or arrangement.

are long, slender coiled cells of 4 μm to 500 μm in length. The three main shapes in which spirochetes occur are those of the Leptospira, Treponema, and Borrelia (Figure 13.1).

Staining and Colony Morphology

Most stains are organic salts that combine with the components of bacteria. The basic stains are composed of a colored cation and a colorless anion. The chloride salt of methylene blue, for example, reacts with the acidic RNA or DNA, of the bacteria staining them blue.

The Gram stain devised in 1884 by Christian Gram permits most bacteria to be placed into one of two groups based on fundamental attributes of the bacterial cell wall. Whether or not a bacterium can retain the crystal violet-iodine complex produced by the Gram procedure when exposed to an alcohol wash determines if the organism is Gram-negative or Gram-positive (Table 13.1).

The acid-fast stain is used to identify a few important bacteria that retain basic fuchsin despite an acid treatment. These organisms are difficult to stain by other methods. They have an unusually high lipid content (40 percent) that inhibits penetration by most stains but also prevents loss of basic fuchsin during treatment with a mixture of dilute hydrochloric acid in alcohol. The initial staining with basic fuchsin requires a solvent containing phenol. The acid-fast property is possessed by a few species that are hard to grow in culture, such as the mycobacteria that cause tuberculosis and leprosy and the actinomycetes. The staining procedure is often done on tissue specimens since it provides a strong contrast between the intensely stained bacteria and the destained tissues.

Morphology of bacterial colonies can be observed when individual bacterial cells are allowed to multiply in place in or on a solid medium such as agar. The size, shape, texture, and color of the colonies formed under various conditions of incubation are characteristic for many bacteria. Streptococcal colonies, for example, are usually smaller than staphylococcal colonies. The edge of the microbial colony may be smooth, serrated, raised, or flat. The texture of the colonies ranges from dry to butterlike; some colonies are viscous and sticky. Often the smooth, viscous colonies are formed by encapsulated bacteria, whereas the nonencapsulated variants form a dry colony that has a rough texture. The color of some bacterial colonies is due to pigments produced by the bacteria but seen only when a mass of bacterial cells are together. *Staphylococcus aureus* colonies, for example, are characteristically gold, and *Serratia marcescens* is bright red.

Some differential media are used to detect physiological properties expressed best by the bacterial mass in a colony. The most widely used differential medium is blood agar; by its use various types of hemolysins can be detected. Some examples of the morphology of colonies of pathogenic bacteria are shown in Figure 13.2.

Structural Components

Certain structural properties of bacteria serve as virulence factors. These were described in Chapter 12. Other structural components are important because they

Table 13.1 CLASSIFICATION OF SOME IMPORTANT PATHOGENIC BACTERIA THAT CAUSE COMMON DISEASES

Characteristics	Genus	Common disease
Gram-negative rods, aerobes	*Pseudomonas*	Opportunistic infections
	Legionella	Acute atypical pneumonia
	Bordetella	Whooping cough
	Brucella	Undulant fever
Gram-negative rods, facultative anaerobes	*Klebsiella*	Bacterial pneumonia
	Escherichia	Gastroenteritis, meningitis
	Shigella	Dysentery
	Salmonella	Typhoid fever
	Yersinia	Plague
	Vibrio	Cholera
Gram-negative, pleomorphic anaerobes	*Bacteroides*	Trench mouth and gingivitis
	Fusobacterium	
Gram-positive rods, spore-forming	*Bacillus*	Anthrax
	Clostridium	Tetanus, gas gangrene, food poisoning
Gram-positive rods, non–spore-forming	*Listeria*	Meningitis, fetal infections
Spirochetes, endoflagella	*Treponema*	Syphilis
	Borrelia	Relapsing fever
Gram-positive cocci	*Staphylococcus*	Pyogenic infections, toxic shock syndrome, food poisoning
	Streptococcus	Pneumonia, glomerulonephritis, carditis, dental caries
Gram-negative cocci	*Neisseria*	Gonorrhea, meningitis
Actinomyces, branching, irregular	*Actinomyces*	Gingivitis
	Corynebacterium	Diphtheria
	Propionibacterium	Acne
	Mycobacterium	Tuberculosis, leprosy
Mycoplasma, no cell wall	*Mycoplasma*	Atypical pneumonia
Rickettsias	*Rickettsia*	Typhus fevers, Rocky Mountain spotted fever
	Chlamydia	Psittacosis, trachoma

are used for differentiating among the bacteria and therefore provide a basis for identification. Many of the bacterial components are the targets of the host immune response. A few of the major structural components of bacteria are illustrated in Figure 13.3.

Cell Envelope The boundary of the bacterial cell is referred to as the *cell envelope*. It includes the cell wall, one lipid bilayer membrane and, in Gram-negative bacteria, a lipid bilayer outside of the cell wall. These layers have a variety of components, some of which control the transport of nutrients and the flow of ions in and out of the cell. In addition, some envelope components serve as sites for attachment

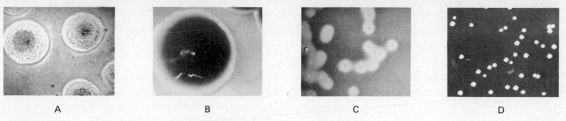

A   B   C   D

Figure 13.2 Some common types of colony morphology displayed by pathogenic bacteria. (A) *Mycoplasma* colonies, showing typical "fried egg" appearance, photomicroscopic courtesy of N. Sommerson, Dept. of Microbiology, The Ohio State University. (B) Single large *Serratia marcescens* colony. (C) Small shiny *Streptococcus pyogenes* colonies on blood agar. Each colony is surrounded by a broad band of hemolysis. (D) Small *Neisseria meningtides* colonies on blood agar. The organism does not produce a hemolysin and thus the colonies are not surrounded by a band of hemolysis.

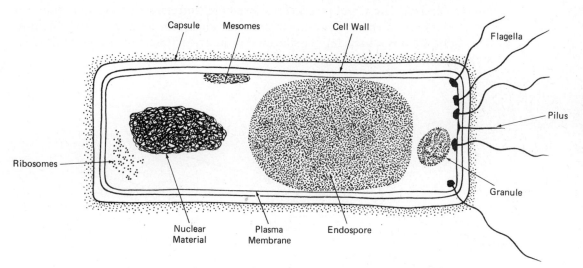

Figure 13.3 Schematic drawing of a bacterial cell showing the major structural components. Not all of the structures shown are present in bacteria of any one species.

to host cells. Some cell envelope components may be toxic for human and animal cells; the lipopolysaccharide of Gram-negative bacteria is an example of such a material.

Bacteria, with the exception of the mycoplasmas and some forms produced by antibiotic treatment, have cell walls that provide the cell with a fixed, rigid shape as well as protection from osmotic pressure. The cell wall has a complex, rigid three-dimensional structure composed of cross linked peptidoglycan. The peptidoglycan molecules are composed of repeating units of N-acetylglucosamine and N-acetylmuramic acid. These repeating units are held together by cross linking by pentaglycine residues (Figure 13.4). As animal cells lack these cell walls, antibiotics such as penicillin that act on cell walls are not toxic for animal cells. The penicillins inhibit bacterial wall synthesis and as a result the bacteria cannot resist osmotic lysis.

As noted earlier, differences in the reaction of cell envelopes with the Gram stain provide the basis for separating bacteria into Gram-positive and Gram-negative groups. The cell envelopes of Gram-positive cells are structurally simpler than Gram-negative cell envelopes even though they are generally thicker. Starting with the inner surface, the Gram-positive bacteria possess a cytoplasmic membrane, a very thick peptidoglycan layer, and an outer layer that is a capsule or glycocalyx (Figure 13.5). Gram-negative bacteria contain an inner membrane. There is a periplasmic space between the inner and outer membranes (Figure 13.5). There are more lipids in the Gram-negative cell envelope than in the Gram-positive one: from 15 to 20 percent versus from 2 to 4 percent for Gram-positive bacteria. Sometimes a capsule is also present on the bacterial surface.

The reaction of bacteria with the Gram stain reflects a fundamental difference among bacteria. The Gram reaction, for example, correlates with susceptibility to antibiotics in some cases, Gram-negative bacteria being more resistant to penicillin. The Gram stain is a basis for classification of most bacteria and is used as the first step leading to their identification.

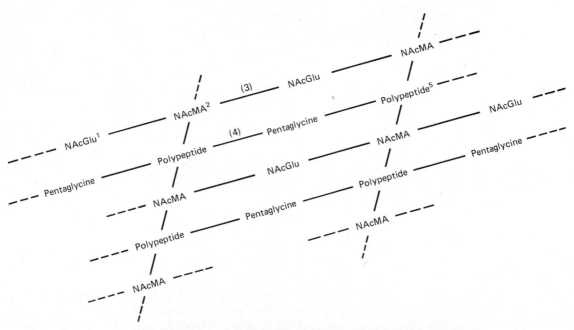

Figure 13.4 The peptidoglycan component of bacterial cell walls consists of long polymers of N-acetylglucosamine and N-acetylmuramic acid cross linked by a mixed polypeptide in one dimension and by pentaglycine in the other dimension. The pentaglycine links the mixed polypeptide units. All bacterial cell walls contain this structural component. The sites of action of penicillin (3) and lysozyme (4) are shown.

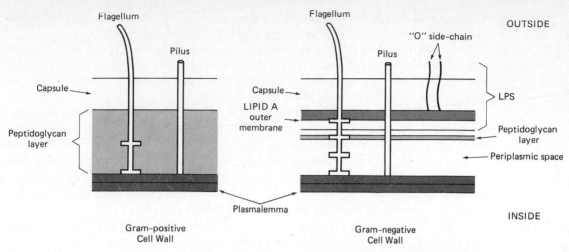

Figure 13.5 Structural features of the cell envelope of Gram-positive and Gram-negative bacteria. One major difference between the two is the greater thickness of the peptidoglycan layer in Gram-positive bacteria. In addition, the Gram-negative cell envelope has a periplasmic space. This is located between the outer membrane, which is not present in Gram-positive bacteria, and the plasmalemma.

The compounds contained in cell envelopes are important in host–parasite interactions. They play a role in pathogenicity and contribute to the uniqueness of the bacterium. Many of the proteins and polysaccharides in cell walls are antigenic or act as haptens in immunological reactions. Detection of these antigens often aids in the diagnosis of bacterial infections. For example, the outer membrane of the Gram-negative cell envelope contains lipopolysaccharide; its detection indicates infection with a Gram-negative bacterium. The Gram-positive cell envelope contains lipoteichoic acid molecules attached to either the cytoplasmic membrane or the peptidoglycan. Antibody to it indicates infection with a Gram-positive bacterium. The presence of such antibody provides some protection to the host.

Lipopolysaccharide (LPS) only occurs as part of the outer membrane of Gram-negative bacteria. The LPS is oriented to the outside of the cell and is in contact with the environment in which the bacterium exists. The major surface antigen of all Gram-negative bacteria is the O-antigen, which is the outermost polysaccharide component of LPS. Differences in the O-antigen of the bacteria determine their serotype. Bacteria of a given species have the same O-antigen. The O-antigen is a side-chain that is attached to a core polysaccharide. This core is antigenically the same in all bacteria of a given genus. The core polysaccharide is attached in turn to the lipid A component of LPS. The lipid A component is embedded in the phospholipid bilayer of the outer membrane of Gram-negative bacteria (Figure 13.5). It is the LPS, especially the lipid A portion of LPS, that is responsible for the endotoxemia associated with infections with Gram-negative bacteria. Antibiotic treatment often results in the liberation of the LPS from the bacteria following their deaths. As a result the clinical signs of endotoxemia may develop after antibiotic treatment.

Capsule and Glycocalyx   A layer of gelatinous material surrounds most bacteria. It is on the outside of the cell envelope and is called the *capsule.* The term *capsule* is most often used to refer to the material around a single bacterial cell, whereas *slime layer* is the term used to describe the same material when it is around a mass of cells. A *glycocalyx* is a capsule composed of carbohydrates and may be used to refer either to a capsule or a slime layer.

Most capsules are thin; however, the capsules around *Klebsiella* and pneumococci are thick, in many cases thicker than the diameter of the cell. Capsules are most often of polysaccharide nature. Their composition may vary widely, with some being made up of simple homopolysaccharides of a single hexose sugar whereas others may be branched heteropolysaccharides. The capsules of the bacteria of the genus *Bacillus* are composed of amino acids rather than of polysaccharides; the capsule of *Bacillus anthracis* is a poly-d-glutamate.

Capsules have important functions. They may, for example, provide a means for attachment to surfaces; they may also concentrate nutrients. Many microbes are protected by their capsules. Capsules of pathogenic bacteria, for example, may interfere with phagocytosis or may prevent activation of complement by the alternative pathway. The nonpathogenicity of strains of *Streptococcus pneumoniae, Haemophilus influenza,* and *Bordetella pertussis,* which lack capsules, clearly shows the protective role of capsules.

Flagella   Flagella are long filamentous appendages that are anchored on the inside of the cytoplasmic, or inner, membrane of bacteria and extend to the surface and beyond (Figure 13.5). Some flagella are up to 25 μm long. Bacterial flagella have a specialized "hook" embedded in a basal body in the envelope. The flagellum is a hollow tube composed of intertwined fibers of an alpha-helical form of the protein flagelin. Some bacteria have one flagellum (monotrichous); others have several flagella in a tuft at one end of the cell (lophotrichous); and others have flagella over the whole surface (peritrichous). The motility conferred by flagella is a result of a rotary movement they make. The movement of the bacterial cell by flagella is directional and is usually in response to chemotactic stimuli.

Pili (Fimbriae)   Pili are very minute or fine filamentous appendages that extend outward from the bacterial cell. They, like flagella, originate in a basal body in the cytoplasmic membrane (Figure 13.5). Pili occur most frequently on Gram-negative bacilli. They are of two basic types. The sex pilus is involved in bacterial conjugation and allows passage of DNA through the pilus into another bacterial cell. The second type of pilus serves to attach the bacterium to host cells, especially mucosal cells. Attachment is necessary in many cases for colonization of a tissue by a microbial pathogen. The gonococcal pili, for example, serve to attach this pathogen to the urethral mucosa and are therefore an important factor in its virulence. Vaccines using pilus protein as antigen are being developed for several diseases, including gonorrhea and various types of bacterial dysentery.

Endospores   Spores are resistant to acids, alkalis, alcohol, and many other chemicals, and to heat and drying. They are produced by bacteria of the genera *Clostrid-*

ium and *Bacillus.* Spores are formed when environmental conditions no longer support vegetative growth. Although spores are not virulence factors *per se* since they permit prolonged survival of the microbe in the environment, they increase the chance of infection. The introduction of spores into a susceptible host quickly results in outgrowth of the bacteria. Humans and most of their domestic animals can be infected with spores of *B. anthracis* and *Clostridium tetani,* for example, and the diseases produced can be quite severe.

SOME MEDICALLY IMPORTANT BACTERIA

Many pathogenic bacteria initiate infection by entering the host through the mucous membranes of the oral, respiratory, ocular, gastrointestinal, or genitourinary tract. The other common route of infection is through breaks in the skin. Infection by some bacteria is restricted to the site of entry, whereas others may disseminate to other sites. In some cases the clinical signs of infection may be widely removed from the original site of initiation of the infection.

The skin is an effective barrier against bacterial invasion. A few bacteria, however, can cause infections of the superficial layers of intact skin or even invade deeper tissues through the hair follicles in the absence of overt injury. Contact with the bacteria is all that is required. However, even with infections caused by these bacteria, a minor break in the skin will greatly increase the chances that the pathogens will pass the barrier.

If the integrity of the skin is broken by wounds, burns, surgery, or animal or insect bites, then a variety of bacterial pathogens that cannot otherwise enter the body may establish an infection. Wound infections are most often caused by *Staphylococcus aureus* and *Streptococcus pyogenes.* Gas gangrene is an infection caused by the growth of *Clostridium perfringens* or closely related clostridia. For clostridial infection to develop, wound contamination with endospores and anaerobic conditions for germination and growth are required. The toxins produced by the clostridia are a group of exotoxins and enzymes with proteolytic activity that literally digest the tissue. If damaged tissue in a wound is removed, anaerobic conditions are unlikely to occur. The bulk of gasses produced in gas gangrene are carbon dioxide and hydrogen.

The term *zoonosis* refers to an infectious disease of humans that is contracted from diseased lower animals. Arthropods are the most common insect vector for transmitting such microbial diseases. Many zoonotic diseases are acquired through the skin, the arthropod providing passage through the skin while feeding.

Many diseases of the oral cavity are caused by bacteria, especially bacteria that are indigenous to the mouth. These infections are among the most common bacterial infections of humans. As the organisms causing them are usually not highly pathogenic, host factors play a role in whether disease develops following infection.

The respiratory tract also provides a convenient portal of entry for many pathogens. The opportunity for infection is great since humans inhale 10,000 l of air each day. Some of the infections remain localized within the respiratory tract and others may disseminate to adjoining tissues or even throughout the body, becoming systemic infections. Airborne transmission of bacterial pathogens occurs when microscopic droplets containing bacteria are transferred between individuals. A few airborne infections such as Legionnaire's disease are a result of infection with bacteria from the environment; more commonly the organisms are derived from exhalations by infected individuals.

The gastrointestinal tract is exposed to large numbers of bacteria ingested with food and water, and also contains a large indigenous population. Two general types of disease of the tract occur. The first is termed *food poisoning* and is the result of absorbing toxin produced by the bacteria. In this type of disease infection or invasion may not occur. The second type of disease is caused by actual invasion of the tissue. It is therefore a true infection.

Food poisoning caused by the ingestion of preformed toxins is commonly caused by *S. aureus* or *Clostridium botulinum,* which grow in food.

Infections associated with diarrhea are commonly caused by *Salmonella enteritidis, Escherichia coli, Shigella sp.,* or *Vibrio cholera. S. enteritidis* causes a gastroenteritis that is quite severe and relatively common. *E. coli* is responsible for a shigellalike dysentery, as well as an enteritis similar to that caused by the cholera and Salmonella bacilli. Pathogenic *E. coli* produce a labile toxin similar in action to that produced by the other pathogenic Gram-negative rods. *Salmonella typhi* is an example of an invasive bacterium associated with a severe enteric fever.

Infections of the urinary tract often occur with opportunistic pathogens that enter the bladder and kidney. These organisms are most often bacteria of the normal flora of the intestinal tract. Sexually transmitted, or venereal, diseases are infections with obligate bacterial pathogens that have acquired the ability to be transmitted during sexual acts.

In the following sections of this chapter we describe a few bacterial diseases that are grouped according to the organ systems in which they produce their major lesions. This is a system of grouping widely used by members of the medical profession since it aids clinical diagnosis. It is a system that may place diseases caused by unrelated bacteria in the same group, however. Moreover, the effect of some diseases is not limited to a single organ system and may encompass the entire body. These diseases can only be considered to be generalized infections.

INFECTIONS OF THE SKIN

Acne

Propionibacterium acnes and *Staphylococcus epidermidis* are two of the bacteria that invade hair follicles in the epidermal layers of the skin. They may not require overt injury to initiate infection. Infection causes excessive secretion by the sebaceous glands at the base of the hair follicles. A pus-filled pimple results from this type of infection. There is some evidence that a cell-mediated immune response to the bacterial components occurs. This response does not appear to significantly aid clearance of the infection. Hormonal changes associated with puberty are a factor in acne, possibly by affecting the skin secretions in such a way as to facilitate microbial survival.

Impetigo

Impetigo is an infection of the skin with *Streptococcus pyogenes* and then superinfection with *Staphylococcus aureus.* The infection is probably initiated at sites of injury, although the sites may be microscopic. Once infection is started, the hyaluronidase produced by *S. pyogenes* facilitates microbial spread in the connective tissue underlying the skin. The infected skin fills with pus. A delayed type hypersensitivity response to the bacterial antigens causes itching of the skin, which causes scratching that in turn spreads the infection.

Pseudomonas Infections

Extensive burns damage the skin and permit opportunistic pathogens to infect underlying tissues. *Pseudomonas aeruginosa* is the cause of the most common fatal infection of burn victims. Many of the *P. aeruginosa* strains are resistant to antibiotics and therefore pose a serious threat to the burned patient. Burning may not only damage the integrity of the physical barrier provided by the skin, it also seems to affect the immune response of the body. Healthy humans are almost never infected with Pseudomonas. Pseudomonads are ubiquitous, growing readily as saprophytes in soil and water.

INFECTIONS OF THE EYE

Conjunctivitis

Conjunctivitis is a bacterial infection of the mucous membrane lining the eye socket. Bacterial conjunctivitis is caused by a variety of bacteria: *Haemophilus aegyptius, S. aureus, S. pneumoniae, P. aeruginosa,* and *Chlamydia sp.* are probably the most common. "Pink eye" outbreaks among children are caused by *H. aegyptius.* A more serious disease, inclusion conjunctivitis, is caused by *Chlamydia trachomatis.* This last organism causes trachoma, in which there is an invasion of the cornea itself. Trachoma can cause blindness.

INFECTIONS OF THE MOUTH

Dental Caries

The growth of streptococci of several species on the tooth surface results in lactic acid production. The acid is highly concentrated on the enamel surface because it is released in the glycan polymer produced by the bacteria on the tooth surface. The bacteria implicated are *Streptococcus mutans, Streptococcus sanguis,* and *Streptococcus salivarius.* Diet and dental hygiene are factors, along with bacteria, in production of tooth decay. In recent years the incidence of tooth decay in the United States has decreased greatly. The reasons suggested for this include widespread fluoridation of water and widespread use of antibiotics; the causes are a matter of active research.

Periodontal Infections

Diseases of varying severity are caused by a variety of bacteria that invade the tissues and bone supporting the teeth. Gingivitis is caused by species of *Actinomyces*, whereas ulcerative gingivitis, or trench mouth, is caused by various species of *Veillonella, Fusobacterium,* and *Campylobacterium.* Trench mouth is an example of synergy since no single bacteria is able to cause this disease.

In periodontitis, or pyorrhea, there is invasion and destruction of gingival tissue by a mixture of bacteria that includes spirochetes, *Bacteroides,* and the bacteria listed previously that cause the milder form of gingivitis. The most common causative agents appear to be *Treponema vincentii* and *Bacteroides melaninogenicoccus.* Eventually the growth of the bacteria can erode the bone holding the teeth, resulting in their loss.

General health is a factor in infection of the gums. People who are fatigued or malnourished are much more likely to develop ulcers in their mouths than others. Trench mouth, for example, was first described in soldiers who were fatigued by prolonged service in trenches in the first world war.

Endocarditis

Infections initiated in the mouth and around the teeth may have consequences widely removed from the initial site of infection. One of the most serious is endocarditis. The inflammation of the membrane that lines the chambers and valves of the heart, called the *endocardium,* is caused by an infection with *Streptococcus viridans.* Since *S. viridans* is part of the normal flora of the mouth, it may enter the blood stream as a result of local infection, accidental tissue injury, or injury resulting from dental procedures. If the bacteria lodge in the heart, they may produce endocarditis. If the infection spreads to the myocardium or muscle of the heart or seriously damages the heart valves, it may be fatal.

INFECTIONS OF THE RESPIRATORY TRACT

Whooping Cough (Pertussis)

Pertussis is the formal name of the disease most often designated by the characteristic cough accompanying the disease. It is caused by *B. pertussis,* which is a Gram-negative coccobacillus. The virulence factors of *B. pertussis* are the several pertussis toxins, as well as the pili and capsule. Immunization with killed *B. pertussis* bacteria, in a triple vaccine that also contains diphtheria and tetanus toxoids, has reduced the incidence of this disease in infants and young children. A factor in pertussis vaccines causes neurological disorders in a small proportion of children who receive it, however. This has caused a decrease in use of the vaccine and an increase in the incidence of whooping cough. Attempts are underway to produce a pertussis vaccine free of this undesirable effect.

Diphtheria

The clinical signs of diphtheria are largely a result of toxin production by lysogenic strains of *Cornyebacterium diphtheriae*. The organism is not very invasive. It usually only causes a localized infection of the mucosal membranes of the upper respiratory tract with formation of scab or pseudomembrane that can block the trachea. The toxins diffuse from the site of local infection and cause widespread damage. The toxin produced is capable of killing most eukaryotic cells. Antibodies to the toxin neutralize it and prevent the disease even though infection may be present and the host becomes a carrier of the organism. Immunization with inactivated diphtheria toxin effectively prevents the disease.

Scarlet Fever and Streptococcal Sore Throats

Scarlet fever is a result of a localized infection of the throat with *S. pyogenes*. The scarlet rash is caused by an exotoxin secreted by the streptococci that diffuses into the body. An antibody-mediated immunity is developed to the effects of the toxin so that once recovered from an infection or immunized with toxoid the individual does not get scarlet fever again. Unfortunately, immunity to the local infection of the throat is not so easy to develop and many people suffer from repeated bouts of streptococcal sore throat. Children who have such repeated streptococcal sore throats often develop rheumatic fever. Rheumatic fever is a serious outcome of such infections. Rheumatic fever is characterized by a complex group of symptoms that include joint pain, fever, and cardiac muscle destruction resulting in a weakened heart. The other major complication of repeated infections with streptococci is poststreptococcal glomerulonephritis that is responsible for a form of renal failure. These serious complications are only caused by hemolytic *S. pyogenes* that belong to the serogroup A. The disease is at least in part autoimmune in nature; the antibodies elicited by the bacteria cross react with the sarcolemma of the heart muscle, resulting in damage.

Pneumonia

Bacterial pneumonia, an infection of the alveoli of the lungs, most often occurs in patients who have an impaired immune system, including the young and the aged. The most frequent causative agent of acute pneumonia is *S. pneumoniae*. It is an encapsulated organism, the capsule of which confers upon it the ability to resist phagocytosis. Pneumococci are often part of the normal flora of the throat and cause no trouble while the host is young or vigorous. Immune serum specific for the capsule permits phagocytosis of the microbe and when it was introduced in the 1930s as a therapeutic agent had a dramatic effect upon the fatality rate resulting from pneumococcal pneumonia.

Other bacteria that can cause pneumonia are *H. influenzae*, *Klebsiella pneumoniae*, and *S. aureus*. Bacterial pneumonia is today successfully treated with antibiotics; for example, penicillin is used for pneumococcal pneumonia.

Pneumococcal pneumonia is an excellent example of an acute bacterial infection. The elderly are particularly at risk from this type of pneumonia and frequently die of their infections. The onset of pneumococcal pneumonia is abrupt. Symptoms include a high fever, chills, and chest pain. Fluid coughed up from the lungs may be blood streaked, giving it a rusty appearance. In response to the lung infection, fluids collect in the air spaces. These fluids contain red blood cells and leukocytes. An x-ray picture of the lungs of an infected individual characteristically shows a congested area within one lobe of the lung. The infection usually clears rapidly as a result of antibiotic therapy.

S. pneumoniae, the causative agent of pneumococcal pneumonia, is a Gram-positive coccus that is usually seen as pairs of lancet-shaped (somewhat pointed) organisms. Once the disease is established, the microbe may be isolated from blood cultures or sputum produced by coughing. When grown in an agar culture medium containing red blood cells, *S. pneumoniae* produces a hemolysin that partially lyses the red cells and causes a greenish color to develop around the microbial colonies. This is an incomplete, or *alpha,* hemolysis. Like other streptococci, the pneumococcus produces a variety of proteolytic enzymes. However, it is the polysaccharide capsule that is clearly the major virulence factor since it protects the microbe from phagocytosis.

Recovery from the infection depends upon production of opsonic IgG antibody against the specific capsular polysaccharide. Type-specific polysaccharides have been developed as vaccines to immunize people in the high-risk populations. Whereas pneumococci may produce over 80 distinct serotypes of capsular polysaccharides, bacterial pneumonias are usually caused by pneumococci of about 23 serotypes; thus vaccines are composed only of a mixture of the polysccharides that most commonly cause disease.

Atypical pneumonias are caused by three very different bacteria: *Mycoplasma pneumonia, Legionella pneumophila,* and *Chlamydia psittaci.* Mycoplasma lack a cell wall and are not sensitive to penicillin, but can be treated with other antibiotics. Legionnaire's disease was first described in 1976 and eventually the etiologic agent was identified as *L. pneumophila,* an inhabitant of water that may become airborne in aerosols from cooling towers. When such contaminated aerosols are inhaled, infection may result. Psittacosis is also called *parrot fever* and is caused by *C. psittaci,* which is transmitted from birds to humans.

Bronchitis and pharyngitis, infections of the bronchial tree of the lungs and the throat, respectively, are caused by many of the same bacterial pathogens causing pneumonia.

Tuberculosis

Tuberculosis is an excellent example of an infectious disease in which the response of the host immune system plays a major role in the disease process. The cell-mediated immune response (see Chapter 9) contributes both to resistance to the organism and to destruction of human tissues. The interplay of cell-mediated immune activity with other host resistance factors (for example, genetic background, age, prior exposure, and diet) determines whether or not the infection will lead to overt disease.

The primary infection starts when mycobacteria are inhaled and reach the lungs, although outbreaks have occurred following ingestion of unpasteurized contaminated milk. The microbes are ingested by lung macrophages in which multiplication, rather than destruction, may occur (see Chapter 12 for the mechanism). The bacteria may be disseminated through the lymphatic system to the regional lymph nodes, and eventually into the bloodstream. The original lung lesions may heal if the infection is controlled or, if infection persists, the delayed hypersensitivity response elicited may result in formation of tubercles.

Hypersensitivity, an indication of exposure or infection, can be detected by the tuberculin skin test. Tubercles occur in the lungs of people with the bacterial pneumonia caused by the tubercle bacillus. Following infection, the disease may be resolved or the microbes may be spread to other organs of the body and even cause death.

Mycobacterium tuberculosis and related mycobacteria are rod-shaped, aerobic organisms rich in lipids, especially a Wax D component. Most likely, the lipids of mycobacteria contribute to its maintenance in the host and to its unique staining properties. The Gram stain is not useful for detection or identification of these bacilli. Instead, the acid-fast stain is used. In this procedure the waxy component prevents the stained mycobacteria from being decolorized by acid alcohol treatment. The ability to retain the acid-fast stain is presumptive evidence that the organisms grown from clinical material or found on smears made of sputum specimens are mycobacteria.

In addition to *M. tuberculosis, Mycobacterium bovis, Mycobacterium avis,* and various atypical mycobacteria cause human disease. The atypical mycobacteria differ from the tubercle bacilli in their growth characteristics and biochemical reactions; they are particularly important in diseases of immunocompromised patients. Bacteria of the *Mycobacterium avium-intracellulare* complex, for example, are a common cause of infection in those with AIDS.

Mycobacteria can remain dormant within the body; they become reactivated as a result of malnutrition and stress. Tuberculosis is generally a chronic, progressive infection unless it is treated with appropriate antibiotics.

INFECTIONS OF THE GASTROINTESTINAL TRACT

Food Poisoning

Food poisoning is a general term referring to gastrointestinal disease caused by ingestion of contaminated food or water. It is caused by various toxin-producing strains of a variety of bacteria. These include *C. botulinum,* which causes botulism, *C. perfringens,* which causes enteritis, and *S. aureus,* which causes staphylococcal food poisoning. All bacteria responsible for food poisoning produce exotoxins that are termed *enterotoxins.* Botulism is caused by neurotoxins released by *C. botuli-*

num. These toxins are rapidly absorbed from the gut and bind to the synapses of motor neurons. As a result of this binding, neural transmission is blocked. Death occurs because of paralysis of the respiratory muscles. Most cases of botulism (90 percent) are caused by eating improperly canned food. Type A or Type B neurotoxins are the predominant forms found in canned vegetables. The endospores of *C. botulinum* found in the soil survive heating in boiling water, and the bacteria grow out at neutral pH. The key for growth is an anaerobic environment, which exists in cans.

Sudden infant death syndrome may be caused by growth of the *C. botulinum* in the nonacid environment of the infant stomach and small intestine. The disease is treated by administration of antibodies to the A, B, and E botulinum toxins. Botulinum toxins are the most potent toxins known, with a lethal dose of 1 μg for humans.

Food poisoning of a less severe nature than that produced by *C. botulinum* is caused by a type A exotoxin released into cooked meats by *C. perfringens.* The exotoxin released from certain strains of *S. aureus* growing in food also causes a form of food poisoning characterized by nausea and diarrhea.

Salmonellosis

Several species of *Salmonella,* especially *S. enteritidis,* cause gastroenterocolitis. These *Salmonella* are surrounded by pili that enable them to attach to gut epithelial cells and reproduce there. The enterotoxins they elaborate cause the disease seen. *Salmonella paratyphi* and *Salmonella typhimurium,* in particular, can invade tissue and cause a bacteremia in addition to gastroenteritis.

Typhoid Fever

Systemic infections caused by *S. typhi* usually occur as a result of transmission from asymptomatic human carriers who contaminate food or water. The classical example of a healthy carrier of *S. typhi* was "Typhoid Mary," a cook who infected members of the families who employed her. *S. typhi* invades the intestinal epithelial cells, passing from these into the lymphatic system, and then it is disseminated throughout the body by the vascular system. Although *S. typhi* is rapidly ingested by neutrophils and macrophages, the bacteria are not killed, but rather multiply in these phagocytic cells. Systemic disease, including high fever, results from the reaction of the body to the widely disseminated organisms. Infection is established in cells in organs such as the kidney, liver, spleen, gallbladder, and the Peyer's patches or lymph nodules of the intestine. It is these infected cells that harbor the *S. typhi* in carriers and serve as the reservoir for the microorganism between epidemics.

Cholera

Vibrio cholerae, a curved, Gram-negative rod, is the causative agent of cholera. *V. cholerae* adheres to the mucosa within the lumen of the intestine, where it multiplies but is unable to invade further. The major clinical sign of cholera is diarrhea, with dehydration resulting from severe water loss. The severe loss of water and the loss of electrolytes that accompanies it is caused by an enterotoxin produced by *V. cholerae.* The cholera toxin stimulates adenylate cyclase production, which increases intracellular levels of cAMP. In turn, cAMP initiates secretion of both water and ions from the gut epithelial cells. It is the loss of water and salt that causes the shock that is characteristic of the disease. From 10 to 15 percent of those infected may die. Treatment is to restore water and electrolyte balance. The patient is made to consume sufficient balanced salt solution to replace the lost water and salt. Infection may be endemic in areas with poor sewage treatment facilities. Transmission occurs by ingestion of food or water contaminated by the diarrheal feces. Between epidemics, the organisms probably survive as a harmless parasite of copepods and other animals living in rivers, ponds, and estuaries. It is probable that the organism came from rivers in northern India.

INFECTIONS OF THE UROGENITAL TRACT

Urinary Tract Infections

Infections of the urethra or bladder, termed *urethritis* and *cystitis,* respectively, can be caused by any one of the Gram-negative bacteria that occur in the intestines. *E. coli* and *Proteus sp.* are the organisms most commonly isolated from individuals with these urogenital infections. When the infection progresses into the kidney from the bladder, it may have serious consequences, including renal failure and death.

   Listeria monocytogenes, a Gram-positive rod, causes a serious type of infection in the urogenital tract because infection with it may result in damage to the fallopian tubes or, in pregnant women, infection of the fetus, causing fetal death or abnormality.

Vaginal Infections

Vaginal infections occur very frequently. They are sometimes caused by bacteria, but the protozoan *Trichomonas vaginalis* and the yeast *Candida albicans* are more frequent causes. These organisms cause annoying, but not serious, diseases. *Neisseria gonorrhea,* discussed in the next section, is a bacterium that not only can cause disease when it colonizes the vagina, but may also persist there as an inapparent infection.

Toxic Shock Syndrome

Toxic shock syndrome is caused by a toxin released by certain strains of *S. aureus* that contain a lysogenic phage. Although the syndrome has been associated with the use of tampons, it also occurs with infections with *S. aureus* at other sites, especially in surgical wounds. The syndrome is essentially an intoxication, as the organism grows in some isolated site and elaborates toxin there. The disease occurs when the toxin diffuses into the surrounding tissues; the organism seldom invades the tissue, however. The condition assumed prominence with the introduction of a new type of highly absorbent tampon. These tampons were sufficiently absorbent that they did not need changing for many hours. The prolonged retention of the blood- and secretion-soaked tampon provided the organisms an opportunity to grow and elaborate toxin. Surgical wounds also provide sites for microbial growth; for example, around stitches or in gauze or other types of drains that remain in the wounds for fairly long periods.

Gonorrhea

Gonorrhea is the most prevalent sexually transmitted disease and requires direct sexual contact for transmission. The causative agent is the gonococcus *N. gonorrhoeae*, which does not survive long outside of infected tissues. The pili of this Gram-negative diplococcus are necessary for attachment to mucosal cells. There may be some invasion of the subepithelial layer of connective tissue. The gonococcus is not, however, a very invasive organism. It grows mostly on the mucosa of the organs it infects. The resulting inflammation may be quite painful. The organism may grow on the mucosa of the throat and the rectum as well as in the genital organs. Gonorrhea may be spread by asymptomatic carriers or by people with frank infection. It may be a serious disease, particularly if it invades the prostate gland or the fallopian tubes. In the latter case it may cause sterility.

Most strains of the gonococcus prevalent today produce a penicillinase and therefore are resistant to the action of penicillin. Newborns receive eye drops containing a 1 percent solution of silver nitrate. This agent kills any gonococci that may have entered the eye during passage through the birth canal. The treatment prevents blindness that may result from gonococcal infection of the eye.

Syphilis

Syphilis is another bacterial disease that may be considered to be a disease of the urogenital tract although the disease is not limited to that organ system. Syphilis is sexually transmitted. It is caused by the spirochete *Treponema pallidum.* Transmission requires direct contact with a syphilitic lesion as the organisms cannot survive long in the environment. *Treponema* penetrate the skin or mucous membranes at the contact site, where they produce a local, ulcerlike lesion. The organisms soon spread throughout the body, however, and may in later stages damage the skin, bones, joints, and nervous system. It can also cross the placenta and infect the fetus.

There are three stages of syphilis. The primary stage is marked by a chancre on the genitals. The secondary stage occurs as long as eight weeks later and involves dissemination of the organism to numerous parts of the body. Lesions that contain treponemes develop throughout the body as a result of this dissemination. The tertiary stage occurs many years later and is characterized by damage to many organs, including the aorta and the brain. Patients in the latent periods between stages have no clinical symptoms, and they are not infectious during these periods. No one spontaneously clears infection. An immunity capable of preventing or curing infection does not develop; however, sufficient immunity does develop to bring about healing of the primary and secondary lesions and to produce prolonged latency. There is considerable interest in the development of a vaccine to prevent syphilis, but to date success is minimal. Treatment with antibiotics is, however, quite successful.

GENERALIZED INFECTIONS

Although it is possible to consider many diseases to be diseases of certain organ systems, others produce such widespread effects as to require consideration as generalized infections. Syphilis could be considered a generalized infection although, as a venereal disease, it is usually grouped with the infections of the urogenital tract. The diseases described in the following parts of this section, while perhaps affecting some organ system more than others, produce sufficiently widespread effects as to warrant their consideration in the category of generalized infections.

Typhus Fever

Several types of typhus fever exist, all of which are caused by rickettsia transmitted to humans by bites of arthropod vectors. The three common forms of typhus fever in humans are epidemic typhus caused by Rickettsia prowazekii, endemic typhus caused by *Rickettsia typhi,* and scrub typhus caused by *Rickettsia tsutsugamushi.*

Epidemic typhus is transmitted between hosts by the body louse and usually occurs in people living in unsanitary, crowded conditions. The disease is common in wartime. Vascular lesions occur in the blood vessels of the heart and kidneys. Untreated, one-half of all patients die. Murine, or endemic, typhus is transmitted to humans by rat fleas and the nature of the disease is similar to, but milder than, epidemic typhus. In Japan and Korea, humans become accidental hosts for scrub typhus, which is a congenital infection of mice; mites are the vectors of scrub typhus. The host responds to rickettsial pathogens with a cell-mediated immune reaction that destroys the infected cells

Brucellosis

Humans are accidental hosts of several *Brucella* species that normally infect farm animals, particularly goats (*Brucella melitensis*), cows (*Brucella abortus*), and pigs (*Brucella suis*). This Gram-negative, nonmotile aerobic rod enters its hosts by many routes. Infection through minor abrasions in the skin; ingestion of food, particularly unpasteurized milk and cheese; and infection through the eye are common routes of infection. Slaughterhouse workers, farmers, and veterinarians are all commonly at risk of this disease. Veterinarians and farmers are infected when they handle aborted animal fetuses or treat cattle who have aborted as a result of infection. Since the fever associated with the infection may rise and fall, the disease is called *undulant fever.* Unless treated, the infection may persist for years. Vaccines have been developed for cattle, but they are not effective for hogs nor are they used for preventing infection in humans.

Plague

Although this disease is now rare, in the Middle Ages it was responsible for the death of up to 25 percent of the human population of Europe. It is caused by *Yersinia pestis,* a Gram-negative pleomorphic rod that is maintained in wild rodents. Humans are infected by the bite of fleas that leave the rodents after they have died of the disease. The bubonic form of plague results when rat fleas inject the agent while feeding. In this form of the disease *Y. pestis* becomes localized in the lymph nodes draining the area of the bite. When the nodes become enlarged they are called *buboes.* The infection progresses throughout the body. Sometimes the lungs become infected. When this happens, the disease may be spread by aerosols produced by coughing. This form is called *pneumonic plague.* The disease is readily treatable with streptomycin, but if untreated may be rapidly fatal in a high proportion of cases.

Anthrax

Humans are accidental hosts for *B. anthracis.* Anthrax occurs most often in sheep and cattle. The infection in humans is most commonly a result of contamination of breaks in the skin of people who handle infected meat but also occurs as a result of inhalation of dust that contains spores. This form of anthrax commonly occurred in people sorting infected wool and is called *woolsorters disease.* Infection also results from ingestion of spores. This is the route of infection most common in domestic animals. The microbes grow first at the initial site of infection and then throughout the body as the organisms spread. The disease is in part a result of toxin released by the microbes. The disease is often fatal. The virulence factors are both a capsule and the toxin. Vaccination of domestic animals has reduced the incidence of the disease among them and, as a result, in humans.

MECHANISMS OF IMMUNITY AND RESISTANCE TO BACTERIAL INFECTION

Infections may be intracellular or extracellular, toxigenic or nontoxigenic, and either local or systemic. Most of the available immunological effector mechanisms are induced to some degree by most infections and can be detected during the course of any one of these types of infection. It is usually only one or two of the induced mechanisms that are primarily responsible for the immunity that develops, however. In the last section of this chapter the immunological effector mechanisms controlling the various types of infection will be described. The mechanisms associated with each infection are summarized in Table 13.2.

Table 13.2   HOST DEFENSE MECHANISMS IMPORTANT IN RESISTANCE TO VARIOUS
TYPES OF BACTERIAL INFECTIONS

Type of infection	Mechanism
Localized extracellular	
In tissue	Opsonization, complement activation, phagocytosis
On mucous membranes	Blockage of attachment by IgA
Systemic extracellular	
Nontoxigenic	Opsonization, complement activation, phagocytosis
Toxigenic	Antibody-mediated neutralization of toxin
Intracellular infection	
In macrophages	Macrophage activation, granulomar formation, action of lymphokines and monokines
In nonphagocytic cells	Granuloma formation, lysis by cytolytic lymphocytes, antibody-dependent cell cytotoxicity, actions of lymphokines and monokines

Extracellular Bacterial Infections

Bacteria that grow extracellularly often cause acute, rapidly spreading infections with development of large microbial populations and, in some cases, toxin production. Some toxigenic bacteria such as *C. tetani,* however, cause severe disease while only forming limited local infections. Some bacteria causing extracellular infections are encapsulated, some are not.

Nonencapsulated bacteria of types causing extracellular infections are seldom very pathogenic. Infection by such bacteria, when it does occur, follows, for example, an injury that breaches the skin or the mucous membrane covering the tissues. The infection may be controlled by constitutive opsonins and phagocytosis. If the infection should progress and exceed the capacity of the nonspecific host defense mechanisms, then control may be accomplished by induced immune mechanisms. In such cases control of the infection is usually by specific IgG antibody, complement activation, and phagocytosis. The opsonized bacteria are ingested primarily by neutrophils.

Many bacteria that cause extracellular infections are encapsulated. The capsules block complement activation by the alternative pathway and thereby prevent phagocytosis. Antibody produced during the inducible response binds to the capsular material, bringing about complement activation and phagocytosis. Bacteria that produce extracellular infections usually lack mechanisms to resist being killed once phagocytized. The pneumococci, streptococci, and staphylococci are examples of such bacteria. Toxins, if produced, are neutralized by antibody.

Extracellular infections at mucosal surfaces are often controlled by the actions of specific secretory IgA. This antibody may prevent attachment to mucosal cells and prevent colonization of the mucosa. Secretory IgA, when complexed with the bacteria, can initiate the complement cascade, and lysis may result. If phagocytes are present, possibly in exudate produced as a result of inflammation, phagocytosis may take place. Exudates may bring IgG antibody onto the mucosal surface, supplementing the actions of IgA.

Toxigenic Bacterial Infections

Strongly toxigenic bacteria provide the host with special problems. The toxins they secrete must be neutralized before they can do harm. Toxin neutralization is often more vital than elimination of infectious bacteria.

C. tetani produces a local infection at the site of an injury. The disease tetanus is the result of an exotoxin that diffuses from the site. Immunization against tetanus is carried out by injection of pure toxoid; injection of pure antitoxin alone will prevent the disease from developing. The infection itself is adequately controlled by antibody produced during the primary immune response if the effects of the toxin are blocked by transferred antibody or by antibody produced in the secondary immune response in individuals immunized with toxoid.

S. pyogenes and *C. diphtheria*, like *C. tetani*, may also produce diseases by the actions of exotoxins diffusing from a local site of infection. The clinical signs of scarlet fever, caused by a local infection with *S. pyogenes*, usually in the throat, and of diphtheria, caused by a local infection with *C. diphtheria*, also in the throat, are controlled by elaboration of antitoxins. If the toxins are neutralized by antitoxin promptly, the host can usually control the infection later, with the aid of opsonic antibody and phagocytosis. The local infections caused by these bacteria are, however, more severe than those caused by *C. tetani*. People may develop many *S. pyogenes* infections in the throat, but they can only develop scarlet fever once.

Infections with Gram-negative bacteria may result in endotoxemia. Antibodies to endotoxins will precipitate them *in vitro* but do not neutralize their toxicity. The enzymes released by the complement system following its activation effectively degrade endotoxins.

Intracellular Bacterial Infections

Many bacteria and other parasites that normally grow inside of phagocytes are readily phagocytized but have mechanisms to resist destruction once inside. The mycobacteria causing tuberculosis and leprosy are such intracellular parasites. Opsonic antibody that facilitates phagocytosis is of little use in control of such organisms; rather, macrophage activation induced in the course of the development of the inducible immune response is a major factor in their control. The chronic granulomatous reaction that results from the delayed hypersensitivity reaction provides a barrier to the spread of the infection. Various lymphokines such as gamma-interferon and cachectin (tumor necrosis factor), and the reactive oxygen intermediates and enzymes released by cells activated during the inflammatory process also contribute to the control of microbes growing inside phagocytes.

Intracellular parasites growing in nonphagocytic cells may also induce granulomatous reactions. Cytotoxic lymphocytes in the granulomas may destroy the host cells and, with them, the parasites. For the cytotoxic lymphocyte to be able to determine which cells are infected, however, the host cell membrane must contain parasite-derived molecules.

SUGGESTIONS FOR FURTHER READING

R. M. Atlas. *Microbiology: Fundamentals and Applications,* 2nd edition. Macmillan, New York, 1988.

B. A. Freeman. *Burrows Textbook of Microbiology,* 22nd edition. W. B. Saunders, Philadelphia, 1985.

E. Jawetz, J. L. Melnick, and E. A. Adelberg. *Review of Medical Microbiology,* 17th edition. Appleton & Lange, Norwalk, Connecticut, 1987.

G. P. Youmans, P. Y. Paterson, and H. M. Sommers. *The Biologic and Clinical Basis of Infectious Disease,* 3rd edition. W. B. Saunders, Philadelphia, 1985.

Chapter 14

The Viruses

PAUL J. COTE

Division of Molecular Virology and Immunology
School of Medicine
Georgetown University

INTRODUCTION

Viruses pathogenic for humans and animals were initially identified as *filterable agents.* The terminology developed because viral infection could be produced with infectious fluids that were filtered to eliminate bacteria. This separation is possible because viruses are much smaller than bacteria. Viruses are in fact small packets of protein and nucleic acid that only reproduce inside a susceptible host cell. The proteins of viruses have structural, enzymatic, and regulatory properties, and their function in the virion (virus particle) is to initiate an infection.

Viruses have no intrinsic means to generate energy so they must rely totally on the metabolic machinery of host cells to synthesize new viral components. During the process of viral replication, the nucleic acid of the virus (its genome) becomes an active functional component within the infected cell. In the host cell, newly produced viral proteins and genomic elements assemble into new infectious virions that are then released. Although we usually say that a virus *replicates inside* a host cell, it is probably more correct conceptually to say that a virus *is replicated by* the host cell or that the virus-infected cell is a new entity.

MORPHOLOGY AND STRUCTURE OF VIRUSES

The simplest viruses are helical viruses. They consist of a rodlike helix or coil of nucleic acid and closely associated structural proteins. There are no known animal viruses with naked helical morphology (that is, lacking an outer envelope); however, an example of one found in plants is the tobacco mosaic virus. The simplest animal viruses are naked icosahedral viruses. They consist of a nucleic acid strand within a protein shell called a *capsid* (Figure 14.1a). The capsid consists of a structure created by the regular arrangement of structural subunits called *capsomers.* Each capsomer is composed of a set of viral structural proteins. Viral nucleic acid strands with bound proteins are called *nucleoproteins* and generally have helical morphology; viral genomes within capsids are called *nucleocapsids* and are characterized by icosahedral morphology.

Nucleoproteins or nucleocapsids are internal components of enveloped viruses. The viral envelope is essentially a membrane derived from the host cell and consists of a lipid bilayer with inserted virus encoded proteins. Such proteins are usually glycosylated by host cell enzymes and appear as "spikes" on the viral surface when viewed by electron microscopy (for example, Figures 14.1b and 14.1c). Except for some members of the poxvirus family (see following section) all enveloped viruses lose their infectivity following extraction of their lipid with ethylether. Naked, nonenveloped viruses are unaffected by treatment with ether.

CLASSIFICATION OF VIRUSES

There are two main groups of viruses based on the type of nucleic acid present in the virion. Viruses contain either DNA or RNA, never both. Viruses are further classified into several families based on morphologic, structural, and genetic charac-

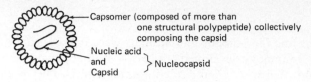

(A) Naked Icosahedral
(e.g., parvovirus, papilloma virus, adenuvirus, picoruavirus)

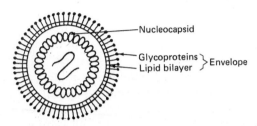

(B) Enveloped Icosahedral
(e.g., herpesvirus, togavirus)

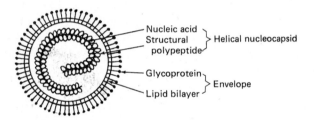

(C) Enveloped Helical
(e.g., Paramyxoviruses, Orthomyxoviruses (segment), Rhabdoviruses)
(round) (pleomorphic) (bullet-shaped)

Figure 14.1 Morphology of viruses. Viruses all consist of either a nucleic acid core and a protective coating of protein or in some cases proteins and lipids. Animal viruses may exist in (a) naked icosahedral, (b) enveloped icosahedral, or (c) enveloped helical forms.

teristics, including the size, structure, and "strandedness" of the nucleic acid (Table 14.1). Viruses are classified further by the organization and function of their genetic coding and regulatory sequences, and also by the functions of specifically encoded enzymes and protein antigens. Some human and animal viruses classified by family are listed in Table 14.1.

Viral pathogens are frequently named after the diseases and the specific symptoms they cause, and the tissues they infect (Table 14.2). This is a poor system because in some cases similar disease conditions may be caused by viruses from different families and in other cases viruses of the same family can cause very distinct diseases.

Table 14.1 CLASSIFICATION AND PROPERTIES OF ANIMAL VIRUSES

Family	Diameter (nm)	CAP	ENV	NA (10^6 D)	Examples
Parvoviridae	18–25	ICH	N	ssDNA (1.8)[a] Linear (+ or −)	Human gastroenteritis viruses, canine parvovirus
Hepadnaviridae	42–45	ICH	E	dsDNA (2.2)[b] Circular (relaxed w/partially SS Region)	Hepatitis B virus, woodchuck hepatitis virus, duck hepatitis B virus, ground squirrel hepatitis virus
Papovaviridae	45–55	ICH	N	dsDNA (3.5)[a] Circular (supercoil)	Human, bovine, and rabbit papilloma viruses
Adenoviridae	70–90	ICH	N	dsDNA (25)[a] Linear	Human adenoviruses
Herpetoviridae	120–150	ICH	E	dsDNA (125)[c] Linear	Herpes simplex I and II, cytomegalovirus, varicella-zoster, Epstein-Barr virus
Poxviridae	200 × 400	Ovoid	C	dsDNA (180)[cd] Linear w/"covalently closed ends"	Smallpox virus, vaccinia virus, myxomavirus
Picornaviridae	20–30	ICH	N	ssRNA (2.1)[e] Linear (+)	Poliovirus, hepatitis A virus, rhinovirus
Togaviridae	40–50	ICH	E	ssRNA (4.2)[e] Linear (+)	Rubella virus, yellow fever virus, Sindbis virus
Orthomyxoviridae	80–90 (PLM)	HEL	E	ssRNA (2.4)[f] Linear (−), 8 segments	Influenza A virus, swine flu virus
Paramyxoviridae	80–120	HEL	E	ssRNA (6.5)[f] Linear (−)	Measles virus, canine distemper virus, mumps virus, Sendai virus
Rhabdoviridae	60 × 225	HEL	E	ssRNA (4.5)[f] Linear (−)	Rabies virus, vesicular stomatitis virus
Bunyaviridae	90–100	HEL	E	ssRNA (5.5)[f] Linear (−) 3 segments	California encephalitis, LaCrosse virus
Arenaviridae	00–300	PLM	E	ssRNA (5)[f] Linear (−), 4 large and 1–3 small segments	Lymphocytic choriomeningitis virus
Coronaviridae	80–160	HEL PLM	E	ssRNA (6.5)[e] Linear (+)	Human respiratory viruses, mouse hepatitis virus

(*continues on page 232*)

A virus that infects and exerts its main pathologic effect in only one primary target tissue is said to have a *restricted tissue tropism*. Viruses that infect many different cell types and produce disease in several organ systems are said to have a *broad tissue tropism*. Viruses that infect and produce disease in a primary target

Table 14.1 (*Continued*)

Family	Diameter (nm)	CAP	ENV	NA (10^6 D)	Examples
Retroviridae	65–150	HEL COIL	E	ssRNA (9)^g Linear (+) (2 copies per virion)	Human T-cell leukemia viruses, human immunodeficiency viruses, mammalian and avian RNA tumor viruses
Reoviridae	70–75	ICH DBL	N	dsRNA (10)^e (10 to 12 segments)	Human reovirus types I, II, and III

CAP = capsid morphology; ICH = icosahedral; HEL = helical; PLM = pleomorphic; COIL = coiled; DBL = double layer of capsid proteins; ENV = presence of envelope; E = classical envelope that is ether-sensitive; N = naked capsid/no envelope; C = complex outer shell of surface proteins that can be considered an envelope based on sensitivity of some members of this family to ether extraction; however, the better known poxviruses are resistant to ether (*e.g.,* examples in table); NA = nucleic acid (with representative molecular weight in megadaltons); ss = single stranded; ds = double stranded; plus (+) refers to polarity of NA strand being the same as that for naturally occurring mRNA codons; minus (−) indicates that the NA strand is present in the opposite polarity from mRNA. DDDP = DNA-dependent DNA polymerase; DDRP = DNA-dependent RNA polymerase; RDRP = RNA-dependent RNA polymerase; and RDDP/RT = RNA-dependent DNA polymerase/reverse transcriptase.

^{a}Uses cellular DDDP and DDRP.

^{b}Has ssRNA intermediate (+) strand transcribed by cellular DDRP; this is made into (−) DNA strand by viral RDDP/RT activity that is then converted to a partially completed dsDNA by endogenous viral DDDP.

^{c}Virus carries or codes for its own DDDP.

^{d}Virus carries or codes for its own DDRP.

^{e}RDRP is synthesized first directly from (+) genomic strand of viral RNA.

^{f}Virus carries and codes for its own RDRP to initiate transcription and replication from (−) genomic strand.

^{g}Virus carries and codes for its own RDDP/RT enzyme to initiate proviral synthesis (see text for details).

tissue, however, may sometimes infect and produce secondary disease in another tissue.

Many viruses are relatively species specific. They cause infection and disease in one or a few specific hosts, whereas others are not species specific and can infect several species in which they may or may not produce disease. Viruses produce a wide range of disorders; these range from acute inflammatory disorders to chronic degenerative disorders; viruses of several families cause cancer or have been implicated as cofactors in the development of cancers.

VIRAL PATHOGENESIS AND ANTIVIRAL STRATEGIES

The cell is the basic unit of biological organization, so most disease processes can be traced to dysfunctions in cells. Many aspects of viral pathogenesis result from the imposition of virus replication on the normal host cell physiology. Cellular malfunctions due to viral infection become manifest when cellular malfunctions disrupt tissue and organ systems. Many of the fundamental processes involved in

Table 14.2 CLASSIFICATION OF PATHOGENIC ANIMAL AND HUMAN VIRUSES

Symptoms/tissue	Viral pathogen	Virus family
Respiratory	Influenza A virus	Orthomyxoviridae (RNA)
	Coronaviruses	Coronaviridae (RNA)
	Rhinoviruses	Picornaviridae (RNA)
	Measles virus	Paramyxoviridae (RNA)
	Adenoviruses	Adenoviridae (DNA)
	Smallpox virus	Poxviridae (DNA)
Neurological	Encephalitis viruses	Bunyaviridae (RNA)
	Encephalitis viruses	Togaviridae (RNA)
	Rabies virus	Rhabdoviridae (RNA)
	Measles virus (SSPE)	Paramyxoviridae (RNA)
	Poliovirus	Picornaviridae (RNA)
	Immunodeficiency virus	Retroviridae (RNA)
	Herpes simplex type I	Herpetoviridae (DNA)
Gastrointestinal/Viscera	Infant gastroenteritis	Reoviridae (RNA)
	Hog cholera virus	Togaviridae (RNA)
	Gastroenteritis virus	Parvoviridae (DNA)
	Smallpox virus	Poxviridae (DNA)
Hepatitis	Hepatitis A virus	Picornaviridae (RNA)
	Yellow fever virus	Togaviridae (RNA)
	Mouse hepatitis virus	Coronaviridae (RNA)
	Hepatitis B virus	Hepadnaviridae (DNA)
	Epstein-Barr virus	Herpetoviridae (DNA)
Skin and mucosal lesions	Rubella virus	Togaviridae (RNA)
	Measles virus	Paramyxoviridae (RNA)
	Papilloma viruses	Papovaviridae (DNA)
	Varicella (chicken pox)	Herpetoviridae (DNA)
	Herpes simplex I and II	Herpetoviridae (DNA)
	Smallpox virus	Poxviridae (DNA)
Lymphoid	Measles virus	Paramyxoviridae (RNA)
	Immunodeficiency virus	Retroviridae (RNA)
	Epstein-Barr virus	Herpetoviridae (DNA)
Tumors		
Leukemia/Lymphoma	Chronic leukemia viruses	Retroviridae (RNA)
	Acute leukemia viruses	Retroviridae (RNA)
	Epstein-Barr virus (?)	Herpetoviridae (DNA)
Mammary carcinoma	Mouse mammary tumor virus	Retroviridae (RNA)
Cervical carcinoma	Human papilloma virus (?)	Papovaviridae (DNA)
	Herpes simplex II (?)	Herpetoviridae (DNA)
Nasopharyngeal	Herpes simplex I (?)	Herpetoviridae (DNA)
Hepatomas	Hepatitis B virus	Hepadnaviridae (DNA)
	Woodchuck hepatitis virus	Hepadnaviridae (DNA)
Polyomas	Simian virus 40	Papovaviridae (DNA)
Myxomas	Rabbit myxomatosis virus	Poxviridae (DNA)

viral pathogenesis have been elucidated using cell culture systems and experimental animals.

Viral infection is initiated following virus adsorption, penetration, and uncoating (Figure 14.2). The nucleic acids of all DNA viruses are reproduced in the cell nucleus, except those of the poxviruses, which are reproduced in the cytoplasm. The nucleic acids of all RNA viruses are reproduced in the cytoplasm, except for retroviruses and certain myxoviruses (for example, influenza A virus). The parental genomic element formed during early nucleic acid synthesis acts as a template for synthesis of new viral genomes and messenger RNA transcription; it is called the *replicative form (RF)*. The RF gives rise to progeny viral nucleic acids, detected

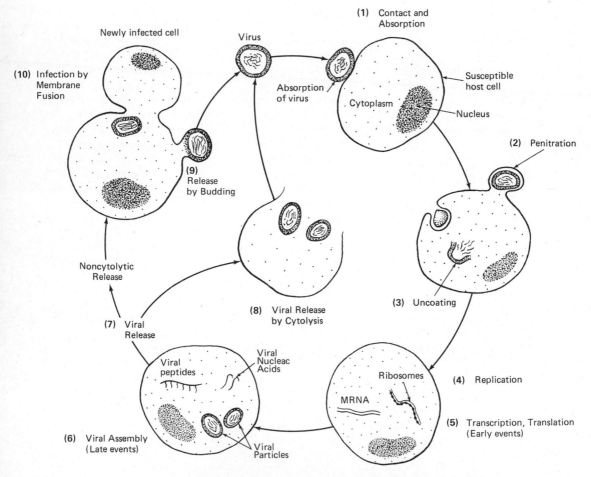

Figure 14.2 Viral replication can be considered to consist of a number of steps. (1) The virus must be absorbed onto the host cell; (2) it must penetrate the cell; (3) it must uncoat inside the cell either in the nucleus or the cytoplasm; (4) it must replicate. In replication there are (5) early events that prepare the cell for virus synthesis and (6) late events that result in production of virus and assembly. Finally the virus must (7) escape from the cell by (8) causing cell lysis; (9) by budding or (10) by moving from one cell directly to another through cell membrane fusion.

as replicative intermediates in addition to viral mRNA. Translation of viral mRNA gives rise to the viral proteins. The processes of assembly, maturation, and release of progeny virions from cells are generally associated with cytopathic effects. These effects include formation of inclusion bodies, cytolysis, and cell fusion.

Many factors determine susceptibility of cells to viral infection. However, the outcome of viral infections in terms of host survival is governed mainly by the host immune response to antigenic viral proteins (Figure 14.3). The pathology of viral diseases may be due to host cell death, chronic inflammation in tissues, or immunopathologic effects associated with infection of cells of the immune system.

Many viruses become latent after infection; viral latency may be a part of the natural life cycle of the virus or may be imposed on the virus as a result of the host's immune response (Figure 14.4). Latency allows the viral genome to persist in a quiescent or inactive state in the host, and frequently leads to the development of recurrent disease. Reactivation of the genome and production of new virus contribute to cellular transformation and the development of malignancies.

Viral infections resolve or persist depending on the efficacy of the total antiviral response of the host, including adaptive immunity and natural surveillance. Although some viral antigens stimulate antibody production independently of help from T-cells, most viral antigens induce immune responses that are dependent on T-helper cells (Chapter 8). Antibodies to the outer viral proteins can neutralize the infectivity of free virus, and antibody to these and other components facilitate viral clearance. Antibodies also aid in the elimination of virus-infected cells by the mechanisms of complement-dependent lysis and antibody-dependent cellular cytotoxicity. Cell-mediated effector mechanisms are active in individuals with many viral infections. Specific killing of virus-infected cells is mediated by cytotoxic T-cells that recognize viral antigens associated with host histocompatibility proteins in the host cell membranes (Chapter 9). Natural killer cells may participate in the elimination of infected or transformed cells, but the recognition processes are poorly understood.

In persistent infections, the infection is not cured and the viral genome remains inside the host cell. The infected cell may or may not express significant amounts of virus or viral antigens, depending on the state of the viral genome (that is, latent

(1) Infection Blocking
   Virus–neutralizing antibody
      Phagocytosis
      Complement–mediated lysis

(2) Fusion Inhibition
   Antibody mediated

(3) Inhibition of Viral Growth in Cells
   Interferons

(4) Destruction of Infected Host Cells
   Cytolytic I–cells
   Antibody–dependent cell lysis
      Killer (K) cells
      Natural killer (NK) cells
      Macrophages

Figure 14.3 Host resistance mechanisms. (1) Extracellular virus may be prevented from entering cells by virus-specific antibody. (2) Virus movement from cell to cell by fusion may be blocked by antibody to virus-produced fusogenes in the cell membrane. (3) Interferons and possibly other substances may inhibit viral growth in cells. (4) Virus may be destroyed or prevented from reproducing by destruction of infected host cells.

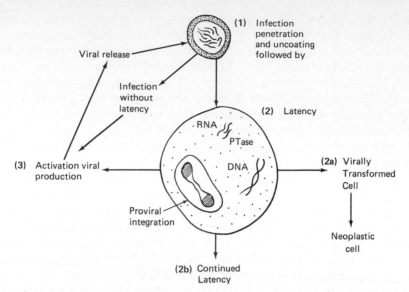

Figure 14.4 Viral latency. After (1) entry into a cell virus may integrate and (2) become inactive or latent. The virus genone may (2a) cause neoplastic transformation of the cell, (2b) continue latent, or (3) become activated and reproduce.

or active). In persistent infections where the viral genome becomes latent, the cell expresses few viral antigens and is less susceptible to immune attack. However, persistent infections in which active viral antigen production occurs frequently result in tissue injury from the deposition of immune complexes and complement on the infected cells. Persistent expression of viral antigen by infected cells can also induce cell-mediated immune responses and delayed type hypersensitivity reactions (Chapter 10), leading to chronic inflammation and tissue damage at the site of infection.

There are only a few drugs presently available that are effective against viral infections. The virus–host cell interactions are so intimate that it is difficult to interfere with viral functions and not damage host cell function. Successful antiviral therapies require drugs that are active against virus-specific targets, such as viral enzymes and regulatory proteins, but not against host cell systems. They may also act by stimulating natural intracellular processes that prevent replication and spread of viruses.

Immunization to prevent infection has been the most important and successful antiviral strategy available. Immunization has been particularly effective against acute viral infections.

A survey of viral diseases and their etiologic agents is presented in the next section and is summarized in Table 14.2. Diseases are grouped by whether the causative virus produces acute infection or persistent infection. The information in Table 14.1 can be referred to as you read the rest of this chapter.

EXAMPLES OF DISEASES RESULTING FROM ACUTE VIRAL INFECTIONS

Smallpox

Smallpox was a very common disease of humans in the fifteenth and sixteenth centuries and was still common in many areas of the world until recently. It was observed in sporadic and epidemic outbreaks with high or low mortality. Jenner developed the first safe vaccination procedure against smallpox (Chapter 17).

The etiologic agent of smallpox was the variola virus, a large and complex DNA virus (Poxviridae, Table 14.1). It naturally infected humans and could also be transmitted to some higher primates. Two distinct forms of the disease occurred in humans: variola major, with 25 to 50 percent mortality, and variola minor (alastrim, or classical smallpox), which had less than 1 percent mortality. Smallpox was a highly contagious disease spread mainly by inhalation of virus. Virus also entered through breaks in the skin, and infection could result from contact with pock fluids or contaminated clothing and bedding (fomites). Poxviruses survived in the environment for a short time because the virion had a protective fibrous protein outer coat. Infection, however, usually was by relatively close contact with people with active cases.

Smallpox produced an acute infection. After inhalation the virus first multiplied in mucosal cells of the upper respiratory tract, and then infection spread to the regional lymph nodes. A mild transient viremia was followed by infection of the liver, spleen, and lungs. In these organs multiplication continued for about 12 to 16 days. Few symptoms were present at this stage, and it was thus referred to as the *incubation period.* The secondary viremia that ensued produced generalized symptoms including fever, pain, headache, malaise, and rash. Epidermal cells then became infected, and the virus multiplied over an additional two-week period. During this phase there was necrosis of epidermal cells and leukocytic infiltration, leading to formation of the characteristic skin pustules, or pocks. Lesions similar to pock lesions may also have formed in the liver and other soft tissues. In nonfatal cases the skin lesions eventually resolved by "crusting" and scarification, and the infection terminated with the development of permanent immunity.

Variola virus differed from other DNA viruses in that it replicated entirely in the cytoplasm of infected cells. The characteristic cytoplasmic inclusion bodies (Guarneri bodies) contained viral antigens, nucleic acids, and maturing virus particles. Virus production ultimately killed the infected cells, and progeny virions were released by cytolysis.

The outer coat of variola virus contained a hemagglutinating protein that mediated virus uptake by cells; this was the main target for virus-neutralizing antibodies. Viral dissemination in the primary viremic phase was prevented by vaccination because vaccination induces virus-neutralizing antibodies. A worldwide vaccination program initiated by the World Health Organization led to the eradication of smallpox in the present century.

Rabies

In early times, rabid animals and humans were thought to be "possessed." However, by 1804 the infectious nature of the disease was well recognized. In the 1880s, Pasteur attenuated the virus in mice by serial passage of brain homogenates from rabid dogs. The passaged material was used as a postexposure vaccine for persons bitten by rabid animals. In 1903, Negri showed that a filterable agent produced the disease in animals and became the first to demonstrate the characteristic cytoplasmic inclusion bodies of rabies, the Negri bodies, in neural cells.

Rabies is caused by a bullet-shaped, RNA-containing virus that has been classed with the Rhabdoviridae (Table 14.1). It can infect virtually all mammals and is transmitted in saliva inoculated by the bite of diseased animals. Rabies may sometimes be acquired by inhalation of aerosols in caves inhabited by large numbers of rabid bats. Rabies virus has a worldwide distribution, and there is a considerable reservoir of the virus in wild animals that continues to frustrate control efforts. The main sources of human rabies infections are unvaccinated pets that contract the virus from wild animals. Most control efforts are directed at the pet population. Attempts to control the infection in wild animals may be possible by use of oral vaccines in bait.

Rabies follows an acute course of infection that causes death in a high proportion of individuals who develop clinical disease. Virus enters a bite wound with infectious saliva and replicates locally in muscle cells and other cells at the site of injury. The incubation period is 20 to 60 days in humans. There is little hematogenous spread of rabies virus. Instead, the virus enters nerve endings and travels in the nerves to the central nervous system. Infection of nerves causes the *prodromal phase,* which is characterized by sensations at the site of injury, fever, and changes in temperament. The *excitative phase* correlates with virus multiplication in the brain, and during this phase there is spread of virus through efferent nerves to the salivary glands. Virus multiplication in the salivary glands is associated with symptoms such as difficulty in swallowing and frothing at the mouth. It is from these symptoms that the term *hydrophobia* is derived. The *convulsive phase* is characterized by seizures and terminates in death within three to five days.

Because the lesions detected in the central nervous system at autopsies are seldom extensive, it is thought that the mortality in rabies is probably caused by the disruption of vital functions mediated by specific neurons. Specific groups of neurons become infected, but the virus does not cause cytolysis of these cells. The virus reproduces in the cytoplasm and matures by budding through the cell membrane. The mechanism of host protection induced by administration of vaccine is not well understood, but it is probably related to cell-mediated destruction of infected cells in the bite wound and to the antibody-mediated neutralization of progeny virions before they invade the nervous system. The currently used rabies vaccines consist of inactivated virus derived from cell cultures and require only a few inoculations to elicit immunity.

The envelope glycoprotein component of rabies virus has been shown experimentally to play a role in the pathogenesis of this disease. The lethal characteristics for mice of rabies virus are determined by a single amino acid in the envelope glycoprotein. Viruses having envelope glycoproteins with isoleucine or glutamine substituted for arginine at residue 333 are attenuated, whereas revertants with arginine at this site are lethal.

Polio

Polio was first described in the eighteenth century. Epidemics occurred until 1955, when attenuated and inactivated polio vaccines came into wide use. The disease still occurs sporadically, usually in unvaccinated people. Poliovirus was one of the first viruses propagated in cell culture, and its complete crystallographic structure is known today.

Poliovirus is a relatively small, naked icosahedral virus with a single stranded RNA genome. Its family, the Picornaviridae (Table 14.1), includes the rhinoviruses, which cause the common cold, and the hepatitis A virus, which causes acute liver disease. Humans are the natural hosts of poliovirus. The virus infects primarily intestinal mucosal cells but may infect other cells, including neurons. The virus can be transmitted to the chimpanzee, and strains are available that infect mice.

In nature the virus spreads from person to person by ingestion of food and water contaminated with fecal material. The virus is stable in the environment and is not inactivated by the stomach acids. Poliovirus infection in humans can be unapparent. This is the most common form of infection. Poliovirus infection can also cause acute mild illness, acute nonparalytic aseptic meningitis, or paralytic poliomyelitis. The paralytic disease results in permanent paralysis and occurs more often in older than in younger children. Between 1940 and 1950, improved infant health care practices in developed countries prevented infections of young children. Infection then occurred when the children were older, and there was therefore a greater incidence of paralytic disease.

Early in the infection, poliovirus replicates in the oropharyngeal and intestinal mucosal cells and is shed into the throat and feces. The virus then infects the tonsils and Peyer's patches, and the cervical and mesenteric lymph nodes. After from 7 to 14 days, a transient viremia develops and is sometimes followed by clinical recovery. In other individuals there is further dissemination of virus to susceptible nonneural tissues. This gives rise to systemic illness. By 15 to 20 days after infection, the virus may enter the central nervous system and cause neurologic effects. Virus replication in the central nervous system results in the death of neurons. This is fatal in cases of infection of the medullary portion of the brain but gives rise to variable degrees of paralysis when the infection is in the cortex or spinal cord. Partial or complete recovery from paralysis depends on host factors such as compensatory muscle hypertrophy and use of alternate efferent motor circuits. Only from 1 to 2 percent of all poliovirus infections result in central nervous system involvement, but during epidemics the overall number of individuals with paralytic disease can be quite high.

Poliovirus has a relatively simple method of replication. The virus enters susceptible cells following attachment to cellular lipoprotein receptors. New virus production occurs within the cytoplasm, and cells are lysed to release the progeny virions. The single-stranded RNA genome is plus-stranded, as is cellular messenger

RNA. This enables the viral RNA to be translated directly after uncoating. The result of translation is a single large protein that is cleaved into an RNA-dependent RNA polymerase, and also into four polypeptides that form the individual capsomers of the nucleocapsid. The genomic RNA is copied by the viral polymerase into a complementary strand of RNA that serves as the replicative form of the virus. New virions assemble in the cytoplasm within inclusion bodies and are released following cytolysis.

The attenuated Sabin vaccine and the inactivated Salk vaccine contain the capsid proteins of the three major serotypes of poliovirus. Immunity is conferred by the induction of virus-neutralizing antibodies to the capsid proteins. Infection of neurons is prevented by these neutralizing antibodies. Compared to inactivated vaccines, attenuated live vaccines require smaller initial quantities of virus, and viral replication is required for induction of immunity. They must therefore be handled carefully during distribution and use to prevent inactivation and ensure infectivity. The major advantage of the inactivated vaccine, despite the need for larger initial amounts of virus, is that activation eliminates the possibility of reversion to the wild type virus.

Influenza A

Flulike symptoms can be produced by several viruses and by other infectious agents, including bacteria. Influenza imposes a significant disease burden on the population because it occurs in large epidemics every two to four years. The pandemics of 1743, 1889–1892, and 1918–1919 were widespread and caused particularly serious disease. During the last worldwide influenza pandemic (1918–1919) over 80 million people became ill and there were many deaths. In this pandemic *Hemophilus influenza* was a common cause of a secondary bacterial pneumonia and was initially thought to be the cause of the pandemic. Many of the people who died, however, did so without secondary bacterial infection. In 1933 the pandemic was shown to be caused by a filterable agent, later named influenza virus, type A. Type A influenza viruses are genetically distinct from type B and C influenza viruses and are distinguishable and classified on the basis of serologic differences among their nucleocapsid antigens.

Human influenza A virus is a typical enveloped virus with a helical RNA-containing nucleoprotein (Orthomyxoviridae, Table 14.1). Related influenza A viruses also infect animals of a variety of species; one is the cause of swine flu. Influenza virus is normally inhaled and multiplies initially in mucosal cells of the upper respiratory tract. There is no viremic phase, but the acute disease is nonetheless associated with general symptoms such as malaise and fever. Virus replication kills mucosal cells and results in necrosis and desquamation of the mucosa. The virus may spread to the lungs, where it can cause moderate to severe damage, including bronchial necrosis, hemorrhage, and edema. As free virus inhibits the uptake of bacteria by phagocytes, severe secondary bacterial pneumonia may sometimes develop.

The neuraminidase enables influenza virus to penetrate mucous secretions by virtue of its enzymatic activity. Neuraminidase also promotes the release of the virions as they bud from the cell surface. The envelope hemagglutinin serves to attach the virus to cells by binding to cell receptors. The virus then enters the cell in an endosomal vesicle. As the pH of the vesicle becomes acidic, the hemagglutinin causes fusion of the viral envelope with the endosomal membrane, resulting in uncoating and release of the viral nucleocapsid into the cell cytoplasm. Influenza viruses, unlike most RNA viruses, replicate in the cell nucleus rather than in the cytoplasm. The influenza virus has a negative-stranded RNA that is not translated directly by the host cell. Initiation of replication is possible because the virus encodes and packages its own RNA-dependent RNA polymerase. The viral RNA consists of eight different single-stranded segments, each coding for at least one of the major viral proteins. If two strains of influenza A virus infect the same cell, an interchange of entire genomic segments can occur; this is referred to as *high-frequency recombination.* Unlike classical genetic recombination, splicing and rejoining of the nucleic acid is *not* required in this process.

At least 12 different hemagglutinin (H) and 9 different neuraminidases (N) occur in influenza A viruses and give rise to a number of parental serotypes. The great flu pandemic of 1918–1919 was apparently caused by a recombinant type A virus that contained the human type 1 neuraminidase and the swine flu hemagglutinin. Other epidemics have also resulted from viruses produced by high-frequency recombination because the new protein alters viral infectivity and pathogenicity. This process is referred to as *antigenic shift.* The possibility that the highly virulent "swine flu variant" was present in 1976 led to the vaccination of over 40 million people. However, the 1976 outbreak turned out to be caused by a swine flu virus that was not highly virulent in humans.

In addition to changes in the set of envelope proteins brought about by antigenic shift, the viral envelope genes can undergo small mutational changes resulting in amino acid sequence divergence in the envelope protein. These changes are called *antigenic drift* to imply that they occur *within* a given parental HN serotype. The changes in serotype resulting from antigenic drift frequently enable the variants to evade neutralization by humoral antibody to the parent type and may permit reinfection of a previously exposed host.

EXAMPLES OF DISEASES RESULTING FROM VIRAL INFECTIONS THAT MAY EITHER RESOLVE OR PERSIST

Measles and Subacute Sclerosing Panencephalitis

Measles was first described in the seventeenth century and was shown to be infectious in 1758 by transmission to human volunteers. The disease was transmitted to monkeys in 1911, and in 1954 Enders isolated and grew the causative virus in cells in culture. The virus belongs to the Paramyxoviridae family of large enveloped RNA viruses (Table 14.1). The acute disease caused by measles virus is called *rubeola.* Rubeola is distinct from rubella, or German measles, which is caused by a Togavirus (Tables 14.1 and 14.2). The measles virus is related to the distemper virus of dogs, the Sendai virus of mice, and the rinderpest virus of cattle. Other members of the Paramyxoviridae include mumps virus and parainfluenza virus.

Measles is one of the most infectious diseases known. It is present in respiratory secretions before the development of symptoms. In children, in which it usually occurs, it causes an acute illness that confers permanent immunity. The measles virus multiplies first in the mucosal cells of the upper respiratory tract and in cells in the regional lymph nodes. It is then shed into the secretions and bloodstream. The prodromal phase, characterized by respiratory symptoms, fever, and the presence of red macules called *Koplik spots* inside the cheeks, occurs when the virus is in the blood. Following the prodromal stage, the virus is disseminated to previously uninfected lymphoid tissues and to basal epidermal cells. Infection of the latter cells results in the measles rash.

Measles virus infection of cells of the immune system, particularly of B- and T-lymphocytes, causes transient immunosuppression. Natural killer cell activity is also depressed during acute measles virus infections, but the mechanism of this suppression is less clear.

The virus infects cells of numerous types and replicates in the cytoplasm. It is noncytolytic and matures by budding from the plasma membrane. The virus has a single-stranded unsegmented RNA of negative polarity. This RNA codes for a matrix protein, a nucleoprotein, a phosphorylating protein, an RNA-dependent RNA polymerase, and two envelope structural proteins. One envelope protein is a combined hemagglutinin and a neuraminidase, and the other induces membrane fusion. The neuraminidase-hemagglutinating protein mediates attachment of virus to cells and the fusion protein mediates penetration.

In people with measles, multinucleated giant cells are frequently found in respiratory secretions. Antibodies to the neuraminidase-hemagglutinating proteins and some antibodies to the fusion protein neutralize virus infectivity; however, only antibodies to the fusion protein inhibit virus-mediated fusion of cells.

There is only one serotype of measles virus, so a monovalent vaccine is all that is needed. An attenuated strain of the virus is used. Vaccination against measles should not take place before nine months of age. Passively acquired maternal antibody to measles virus normally protects young children from infection, but for reasons not fully understood, the maternal antibody appears to impede or alter the child's immune response to the vaccine. In such individuals the course of subsequent infection may be altered to favor persistent viral infection in lymphoid tissues and the central nervous system. These infections can persist for a long time and cause the development of the debilitating condition known as *subacute sclerosing panencephalitis.* In children with this type of measles infection, there may be progressive destruction of the nervous system that is ultimately fatal.

Warts and Papillomatous Tumors

A filterable agent was demonstrated to transmit human warts in 1907. Warts rarely become malignant in humans. In the 1930s Shope demonstrated that myxoma virus, a papilloma-inducing virus of rabbits, could cause malignant squamous cell carcinoma. He showed that domestic rabbits infected with myxoma virus developed malignancy more frequently than did wild cottontail rabbits and that topical application of certain chemicals increased the incidence of malignancy. Thus, both host genetic factors and environmental agents were shown to act as cofactors in the development of the virus-induced malignancy.

Papilloma viruses are small naked icosahedral viruses composed of a capsid and a closed circular double-stranded DNA molecule with superhelical conformation (Table 14.1). These viruses occur in a variety of mammals. Infection that results in production of complete virus is generally species specific. Transmission of virus occurs by contamination of mucosal surfaces or injured skin. The viruses have not been grown in culture and therefore must be obtained from susceptible animals. The bovine papilloma virus is a prototype of this group of viruses.

A variety of different serotypes of human papilloma virus that differ in their major capsid antigens exist. Most cause benign warts, including the familiar skin wart and the deeply recessed plantar wart. The viral DNA replicates as an episomal element in dermal cells, enhancing host cell proliferation and differentiation into keratinized cells. It is during the keratinization process that new viral components are expressed and assembled.

Warts usually regress spontaneously, and regression may occur in several locations at once. This pattern of rejection suggests an immune-mediated mechanism. This suggestion is further supported by the observation that rabbits cured of benign papillomas are resistant to subsequent challenge with the virus that caused them.

Papilloma viruses may be transmitted during sexual contact. The mucosal infections that result can be asymptomatic or can give rise to characteristic lesions in the ano-genital and cervical areas. Development of papillomas in these areas has been linked epidemiologically with an increased risk of developing genital tumors and cervical carcinomas.

Acute and Chronic Type B Hepatitis and Hepatocellular Carcinoma

Yellow jaundice associated with inflammation of the liver was previously classified by the mode of acquisition, length of incubation period, and course of disease. Infectious hepatitis occurred epidemically, was transmitted by fecal contamination of food and water, and had a short incubation period that was followed by acute liver disease and recovery. In contrast, serum hepatitis was transmitted by blood transfusion or contact with infected body fluids and had a longer incubation period that was followed by acute disease and occasional progression to chronicity. Since the discovery of the etiologic agents, these names are no longer used. Infectious hepatitis is now referred to as *type A hepatitis* and is caused by hepatitis A virus, a RNA-containing picornavirus (Table 14.1). Serum hepatitis is now known as *type B hepatitis* and is caused by the hepatitis B virus , which is a small DNA-containing virus belonging to the Hepadnaviridae (Table 14.1).

Hepatitis B virus is a double-shelled structure. It consists of an inner nucleocapsid core and an outer shell of coat proteins with some associated lipids. During infection, hepatocytes produce virions as well as noninfectious subviral structures consisting of the outer surface proteins. Blumberg discovered the subviral particles in the mid-1960s, but the virion was not discovered until the 1970s by Dane. There are 10^4 to 10^6 subviral particles for each virion in the blood. Chronic carriers of the hepatitis B virus who have no overt symptoms can have up to 500 μgs of total viral surface protein per milliliter of plasma. The spread of hepatitis B virus by blood and blood products used in therapy was common before the development of serologic assays for detection of the viral surface antigen.

Hepatitis B virus induces a broad spectrum of liver diseases in humans. There is no correlation between the form of the disease produced and the subtype of the virus present. The virus is not particularly cytolytic. Both host inflammatory responses and viral effects appear to contribute to cell and organ damage.

The modes of transmission and the nature of the liver disease caused by infection vary from region to region. For example, in Western societies, most infections occur in adults as a result of contact with infectious body fluids such as blood or semen. The infection is common among intravenous drug abusers and among male homosexuals, for whom it is a common venereal disease. The infections are either inapparent or produce acute hepatitis. Recovery follows production of antibodies to the viral surface antigens. Fulminant acute hepatitis may occur, resulting in death, but this is rare. In contrast, in the Orient and sub-Saharan Africa the infections occur in the young. Infants mainly acquire infections from mothers who are chronic carriers of the virus. There is no clear evidence for infection of the fetus, so it is probable that transmission from mothers usually occurs sometime during or shortly after birth.

Infections in the very young often result in persistence of infection throughout the lifespan of the individual. In persistently infected people, the virus may replicate in the hepatocytes, exist in a quiescent episomal state, or be integrated into the host cell DNA. Integrated viral DNA is frequently incomplete and no longer gives rise to new virus, but may still program production of surface antigens. Persistent infection may be asymptomatic or may cause liver inflammation, which frequently results in liver cirrhosis and, after many years, hepatocellular carcinoma. At present, there are over 250 million chronic carriers of hepatitis B virus worldwide.

Hepatitis B virus infects only humans and a few higher primates, including the chimpanzee. The hepadnaviruses are essentially hepatotropic, although recent evidence indicates that they can also infect lymphocytes *in vivo.* The duck hepadnavirus also infects pancreatic cells. Although the chimpanzee is useful for study of hepatitis B virus infection, the disease produced in this animal is less severe than that produced in humans. However, studies of hepatitis B virus infection in the chimpanzee were directly responsible for the development of a safe and effective vaccine.

The naturally occurring woodchuck hepatitis virus and its rodent host, the eastern woodchuck (*Marmota monax*), are used to study both acute and chronic hepatitis. Persistent infections with the woodchuck virus invariably result in chronic hepatitis and hepatocellular carcinoma within two to four years, so that it is now possible to study hepadnavirus-induced liver cancer within a realistic time span. Woodchucks are also being used for the development and testing of therapies for chronic viral infection and disease.

Hepadnaviruses replicate their DNA by a complex and unique mechanism involving a virally encoded DNA-polymerase having both DNA-dependent and RNA-dependent polymerase activities (Table 14.1, footnote *b*). Hepadnaviruses make highly efficient use of their small genome for encoding proteins. The genome has overlapping coding sequences in two of the three possible reading frames. One of the major reading frames encompasses most of the viral genome and encodes the viral polymerase. The other reading frame contains at least three genes for other viral proteins; the surface and core protein coding sequences each have two or three different starting codons in the same reading frame. These give rise, respectively, to sets of structurally and antigenically related surface proteins and to core proteins that form the nucleocapsid and other soluble products.

The first hepatitis B virus vaccine consisted of plasma-derived surface antigen particles, cost about $100 per person, and was too costly for application on a worldwide scale. The surface antigen particles are now produced more cheaply in cultures of yeast into which the viral surface protein gene has been introduced by recombinant DNA technology. All of the vaccines function by stimulating production of antibodies to viral surface proteins. These antibodies neutralize the virus and promote its phagocytosis. Male homosexuals and children born to chronic hepatitis B virus carriers are currently being vaccinated in an effort to prevent infection.

DISEASES ASSOCIATED WITH PERSISTENT VIRAL INFECTIONS

Recurrent Herpes and Epithelial Cell Carcinomas

Herpes simplex viruses (HSVs) are responsible for the recurrent "cold sores" many individuals develop on their lips and for similar sores in the genital region. The introduction of the birth control pill and the relaxation of sexual mores in the United States in the late 1960s ushered in the great herpes epidemic of the 1970s. The HSVs have been implicated in the etiology of several human tumors.

The HSVs are large enveloped DNA viruses that are members of the Herpetoviridae (Table 14.1). The ability to produce latent infections is a property of all members of the Herpetoviridae, including cytomegalovirus, varicella/zoster virus, and Epstein-Barr virus.

In latent infections, the primary symptoms resulting from virus replication resolve, and viral genomes become quiescent and persist in only a few cells. In fact, when quiescent, viral genomes and antigens are extremely difficult to detect in host tissues. In latent infections, the virus occasionally reactivates and new progeny virions are produced. Stress may play a role in viral reactivation. Virus reactivation results in the development of recurrent lesions near the site of the initial infection.

Serological criteria are used to classify HSVs into the two types that occur, called *HSV I* and *HSV II.* Viruses of the two serotypes cause lesions in different areas of the body because they infect different nerve ganglia and are transmitted by different forms of contact. HSV I is usually transmitted orally, whereas transmission of HSV II is usually venereal. Both viruses can infect and produce lesions in both areas, however.

Primary infection with HSV 1 is generally inapparent; however, 15 percent of infections result in gingivostomatitis, with multiplication of virus in oral mucosal cells. The virus also replicates in regional lymph nodes and may cause viremia and disseminated disease. In some cases, HSV I causes fatal encephalitis. This results from spread of virus into the cortex, where it precipitates inflammatory disease. More often the virus enters peripheral nerve endings in the oral region and migrates to the trigeminal ganglion, where it becomes latent. HSV I has been implicated as a cause of nasopharyngeal carcinoma. HSV II infects mainly the genital or ano-rectal mucosa and ultimately becomes latent in the sacral ganglion. Generalized herpes infections often occur in children born to women with recurrent genital herpes lesions. There is a higher risk than normal of cervical cancer in women that develop recurrent herpetic lesions on the cervix.

The nucleic acids and nucleocapsids of herpesviruses are assembled in the cell nucleus and bud through the nuclear membrane. They acquire their envelope during budding. The mature virion is not directly cytolytic. It spreads from cell to cell by a process of cell fusion or after release by exocytosis. The recurrent lesions on the oral and genital mucosa result from the host immune response to virus released from neural endings.

Replication of herpesvirus DNA is a complex process. It involves the formation of four types of DNA and the controlled sequential expression of viral genes. In the latent state, the viral genome may be an episome or may be partially or entirely integrated into the host genome. Only a very few cells in the ganglia become latently infected, perhaps with as few as 1 viral genomic equivalent per 10 neurons. During latency the majority of the genome is not transcribed into RNA. However, at least one of the genes may be expressed at very low levels. The product of this gene may promote the expression of other viral genes and down-regulate its own activity. It may also regulate the function of the infected neuron.

Infectious Mononucleosis and Malignant Lymphomas

''Kissing disease'' is one name for an acute illness of adolescents and young adults referred to more correctly as *infectious mononucleosis.* The disease is character-ized by lymphadenopathy, mild hepatitis, abnormal mononuclear lymphocytes, and large amounts of heterophile antibodies in the blood. Infectious mononucleo-sis is caused by the Epstein-Barr virus (EBV), a member of the Herpetoviridae (Table 14.1). EBV is transmitted with infectious body fluids, most commonly saliva. The virus is lymphotropic, infecting B-cells. Primary infection in early childhood is usually asymptomatic, but 30 to 50 percent of individuals infected in early adolescence develop clinical disease. Most people possess antibodies to EBV, indicating prior exposure, but only about 15 percent of seropositive persons shed virus in the saliva.

The virus first infects cells of the buccal mucosa or the salivary glands and then infects B-cells in pharyngeal lymphoid tissue. The virus then disseminates to B-cells throughout the body. After dissemination the virus may continue to replicate or may become latent. Lymphocytes carrying the latent viral genome in episomal form become transformed, or immortalized, and can be propagated in long-term culture. In infected people, the proliferation of transformed B-cells is limited in most cases by the host immune response, but latently infected cells that do divide serve as a reservoir for the virus. The host defenses to EBV include the actions of natural killer cells, virus-specific cytotoxic lymphocytes, and antiviral antibodies. Most of the abnormal mononuclear cells present in the blood early in the course of EBV infection are cytotoxic lymphocytes that specifically kill virus-infected B-cells. The EBV causes polyclonal activation of B-cells that results in production of heterophile antibodies that agglutinate sheep red blood cells. Although during the acute phase of infection there is polyclonal B-cell activation and activation of virus-specific B-cells, there is a transient suppression of cell-mediated immunity to many antigens.

EBV infection is associated with a high incidence of Burkitt's lymphoma among certain peoples of Africa. Host genetic factors may be responsible, for the virus is not always present in people with Burkitt's lymphoma who live in other parts of the world. Generalized lymphomas of various types may develop in immunosuppressed people who carry the EBV. Burkitt's lymphoma in Africans may therefore be a result of immunosuppression caused by other infections. Malaria is often suggested in this context.

Human T-Cell Leukemias

The first demonstration that a tumor could be induced by a viral agent occurred in 1908. Ellerman and Bang caused leukemia in healthy chickens by inoculation of a cell-free filtrate of blood from leukemic chickens. Since then, leukemia-, sarcoma-, and carcinoma-inducing viruses have been discovered in a number of species of animals. The virion of the leukemia-inducing viruses contains two copies of plus-stranded RNA. In 1964, Temin showed that specific inhibitors of DNA synthesis blocked the replication of these RNA viruses in cultured cells and proposed that their replication required DNA synthesis.

In 1970 Temin and Baltimore independently demonstrated a virally encoded enzyme that transcribes RNA into DNA. This enzyme, RNA-dependent DNA polymerase, is a reverse transcriptase. Prior to this, it had generally been accepted that cellular and viral DNA was the template for production of messenger RNA. The only known exception to this pattern occurred in the nontumorigenic RNA viruses that produced their new genomic RNA on their old genomic RNA and transcribed their messenger RNA by the virus-specific, RNA-dependent RNA polymerase.

The replication process in the RNA tumor viruses is unique. The single-stranded viral RNA template is used to produce an initial DNA–RNA hybrid, which is then converted by DNA polymerase into a double-stranded DNA provirus. The provirus integrates into the host cell DNA and is transcribed into both viral messenger and viral genomic RNA. The RNA viruses containing reverse transcriptase were named the *Retroviridae* (Table 14.1) in recognition of the retrograde flow of genetic information from RNA into DNA. The hepadnaviruses are the only other viruses known in which reverse transcriptase activity is needed during the replication cycle (Table 14.1).

The search for cancer-causing human retroviruses was unsuccessful until the early 1980s when Gallo and his colleagues isolated the human leukemia viruses from patients with T-cell leukemias. These viruses were exogenous retroviruses because, unlike the endogenous retroviruses, their proviral DNA is not transmitted as part of the human genome. The new viruses were initially named *human T-cell leukemia viruses, type I and type II (HTLV–I and HTLV–II)*; the abbreviation *HTLV* was later considered to stand for *human T-cell lymphotropic viruses* so that the related AIDS viruses (HTLV–III and IV) could be included in this group.

Chronic leukemia viruses such as HTLV–I and II infect CD4$^+$ helper T-cells. Infection is followed by long periods of latency. Cancer may develop years after infection, but the observed frequency of cancers in infected individuals is low. Whereas the classical acute leukemia viruses are replication defective and require coinfection with a helper virus to initiate a productive infection, the chronic leukemia viruses are replication competent. The classical acute leukemia viruses carry a viral oncogene that rapidly confers tumor-inducing potential. In contrast, the chronic leukemia viruses do not carry a viral oncogene. Therefore, although chronic leukemia viruses are implicated as the cause of malignancy, the precise mechanism of cellular transformation is not fully understood at present. The integrated provirus of a chronic leukemia virus is believed to initiate a cancer in some instances after a prolonged incubation period when limited rounds of replication and infection lead to the insertion of a viral promoter element near a cellular oncogene.

When the leukemia viruses multiply, the genomic RNA is packaged in the capsids in the cytoplasm. The virus becomes mature when it buds through the cell's plasma membrane, where it acquires the major envelope protein. The envelope protein is the virus receptor for the cellular T4 molecule, which is expressed on target cells (for example, helper T-cells). The viral envelope protein–T4 interaction can initiate membrane fusion and thus aid in penetration of free virus into cells as well as permit cell-to-cell spread of the virus.

Transmission of free virus and cell-associated virus occurs mainly with transmission of contaminated blood and by sexual contact, but may also occur from mother to child at birth or possibly during nursing. Malignancies due to HTLV–I and II are rare at present, but the prevalence of antibodies to HTLV–I and II among intravenous drug abusers and prostitutes is increasing. The chronic leukemia viruses persist even though they initiate host immune responses. Immunization against acute retroviral infection has thus far only been demonstrated in rodents. The procedures often require the use of elaborate envelope antigen preparations and immunization protocols. Immunization against chronic feline and bovine leukemia viruses has been accomplished (Chapter 19).

Acquired Immunodeficiency Syndrome

The present acquired immunodeficiency syndrome (AIDS) epidemic is a complex phenomenon. Many years have passed since we as a society have been threatened by a transmissible disease that is uniformly fatal. AIDS was first described in 1981 by Jaffe and co-workers. These physicians observed that sexually active young adult male homosexuals frequently developed an unusually aggressive Kaposi's sarcoma, normally a rare disease in people of this age group. They also observed many opportunistic infections of types that occur in people in an immunosuppressed state. The syndrome also occurred occasionally in people who had received transfusions, in hemophiliacs, in intravenous drug users, and in Haitians. Evidence accumulated rapidly between 1981 and early 1983, suggesting that an infectious agent was involved, most likely a virus. Several known viruses were suspected, including hepatitis B virus, EBV, cytomegalovirus, and, not surprisingly, HTLV–1 and II.

In May of 1983, a group at the Pasteur Institute in France headed by Montagnier and Chermann published a paper in which they described a new retrovirus. The virus was isolated from a patient with a lymphadenopathy of a type that frequently occurs in patients who will develop AIDS. The virus was called *lymphadenopathy associated virus (LAV)*, and was eventually shown to be the causative agent of AIDS. The virus is a member of the Retroviridae and is closely related to retroviruses of the lentivirus subgroup, which include visna virus of sheep. The AIDS virus has been referred to by many names (for example, LAV, HTLV–III, ARV), but was officially named *human immunodeficiency virus (HIV)* in 1986. At present, two viruses, called *HIV–1* and *HIV–2,* are considered to cause AIDS in humans.

HIV–1 probably arose in central Africa and spread from there to other parts of the world. HIV–2 is presently endemic mostly in West Africa. Most HIV infections occur as a result of sexual contact. In Africa, heterosexual intercourse is the common means of transmission. In America and Europe, anal intercourse among homosexual men is the common mode of spread, but some cases resulting from heterosexual intercourse are also being reported in Western countries. Injection of contaminated blood and blood products is also a cause of infection. Infection in intravenous drug users results from use of needles contaminated with infected blood. The screening of blood by serologic tests for antibodies to HIV has reduced the frequency of infection in people requiring transfusions.

Following infection, there is a long incubation period. Years may pass before the development of disease; however, during this time, the virus can still be transmitted. HIV is transmitted as free virus or as cell-associated virus; this usually requires that contaminated blood or semen be introduced into the blood stream of the person at risk. HIV is *not* transmitted by casual contact with an infected individual.

The cells infected by HIV are mainly T-helper lymphocytes that express the CD4 protein on their surfaces. The CD4 protein is the host receptor molecule to which the viral envelope protein binds. Other cells, including macrophages and brain cells, that express small amounts of the T4 protein can also be infected. After the virus enters the cell, it undergoes a limited amount of replication and then integrates a copy of its provirus into the host genome. The virus remains latent until the host cell is activated or stimulated to divide, usually by antigens and cytokines. The virus then reproduces in activated or dividing host cells and, in the case of T-cells, this leads to syncytium formation and cell death.

The eventual depletion of $CD4^+$ helper cells leads to immunodeficiency, thus permitting opportunistic infections. A severe, often fatal, pneumonia caused by

Pneumocystis carinii—an organism, possibly either a fungus or a protozoan, not usually associated with disease in immunocompetent hosts—is common among AIDS patients. Other common diseases among AIDS patients include diarrhea, thrush (caused by *Candida albicans*), tuberculosis, Kaposi's sarcoma (an endothelial cell cancer), and malignant B-cell lymphomas. At present there are no effective treatments for the opportunistic diseases that occur in the immunosuppressed AIDS patients.

HIV has been transmitted to the chimpanzee, but disease has not occurred in animals of this species. Disease-producing immunodeficiency viruses have been identified that infect simians and felines. The pathology of the diseases produced in these animals is being studied in an attempt to obtain knowledge possibly useful in control of the human infection. Through massive research efforts and the application of new biotechnologies, HIV has become one of the most studied and characterized viral agents, all within three to four years of its discovery. These studies have not yielded information useful for immunization against infection or treatment of infected individuals, but have contributed to the development of diagnostic and screening tests. The screening of blood used in transfusions and the use of prophylactics if sex is engaged in are at present the best means available to prevent AIDS infections.

SUGGESTIONS FOR FURTHER READING

B. D. Davis, R. Dulbecco, H. N. Eisen, H. S. Ginsberg, and W. B. Wood. *Microbiology.* Harper & Row, New York, 1969.

E. Jawetz, J. L. Melnick, and E. A. Adelberg. *Review of Medical Virology.* Lange Medical Publications, Los Altos, California, 1982.

W. Murphy. *Coping with the Common Cold.* Library of Health, Time-Life Books, Chicago, 1981.

A. L. Notkins and M. B. A. Oldstone, eds. *Concepts in Viral Pathogenesis.* Springer-Verlag, New York, 1984.

A. L. Notkins and M. B. A. Oldstone, eds. *Concepts in Viral Pathogenesis, Vol. 2.* Springer-Verlag, New York, 1986.

Chapter 15

The Parasitic Worms, Protozoa, and Arthropods

FRANK KAPRAL

Department of Medical Microbiology and Immunology
College of Medicine
The Ohio State University

THE PARASITIC TREMATODES
          The Schistosomes (Blood Flukes)
THE PARASITIC ARTHROPODS
SUGGESTIONS FOR FURTHER READING

INTRODUCTION

The organisms commonly referred to as parasites can be divided into three main groups: These are the single-cell organisms, or protozoa; the parasitic multicellular worms, or helminths; and the multicellular parasitic insects, or arthropods. The protozoa causing disease in humans usually fall into one of four classes: These are the amoebas (Sarcodina), the flagellates (Mastigophora), the ciliates (Ciliata), and the sporozoa. The parasitic helminths are found among the round worms (Nematodes) or the flatworms (Platyhelminthes). The parasitic flatworms are either tapeworms (Cestodes) or flukes (Trematodes). All of the organisms commonly called *parasites* are eukaryotes, and thus they more closely resemble the mammalian host biochemically and physiologically than do bacteria and viruses.

THE PARASITIC PROTOZOA

Entamoeba histolytica

This organism, the cause of amoebic dysentery, occurs in two forms, the trophozoite form and the cyst form. The term *trophozoite* refers to any motile and feeding stage of a protozoan, and in this case is synonymous with the amoebic form. *Entamoeba histolytica* trophozoites are from 15 to 30 μm in diameter and possess a single nucleus. They are passed only in liquid or semiliquid stools. The cyst is the resistant form of the organism. *E. histolytica* cysts are round, thick-walled structures from 5 to 20 μm in diameter and typically contain four nuclei (Figure 15.1). They are passed in formed stools.

The life cycle of *E. histolytica* is fairly simple. Mature cysts, when ingested, excyst in the small intestine; each cyst gives rise to eight trophozoites, which grow on the colonic mucosa. Normally they live on desquamated cells and bacteria. Some may invade the colonic mucosa, however, and after proliferation may cause the formation of flask-shaped ulcers. Some trophozoites encyst after a period of growth in the intestinal lumen and are passed in the feces.

The symptoms of dysentery (blood and mucus in the feces) result from the ulceration of the colonic mucosa that is caused when amoeba invade (Figure 15.2). Secondary bacterial infection of the lesions initiates an inflammatory response and leads to the appearance of neutrophils in the lesions. A concomitant loss of water

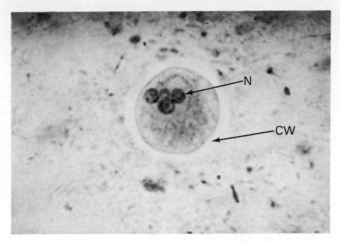

Figure 15.1 Photomicrograph of an *Entamoeba histolytica* cyst. The mature cyst has four nuclei (N) and a surrounding wall (CW) that protects it during passage from one host to another.

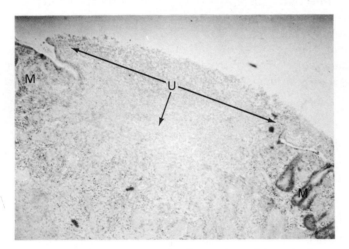

Figure 15.2 Photomicrograph of a section of intestinal mucosa with an *Entamoeba histolytica*–induced ulcer. Fairly normal mucosa (M) can be seen on each side of the ulcer. The ulcer (U), which does not penetrate completely through the mucosa, is characterized by a granular appearance.

and electrolytes through the denuded surface can also occur, and is clinically manifest as diarrhea.

In some cases the amoeba penetrate beyond the submucosa and disseminate throughout the body. The liver is the organ most commonly involved; such invasion may give rise to multiple or single liver abscesses. Secondary lesions in other organs such as the lungs and brain also occur.

It is generally agreed that there are both virulent and avirulent strains of *E. histolytica*. Most infections are due to avirulent strains and do not result in overt disease in otherwise healthy individuals. Infected individuals who do not have clinical symptoms are referred to as *asymptomatic carriers*. Strains may increase in pathogenicity, or weakly pathogenic strains may infect a nonimmune or weakened individual. Under such conditions the amoeba may be invasive and cause severe intestinal disease and liver involvement. When examined in the laboratory, it is apparent that virulent strains are better able to ingest human erythrocytes than are avirulent strains. Trophozoites of virulent strains can also be distinguished by their ability to be agglutinated by concanavalin A. In addition, the two types of strains exhibit different isoenzyme patterns when analyzed by electrophoresis.

The mechanism leading to cytopathology appears to involve three steps. The first is adherence of virulent amoeba to the host cell. This is mediated by the interaction between a lectin on the surface of the amoeba and the appropriate carbohydrate on the target cell membrane. This is followed by a cytocidal process that may involve the release of a protein by the amoeba that can form transmembrane pores in the target cell and thus disrupt ion gradients essential for cell viability. Finally the lysed cell can be phagocytized by the amoeba.

Although infection with *E. histolytica* frequently results in the production of antibodies to numerous antigens of the organism, there is presently no evidence that these antibodies function as a host defense mechanism. Whereas delayed hypersensitivity develops less frequently than do antibodies, its occurrence appears to be correlated with recovery from infection. This suggests that cell-mediated mechanisms are the principal means of host resistance to *E. histolytica*.

Malaria

The sporozoa responsible for malaria belong to the genus *Plasmodium*. Four species can infect humans: *Plasmodium vivax*, *Plasmodium malariae*, *Plasmodium ovale*, and *Plasmodium falciparum*. A variety of other species infect other primates, birds, and reptiles. There is a high degree of species specificity, and only a few of the monkey malarias can infect humans. The plasmodial life cycles are complex; that of *P. vivax* will serve as an example.

While feeding, an infected mosquito injects saliva containing the sporozoites (Figure 15.3*a*). These forms travel via the blood to the liver, where they enter the parenchymal cells and divide by merogony (a form of division where the cytoplasm enlarges, the nucleus divides repeatedly, and the cytoplasm becomes partitioned about each nucleus). The end result of this form of multiplication is the meront (Figure 15.3*b*), a collection of daughter cells within a single host cell. Upon maturation the meront ruptures, releasing the daughter cells (merozoites) into the circulation. Whereas the original sporozoites only infect liver cells, the merozoites from the liver only infect erythrocytes. The merozoites attach to the erythrocyte membrane, which then invaginates and causes the parasite to be enclosed within a vacuole.

Repeated cycles of merogony occur within the erythrocytes; each cycle requires

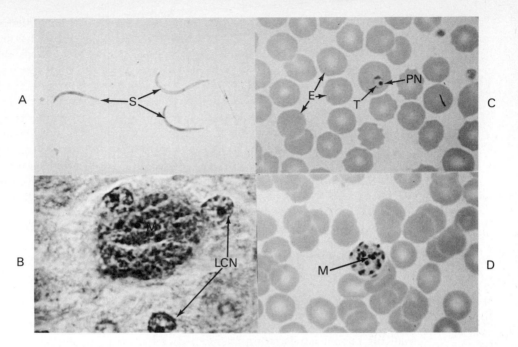

Figure 15.3 (A) Photomicrograph of plasmodial sporozoites. These are the form of the organism injected when the mosquito feeds. (B) Photomicrograph of a plasmodial meront in liver tissue. The large body with many small dots in the center of the picture is the meront (M). The dots are the nuclei of the developing merozoites. The deeply staining vesicular structures are liver cell nuclei (LCN). (C) Photomicrograph of an early stage of plasmodial infection in an erythrocyte (E). This is called a ring form trophozoite (T). The intensely staining dot is the parasite nucleus (PN). (D) Photomicrograph of a plasmodial meront (M) in an erythrocyte. When the many merozoites forming in this erythrocyte are mature, the erythrocyte will burst and the merozoites will infect other erythrocytes.

about 48 hours for completion. An early ring form (Figure 15.3*c*) and a mature meront (Figure 15.3*d*) are shown. Unless multiple infections have taken place in the same host, the erythrocyte cycles remain in phase and the new merozoites are released from all the infected erythrocytes at about the same time. The process of releasing a crop of merozoites at the end of merogony causes disruption of the erythrocyte. The products liberated during this process trigger the episodes of chills and fever associated with this disease (the paroxysm). The reaction is probably immunological and thus a form of allergy.

After several cycles, some of the merozoites differentiate into still other forms, the male and female gametocytes. These are the early sexual stages of the parasite. If the patient is now bitten by an uninfected mosquito, the gametocytes may be ingested with the blood meal. Within the mosquito's stomach, the gametocytes mature into the male and female gametes, and fertilization occurs. The resultant zygote differentiates into the ookinete, which penetrates the gut wall and enters the haemocoel.Here it enlarges into the oocyst, which becomes filled with many nuclei. Each nucleus receives a portion of cytoplasm and is released as an elongated sporozoite. The sporozoites migrate to the mosquito's salivary glands and can then be transmitted to another individual at the next feeding.

Whereas with *P. vivax, P. ovale,* and *P. falciparum* infections the paroxysms occur every 48 hours, in *P. malariae* infections schizogony within the erythrocytes requires 72 hours for completion; thus the chills and fever occur every third day.

In the case of *P. vivax,* some of the organisms in the liver may become dormant even though other organisms in the same patient have infected the erythrocytes and have resulted in a full-blown case of malaria. Later, after recovery from the disease, these dormant organisms may be stimulated to complete their life cycle and give rise to a new attack of malaria. Such relapses can occur repeatedly over a period of several years after the initial infection.

Infection with *P. falciparum* is associated with higher case-fatality rates than are infections with Plasmodia of other species. The severe clinical manifestations frequently seen in *P. falciparum* infections are due at least in part to tissue anoxia induced by plugging of the capillaries resulting from the sequestration of infected erythrocytes in the capillary bed. Erythrocytes infected with *P. falciparum* exhibit electron-dense knobs on their surfaces during the period of meront development. These knobs possess structures that can bind to venous endothelial cells, thus resulting in the sequestration of infected cells in the venules of the brain, heart, lung, kidney, and spleen (Figure 15.4). This phenomenon is responsible for the fact that, contrary to the situation in *P. vivax* malaria, *P. falciparum* meronts are rarely found in blood smears.

Recent studies have shown that antibody directed toward certain sporozoite antigens can be protective by preventing the penetration of the liver cells by the parasite. Immune responses to merozoite antigens can also occur: Antibody to

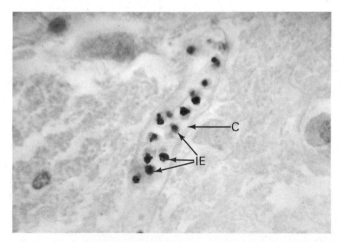

Figure 15.4 Photomicrograph of a histological section of tissue from a patient dead of *Plasmodium falciparum* malaria. The capillary (C) in the center of the micrograph is completely plugged by infected erythrocytes (IE).

merozoites may block entry into erythrocytes and antibody to knob protein in erythrocytes may block attachment to vascular endothelium. Antibody may also aid clearance of parasite debris from the blood. The spleen plays an important role in the host's defense against malaria, and splenectomy can markedly diminish the host's ability to control the organism. The exact role of the spleen in this regard is unknown, but it has been suggested that the spleen may be involved in the clearance of infected erythrocytes from the circulation.

Susceptibility to malaria is genetically determined. Blacks are usually more resistant to *P. vivax* than are people of other racial groups. They lack the molecule on the red cell required by *P. vivax* merozoites for penetration into erythrocytes. Individuals with sickle hemoglobin are more resistant to *P. falciparum* infection than are individuals without sickle cell trait. The evidence suggests that persons with glucose-6-phosphate dehydrogenase deficiency and thalassemia likewise may be more resistant to *P. falciparum.* This could account for the prevalence of these genetic variants in geographic areas in which *P. falciparum* is endemic.

The Trichomonads

Three species of this genus infect humans. *Trichomonas tenax* is found in the oral cavity, *Trichomonas hominis* resides in the intestine, and *Trichomonas vaginalis* occurs in the vagina or urethra of human females and males, respectively. Only the *T. vaginalis* organism is capable of producing disease. These organisms possess both flagella and an undulating membrane, and are highly motile (Figure 15.5). They can be cultured in media with or without the presence of bacteria. All are anaerobes, although *T. vaginalis* is facultatively aerobic.

The optimum pH for growth of *T. vaginalis* is between 5.5 and 6.0; viability is lost below pH 5.0. The pH in the normal vagina of the young adult is between 3.8 and 4.4, and thus will not support the organism. Trichomonal vaginitis usually occurs after the onset of puberty and before menopause, with a peak incidence

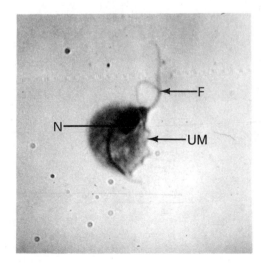

Figure 15.5 Photomicrograph of *Trichomonas vaginalis.* The organism is actively motile because of the activities of flagella (F) and an undulating membrane (UM). The parasite nucleus (N) is prominent in this micrograph.

during pregnancy. Present evidence suggests that some alteration in the vaginal environment is usually necessary, increasing the pH either directly or indirectly, before *T. vaginalis* infection occurs. Although infection rates appear high (20–40 percent), only from 10 to 20 percent of women harboring the organism actually develop vaginitis.

Symptoms usually include burning and itching, as well as a copious frothy, yellowish discharge. The vaginal wall is usually hyperemic and may show punctate lesions or extensive erosion, and petechiae. Males are for the most part asymptomatic carriers, and any discharge from the urethra is usually scant.

T. vaginalis is transmitted primarily through sexual intercourse, although transmission by fomites is possible since the organism can survive a few hours outside the body.

African Trypanosomes

The three species of African trypanosomes, *Trypanosoma brucei brucei*, *Trypanosoma brucei rhodesiense*, and *Trypanosoma brucei gambiense* are morphologically indistinguishable (Figure 15.6) and biochemically closely related. The first infects a variety of African animals, causing the disease Nagana, but does not infect humans. The other two (*T. brucei rhodesiense* and *T. brucei gambiense*) infect humans as well as various other animals. They are the cause of African sleeping sickness in humans. The trypanosomes are slender flagellates approximately 3 × 15–32 μm in size. The flagellum runs the length of the cell body and is attached to it by an intervening undulating membrane. At the anterior end the flagellum may extend beyond the end of the cell as a free structure.

The life cycle is complex and involves two host species, the tsetse fly and the

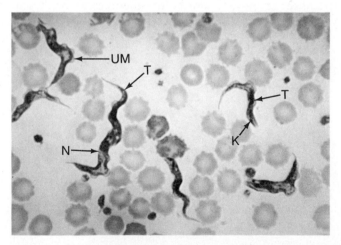

Figure 15.6 Photomicrograph of *brucei* type trypanosomes (T) in blood. The nuclei and undulating membranes of these blood stage trypanosomes are prominent. The kinetoplast (K), a small, round deeply staining body, is visible in the posterior end of the organism.

mammalian host. Organisms in the blood of the mammalian host are ingested by the tsetse fly while feeding. Multiplication takes place first in the mid-gut and then in the salivary glands. During their sojourn in the fly, the organisms undergo various transformations, first becoming procyclic trypomastigotes, then epimastigotes, and finally metacyclic trypomastigotes. The latter are then passed to another mammalian host at the time of the next feeding. The organisms first multiply in the tissues in the vicinity of the bite and, after about a week, appear in the blood, from which they can be picked up by another tsetse fly to complete the cycle.

In the human there may be an initial inflammatory response at the site of the bite, but generally the patient remains asymptomatic for several weeks or a few months, depending upon the subspecies of trypanosomes involved. As the organisms proliferate in the blood vessels and lymph nodes, the host develops a fever and rash. During this time the immune system is stimulated, and antibodies to surface antigens in the organism are elicited. With the advent of antibodies, the trypanosome population is dramatically reduced and the patient again becomes asymptomatic. After about a week, the trypanosome population has risen again and another febrile episode occurs. New antibodies appear, and the trypanosome population again diminishes. This process of growth and elimination may be repeated numerous times; however, eventually some organisms manage to invade the central nervous system, where they can proliferate unchecked, thus leading to coma and death.

The antigen to which the protective antibodies are produced is called the *variable surface glycoprotein (VSG).* The VSG is present in a thick layer covering the entire trypanosome membrane. As antibodies specific for the particular VSG appear, they result in the elimination of about 99 percent of the trypanosome population. Among the remaining 1 percent, however, are organisms that have "switched on" another VSG gene, making their VSG coating nonreactive with the antibody already produced by the host. As organisms with the new VSG variant proliferate, the immune system is again stimulated, this time to produce antibody reactive with the new VSG variant. Again the vast majority of the population is eliminated, and parasites with yet another VSG specificity develop.

Trypanosomes possess several hundred distinct VSG genes that can be recombined in turn to produce yet an even larger array of VSG specificities. Only one VSG can be expressed at a time. These organisms have evolved an extraordinarily effective means of circumventing the host's immune defenses.

THE PARASITIC NEMATODES

Most nematodes are free-living organisms; only about a dozen species are known to parasitize humans. Some species also parasitize various animals, some the roots of plants. Nematodes are cylindrical with tapered ends and are not segmented. The digestive tract is well developed, with the mouth at the anterior end. The sexes are separate, and the female is usually larger than the male. Brief descriptions of the more common nematodes infecting humans follow.

Ascaris lumbricoides

Adult *Ascaris lumbricoides* are substantial in size: The males are 0.3 cm × 15–30 cm and the females are 0.5 cm × 20–35 cm.

The life cycle involves only one host, the human. Adults residing in the jejunum copulate, and females release their ova, which pass from the body with the feces. The ova (Figure 15.7) mature in the soil over a period of from 10 to 15 days. Upon ingestion, the ova hatch in the small intestine and release larvae that penetrate the gut wall and enter the lymphatics. These larvae are transported via the blood to the lung parenchyma, where they molt. From there they enter the alveoli, migrate up the respiratory tract to the pharynx, and are swallowed. Maturation then takes place in the jejunum.

The average worm load is about six adults per infected individual, and the residence of even a few dozen worms seldom causes any marked symptoms. Since the life-span of the worms is approximately one year, infection is usually self-limiting unless reinfection occurs. With repeated infections, however, an individual is apt to become sensitized to worm antigens and may subsequently respond allergically to the migration of larval forms through the body.

A single fertile female worm can produce about 240,000 ova per day. In the temperate zones the ova may survive in the soil for several years, but in the tropics survival time may be shorter. Because of the resistance of the ova to environmental factors, a high rate of reinfection is possible unless extreme care is taken to avoid contamination of food and water.

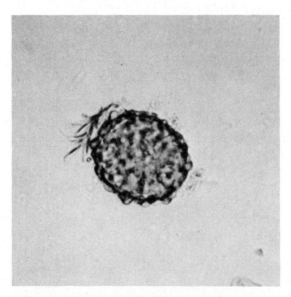

Figure 15.7 Photomicrograph of an ascarid egg. This is the infective form of the parasite; it may persist in the soil for long periods of time. If ingested, it hatches and initiates infection.

The ascaris allergen is probably the most potent parasite allergen known. Coupled with the intimate contact between the larval forms and the host's tissues that the organism's life cycle provides, this readily explains why sensitization occurs so frequently upon repeated reinfection. Although the sensitized host responds allergically to the larvae regardless of where they are located, the most obvious and serious manifestation of this phenomenon occurs in the lungs. Here the condition is referred to as *ascaris pneumonitis* and may consist of consolidation by allergically induced exudates.

Although some degree of immunity appears to result during infection, it is manifest only by a reduction in the worm load. The mechanisms whereby this effect is mediated are not known, but it has been postulated that antibody may interfere with hatching in the intestine, may interfere with penetration of the intestinal mucosa, or may destroy larvae while they are migrating through the tissues.

A disease that can occur in humans and is caused by related organisms is visceral larval migrans. The ascarids of the dog and cat (genus *Toxocara*) have a life cycle similar to that of *A. lumbricoides* in humans. If ingested by humans, *Toxocara* ova can hatch but cannot develop into adult worms. Finding themselves in an abnormal host, the larval forms continue to migrate throughout the body until they finally succumb. During this migration, allergens in the larvae stimulate the immune system and elicit various immunoglobulins, including IgE antibodies. When these appear, the presence of the parasite elicits an inflammatory response, and this eventually produces an eosinophilic granuloma about each larva. Visceral larval migrans is most commonly seen in small children because of their closer association with cats and dogs, and the greater opportunity to ingest infective ova found in their environment.

Hookworms

The principal hookworm species infecting humans are *Necator americanus* and *Ancylostoma duodenale. Ancylostoma ceylonicum* can also infect humans, but is seldom found in the absence of other species. The adult worms are relatively small: approximately 0.3×10 mm, with females slightly larger than males. The anterior portion of the organism is sharply flexed, creating the appearance of a hook (Figure 15.9A), this is responsible for the name of this group of helminths.

Mature adults in the intestines mate, and the females produce ova that are deposited in the soil with the feces (Figure 15.8). The ova hatch and produce free-living rhabditiform larvae that, under appropriate conditions (ample moisture and temperatures above 10°C), can feed on bacteria and organic material in the soil. Eventually these forms mature into the infectious filariform larvae. Following contact with exposed parts of the body, the larvae penetrate the skin and enter capillaries. They are carried in the blood to the lungs. They leave the blood in the lungs and penetrate into the alveoli. From there they migrate to the pharynx and are swallowed. Maturation occurs in the intestines, where they anchor and feed on the mucosa. In the case of *A. duodenale,* ova ingested before reaching the soil can

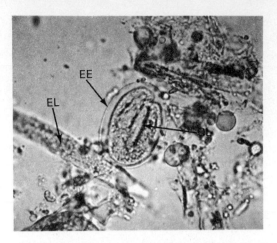

Figure 15.8 Photomicrograph of an embryonated egg (EE) of *Necator americanus,* a common hookworm. A coiled larvum (CL) is present in the egg and will soon emerge. A larvum (EL) that has already emerged is also visible.

hatch and mature into adults in the intestines without going through the migratory phase in the lungs. Worms in the intestines survive about one to five years; thus chronic infections require periodic reinfection.

By virtue of reexposure of the host to larval antigens during reinfections, the immune system is stimulated and produces IgE antibody. Once present, these antibodies can react with migrating larvae and thus elicit allergic reactions, particularly in the skin.

The primary cause of pathology, however, relates to the feeding habits of the adult worms in the intestines. The mouth of the worm is held open by a chitinous ring surrounding the orifice, but jaws are absent. The powerful muscular pharynx of the worm can readily suck mucosal tissue into the mouth (Figure 15.9B), and it is upon this tissue that the organism feeds. This sucking action continues until the mouth reaches the muscularis of the intestinal wall. The worm then releases itself and finds a new site in which to continue its feeding. The vacated site, however, continues to ooze blood for some time before clotting occurs. Since worm loads may reach several hundreds or even thousands in an individual, heavily infected persons may develop severe anemia. The exact circumstances under which anemia will develop in any particular case will depend upon the amount of iron reserves in the patient, the amount of iron in the diet, and the general nutritional state of the host.

Healthy individuals may develop some degree of immunity. This may be brought about by the action of antibodies to worm antigens in the worm's mouth parts. This antibody may interfere with the worm's ability to attach and to digest tissue. Complement and leukocytes may act in concert with the antibody. The migrating immature stages of the parasite are also affected by products of the immune response.

Humans may also become infected by the filariform larvae of dog and cat

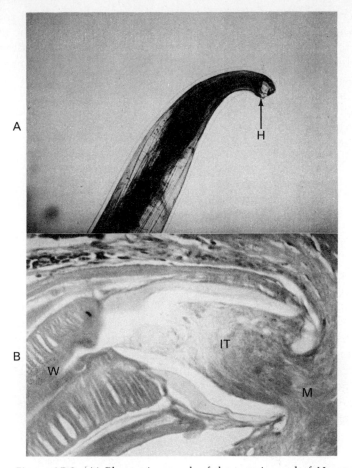

Figure 15.9 (A) Photomicrograph of the anterior end of *Necator americanus* showing the hooked shape (H) from which the name *hookworm* is derived. (B) Photomicrograph of a tissue section showing attachment of a hookworm (W) to the mucosa (M) and ingestion of tissue (IT) into the mouth of the worm. If many worms are feeding in the intestine, much damage and severe bleeding may result.

hookworms. These larvae cannot complete their life cycles in this host, but do migrate in the skin for some time. In the sensitized individual the presence of the larvae may elicit allergic reactions, giving rise to a *cutaneous larval migrans* (also known as *creeping eruption*).

Trichinella spiralis (Trichinosis)

Adult *Trichinella spiralis* worms are quite small, averaging about 1.5 mm × 0.04 mm for the male and about 3.5 mm × 0.06 mm for the female. The life cycle is simple, with the same individual serving as the intermediate host and the definitive host. Any carnivorous mammal may become infected.

Infected muscle (containing encysted larvae) is ingested and the larvae are released in the small intestine, where they immediately invade the mucosa. The sexes differentiate, fertilization occurs, and the females migrate deeper into the mucosa. The viviparous females deposit larvae that enter the lymphatics and the blood. They are carried to the muscles, and there the larvae burrow into the fibers of striated muscle and then encyst (Figure 15.10).

The nature of the symptoms produced depends on the number of worms ingested and may occur in phases corresponding to the periods of intestinal invasion, migration of larvae, and encystment in muscle. Clinical findings usually consist of diarrhea, muscle pain, fever, weakness, and eosinophilia. Death may result from severe infections. The immunological reaction to the worms in the tissue finally results in their encapsulation and resolution of the clinical disease.

THE CESTODES

Cestode worms are flat and ribbonlike in appearance. The adult consists of a head, or scolex (Figure 15.11), that attaches to the intestinal mucosa by means of suckers (and, in some species, also with hooks) and a segmented portion, the body, made up of segments called *proglottids* (Figure 15.12). The body is formed from new segments that are continually produced just behind the scolex. These segments are at first quite small, but increase in size as they mature. There is no digestive tract; nutrients are absorbed directly from the contents of the intestinal lumen. Each proglottid possesses both male and female reproductive organs and is self-fertilizing. The gravid proglottids, which contain numerous ova, eventually separate from the body and are passed with the feces. In order to cure the host of an infestation

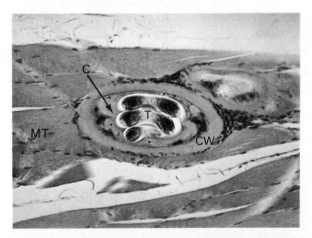

Figure 15.10 Photomicrograph of a section of a trichinella (T) in a cyst in muscle tissue (MT). The worm is coiled up inside the cyst (C), which has a wall (CW) made of connective tissue.

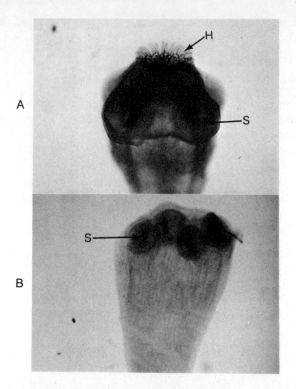

Figure 15.11 Photomicrograph of various types of tapeworm heads. (A) *Taenia solium*, with hooks (H) and suckers (S), and (B) *Taenia saginata* with suckers (S).

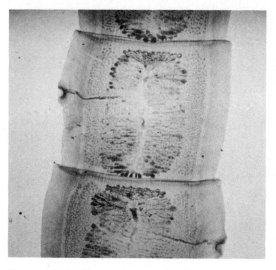

Figure 15.12 Photomicrograph of mature proglottids of *Taenia saginata*.

it is necessary that the scolex be eliminated; otherwise regeneration of the body will occur.

Taenia solium (Pork Tapeworm)

The adult *Taenia solium* may be from 2 to 8 m in length. The scolex is 1 mm in diameter and possesses four suckers and a ring of between 25 and 30 hooks. A mature proglottid is about 12 mm in length and the uterus has from 7 to 12 lateral branches.

Gravid proglottids are passed in feces and then release ova that are subsequently ingested by the hog. Here they hatch in the intestine, enter the blood, and are transported to muscles, where they develop into cysticerci, the larval form of the organism (Figure 15.13). Upon ingestion of uncooked infected pork by humans, the bladder of the cysticercus is digested away and the scolex attaches to the intestine wall, where it develops into an adult worm.

Regardless of the number of cysticerci ingested, an individual almost always harbors only one adult worm in the intestine. The reason for this observation is not known. In any case, irrespective of the length of the worm, most infected individuals exhibit no symptoms and may be unaware of its presence for some time.

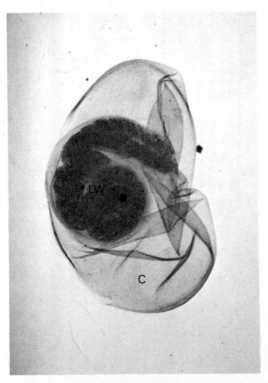

Figure 15.13 Photomicrograph of a cysticercus of *Taenia solium* that has been removed from the muscle tissue. If ingested with infected meat, the larval worm (LW) in the cyst (C) is released and attaches to the intestinal wall.

A far more dangerous situation can occur if humans ingest the ova of this worm. In this case, the ova can hatch and develop into cysticerci scattered throughout the body. These eventually degenerate and calcify, but if located in the brain or other vital organ, they can cause severe disease or death.

Taenia saginata (Beef Tapeworm)

The adult *Taenia saginata* worm is from 4 to 25 m in length and has a scolex from 1 to 2 mm in diameter. The scolex has four suckers but no hooks. A mature proglottid is about 20 mm in length and possesses a uterus with from 15 to 30 lateral branches. Proglottids broken from the terminal portion of the worm frequently exhibit active independent motion.

The cysticercus in the tissues of cattle is ingested by humans. Hatching occurs in the intestine, and adult worms develop. Gravid proglottids release ova in the feces, which are then ingested by cattle. These develop into cysticerci in their tissues.

As in the case of *T. solium,* the host usually harbors only a single adult worm, and its presence generally induces little in the way of clinical response. Also, contrary to the situation seen with *T. solium,* the risk of humans developing cysticercosis from *T. saginata* is extremely slight or nonexistent.

Diphyllobothrium latum (Fish Tapeworm)

The adult *Diphyllobothrium latum* is from 3 to 10 m in length and has a scolex from 1 to 3 mm in size. The scolex has two slitlike suckers (bothria) but no hooks. A mature proglottid is between 3 and 10 mm in length and possesses a centrally located rosette-shaped uterus.

Contrary to the situation with the *Taenia* species, the gravid proglottids do not pass out in the feces intact, but generally disintegrate and release their ova into the intestinal lumen (Figure 15.14). If the ova enter fresh water, they hatch and release a ciliated embryo. These are ingested by copepods in which the larva encysts. If the infected cyclops are ingested by fish, the larva penetrates the intestinal wall and enters various tissues. When infected fish are ingested by humans, the larvae are released from the tissues and adhere to the intestinal wall, where they mature into adult worms.

Infection in the human is usually limited to a single worm. The worm has an exceptional propensity to absorb vitamin B_{12} and thus competes with the host for this nutrient. In cases where dietary factors limit the ingestion of this vitamin, this competition can result in anemia in the host; otherwise, the individual may be totally unaware of the parasite.

Echinococcus granulosis (Hydatid Cyst)

Echinococcus granulosis is the smallest tapeworm to infect humans. The adult consists of the scolex plus only three proglottids (immature, mature, gravid) and has a total length of only 5 mm (Figure 15.15).

The adult worm resides in the intestine of dogs or other canines and releases

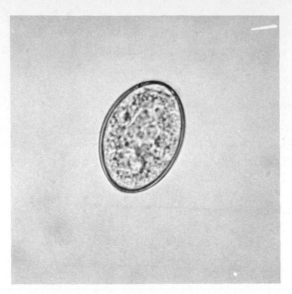

Figure 15.14 Photomicrograph of a free egg of the fish tapeworm of *Diphyllobothrium latum.* These eggs, unlike eggs of other tapeworms, are free in the feces and are not retained in the proglottid.

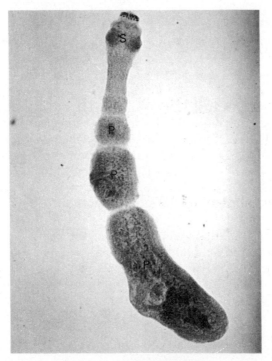

Figure 15.15 Photomicrograph of an entire *Echinococcus granulosis* tapeworm. Only a few proglottids (P) attached to the scolex (S) are present. The entire worm is only about 5 mm in length.

ova in the feces, which are then ingested by sheep or cattle. Upon hatching, the larvae in the tissues develop into a form called the *hydatid cyst*. If infected meat is ingested by a dog, the larvae develop into adults in its intestine.

Humans become accidental hosts by ingesting ova. These hatch in the intestine and the resultant larvae enter the circulation and are disseminated throughout the body. Subsequently, they develop into hydatid cysts. Most are located in either the liver or the lungs.

Hydatid cysts consist of an outer cyst wall, an inner germinal layer that gives rise to numerous scolices, and the fluid filling the cyst. Hydatid cysts may continue to grow for years and may be life-threatening. Symptoms are comparable to those of a slow-growing tumor. Treatment consists of the surgical removal of the hydatid cyst. Care must be taken to prevent release of cyst contents during surgery since severe allergic reactions may occur. Furthermore, each scolex or fragment of germinal tissue spilled in the patient can give rise to a new hydatid cyst. To prevent such complications, formalin or iodine is usually injected into the cysts during surgery.

THE PARASITIC TREMATODES

Parasitic trematodes (flukes) are generally hermaphroditic and have a flattened, leaflike appearance. They possess two suckers and an abbreviated digestive tract. All require a mollusc as an intermediate host. Depending on the fluke species, adults may reside in various organs of humans such as the intestine, liver, lung, or blood. Lung and liver flukes occur in many domestic and wild animals, also. Medically, the blood flukes (schistosomes) are important and are discussed further in the next section.

The Schistosomes (Blood Flukes)

The schistosomes differ from typical flukes in that the sexes are separate and the adults are thin and cylindrical (Figure 15.16*b*). They also differ from other flukes in that their life cycle does not include a separate metacercarial stage. Four species, *Schistosoma mansoni, Schistosoma hematobium, Schistosoma japonicum,* and *Schistosoma mekongi,* infect humans. Adult worms are 6–20 mm $\times$ 0.5 mm in size.

The eggs passed in feces hatch in fresh water. The resultant ciliated miracidium penetrates the appropriate species of snail and undergoes developmental stages in its tissues. The forked-tailed cercariae (Figure 15.16*a*) leave the snail and swim about in the water until they can penetrate the skin of humans. Then they shed their tails and burrow through the tissues until they enter the circulation. The worms mature in the portal system of the liver and then migrate back into the nearby venules during egg laying. In the case of *S. mansoni, S. japonicum,* and *S. mekongi,* egg deposition usually occurs in venules near the intestines; *S. hematobium* prefer vessels near the bladder. The release of lytic enzymes from the larvae within the eggs, together with the peristaltic action of host organs, assist the eggs in their passive migration through the tissues. Because of the location where

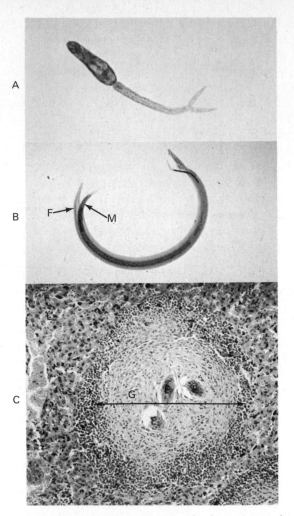

Figure 15.16 (A) Photomicrograph of a cercariae of *Schistosoma mansoni.* This form of the parasite develops in the snail host and is released into water. The form in water is infective for her mans. (B) Photomicrograph of a pair of adult *Schistosoma mansoni.* The larger female (F) is wrapped around the smaller male (M); the pair remain united for life. (C) Photomicrograph of a granuloma (G) in the liver (L) of a person with schistosomiasis. Degenerating eggs (E) are present in the center of the granuloma.

the eggs are deposited, *S. hematobium* ova commonly leave the host from the bladder in the urine whereas the ova of the other species usually leave through the intestinal tract, in the feces.

Adult worms can survive from 3 to 30 years, continuously producing eggs. Most eggs do not have the opportunity to leave the body, but give rise to inflammatory reactions and granulomas when they die (Figure 15.16*c*). Since many eggs are swept into the liver, where they become lodged, fibrosis of the liver is a common finding, but fibrosis may occur in other tissues as well. With time, considerable destruction and loss of function may occur in the organs involved.

By residing in the blood for long periods of time, the adult schistosomes are obviously exposed to the products of the immune responses of the host, yet there is no evidence that the organisms are adversely affected by them. The worms seem to be inherently resistant to attack by immunoglobulins and, in addition, it has been shown that the parasites become coated with antigens of the host. These include such entities as blood group antigens and histocompatibility antigens that may fool the immune system into viewing the schistosomes as self and thus obviate the mounting of a response altogether.

Individuals subject to repeated infection with cercariae become sensitized and manifest local allergic reactions about the burrowing parasites. In the northern portions of the United States and in Canada, humans may become infected with cercariae from bird schistosomes. These species of schistosomes cannot complete their life cycle in humans, but repeated exposure can sensitize an individual so that fresh contact with cercariae elicits the allergic manifestations responsible for the condition commonly called *swimmers' itch.*

THE PARASITIC ARTHROPODS

The parasitic worms and protozoa usually complete at least some stage of their life cycles within the host species and are thus endoparasites. The arthropods usually live on the surface of their hosts, and are thus ectoparasites. Some arthropods associate with the host only during the process of feeding; for others the association is more intimate or prolonged. Fleas, lice, bedbugs, flies, mosquitoes, ticks, and mites are parasitic arthropods. Many parasitic arthropods transmit pathogenic bacteria, viruses, protozoa, or worms during feeding, and thus their importance is not just a result of the damage they do to their hosts directly.

SUGGESTIONS FOR FURTHER READING

J. E. Donelson and A. C. Rice-Ficht. "Molecular biology of trypanosome antigenic variation." Microbiol. Rev. *49:* 107, 1985.

G. Kolata. "Avoiding the schistosome's tricks." Science *277:* 285, 1985.

J. P. Kreier and J. R. Baker. *Parasitic Protozoa.* Allen & Unwin, Boston, 1987.

L. H. Miller, R. J. Howard, R. Carter, M. F. Good, V. Nussenzweig and R. S. Nussenzweig. "Research toward malaria vaccines." Science *234:* 1349, 1986.

Z. S. Pawlowski. "Ascariasis: Host–pathogen biology." Rev. Infect. Dis. *4:* 806, 1982.

J. I. Ravdin. "Pathogenesis of disease caused by *Entamoeba histolytica:* Studies of adherence, secreted toxins, and contact dependent cytolysis. Rev. Infect. Dis. *8:* 247, 1986.

D. Trissl. "Immunology of *Entamoeba histolytica* in human and animal hosts." Rev. Infect. Dis. *6:* 1154, 1982.

D. J. Wyler. "Malaria: Host–pathogen biology." Rev. Infect. Dis. *4:* 785, 1982.

Chapter 16

The Fungi, Molds, and Yeasts

JOHN A. SCHMITT, JR.

Department of Botany
The Ohio State University

INTRODUCTION

You may have the impression that fungi are of little importance as disease-producing organisms in human beings. To many microbiologists, fungi are mysterious because they are reputedly difficult to identify and the diseases they produce are seemingly so similar as to be extremely difficult to differentiate one from another or from disease processes evoked by nonfungal organisms. Indeed, differential diagnosis is an important aspect of successful treatment. But evaluation of all data (clinical, cultural, stained sections of biopsy material, serological) will almost always lead to a definitive diagnosis.

There are from 200,000 to 400,000 species of fungi. Fortunately, most of them are saprophytic (utilizing dead organic material as an energy source) and are never incriminated in human disease. In truth, there are probably not more than 80 species of fungi that are considered to be human pathogens. Many of the currently recognized systemic mycoses were once considered to be rare, invariably fatal diseases since they were diagnosed only at autopsy. As serological techniques for detection of fungal infections emerged and were refined, scientists realized that most of the mycoses are in fact common, rarely fatal problems. We now generally refer to these zoopathogenic fungi as *opportunistic* fungi; that is, organisms that can become established and evoke pathology, but only in a person whose integumental structure or immunologic state has been compromised in one way or another. The intact epidermis is a magnificent barrier to the establishment of a fungal infection. The normal immune system is also an effective barrier to fungal infection; only when it is depressed (either by other diseases or by medication) is the probability of an overt mycosis high.

In human beings, only one zoopathogenic fungus is endogenous. This is *Candida albicans,* a truly versatile fungus in terms of the types of disease it can evoke. It occurs in the gastrointestinal tracts of about 85 percent of healthy adult humans. Infection only comes to light when feces or other specimens are cultured for fungi.

The yeast cell form of *C. albicans* (Figure 16.1*a*) is commonly seen when a pathologist reads a "Pap smear" slide. In fact, vaginal candidiasis is probably the most common form of candidiasis; some gynecologists claim that almost 100 percent of women have problems of varying degrees of severity at some time in their lives with this fungus.

Since *C. albicans* is the only endogenous fungal zoopathogen, all other mycoses are the result of contamination from the environment. The deep mycoses affecting internal organs and tissues are primarily pulmonary diseases: The fungal propagules are inhaled into the bronchi and lungs, from where the organisms disseminate, usually hematogenously, to various other sites, giving rise to secondary, or metastatic, lesions. The subcutaneous mycoses develop following contamination of a puncture wound. The cutaneous mycoses, in which the fungus rarely penetrates beyond the dead layers of the skin, are primarily diseases causing cosmetic problems and minor annoyance; there rarely is any significant lasting damage. In only a few mycoses—for example, genital candidiasis, trichomycosis pubis, and the dermatomycoses—is there direct person-to-person transfer. In the annoying, yet common, mycoses known collectively as the *dermatomycoses,* there may be direct transfer or there may be indirect transfer from person to person by way of the environment. The floors of showers are frequently contaminated with the fungi that cause "athlete's foot." Unless clothing or towels that have been in contact with the disease site are disinfected properly, reinfection is common.

Several of the fungi causing deep mycoses are dimorphic; that is, they can assume one or the other of two different forms, depending on the environment. The usual pattern is for the tissue phase (*in vivo*) and the phase grown *in vitro*

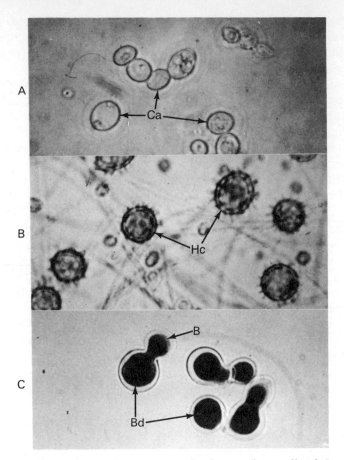

Figure 16.1 (A) Photomicrograph of yeast-phase cells of *Candida albicans* (Ca). The organisms are spherical to subspherical. (B) Photomicrograph of macroconidia of *Histoplasma capsulatum* (Hc). Note the tuberculate macroconidia typical of the beige strains of the organism. (C) Photograph of yeast phase of *Blastomyces dermatitidis* (Bd). Note the broad base of attachment of the bud (B) to the parent cell.

at 37°C to be identical and to be a yeast. The form that develops *in vitro* at room temperature is mycelial (filamentous), producing one or more types of conidia, which are asexual reproductive structures. For some of the dimorphic fungi, the yeast phase (Y-phase) is a more-or-less nondescript yeast cell with few, if any, distinctive features. For identification in such cases, the mycelial phase (M-phase) must be obtained, because only the conidial structures provide a basis for recognition. For example, *Histoplasma capsulatum*, the causal agent of histoplasmosis, can only be identified by examination of its M-phase. During the Y-phase it is a small (2–4 μm), ovate, single-budding yeast; whereas during the M-phase it develops distinctive macroconidia (Figure 16.1*b*). The causal agent of blastomycosis (*Blastomyces dermatitidis*), on the other hand, produces an ambiguous conidial

M-phase; in the Y-phase it becomes a characteristic small, single-budding yeast with a broad bud attachment (Figure 16.1*c*). The exception to the rule that the Y-phase occurs *in vivo* and *in vitro* during cultivation at 37°C is *C. albicans,* in which the reverse is true. *In vivo* and at 37°C in the incubator, *C. albicans* grows as a pseudomycelial organism (Figures 16.2*a* and 2*b*), and only *in vitro* at room temperature (or, at least, at less than 35°C) does it grow as a single-budding yeast. It is important to note that, at least theoretically, to identify a fungus, the interconversion from Y- to M- and M- to Y-phases must be demonstrated; in practice, this probably is not done as part of the routine identification of the causal agent of most fungal infections.

THE MYCOSES

Mycoses are classified, according to the parts of the body affected, as *cutaneous, subcutaneous,* or *deep mycoses.* This classification is artificial. Subcutaneous mycoses may also have a cutaneous manifestation, and deep mycoses usually

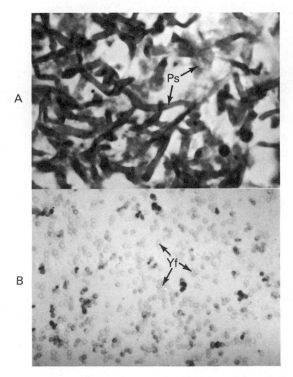

Figure 16.2 Photomicrographs of (A) pseudomycelial and (B) yeast forms of *Candida albicans.* Note the chains of elongate yeast cells constituting the pseudomycelium (Ps); contrast this to the single and single-budding cells (Yf) that form in culture at room temperature.

involve subcutaneous and cutaneous tissues as well as the internal organs. The scheme for the classification of human mycoses is outlined in Table 16.1; the mycoses listed are illustrative, not exhaustive.

Cutaneous mycoses affect only the dead layer of the skin and its appendages, the hair and nails. They cause little damage, but rather are primarily minor diseases, disfiguring and annoying. As stated earlier, most fungi cannot cause disease in a normal, healthy animal or person; cutaneous mycoses are probably the exception to this rule, as they produce infections in many healthy, normal people and animals.

A description of a few of the mycoses is given in Table 16.1. Some of the diseases discussed are selected because of their common occurrence; others to illustrate a diagnostic point or a principle of treatment.

Superficial Mycoses

Among cutaneous superficial mycoses, the one most commonly seen by dermatologists is pityriasis versicolor, which is caused by *Malasezzia furfur.* The macular lesions characteristic of this condition are clearly circumscribed and are located on the smooth skin of the body. As they age, the lesions become scaly. In Caucasions, if the lesion is on a part of the trunk not exposed to sunlight, it will appear tan or fawn colored; that is, darker than the surrounding skin. If it is on an area that is "tanned," the lesion is lighter than the surrounding tissue. Hence on either site the lesion is an obvious cosmetic problem.

Diagnosis of pityriasis versicolor is made during an office procedure that requires about 15 minutes and a moderately good microscope. Scales are collected from a lesion onto a glass microscope slide. They should be defatted with either acetone or ether before one or two drops of 10–20 percent potassium hydroxide are added; a cover glass is placed over the slide. After heating gently to speed the clearing of the host cells, the scales should be viewed at 400× magnification. Evidence of refractive hyphal fragments and thick-walled spores will confirm the presence of *M. furfur* (Figure 16.3). If there is some doubt, the patient should be placed in a darkened room and the lesions examined with the aid of a specially filtered ultraviolet light (Wood's lamp); lesions of pityriasis versicolor fluoresce a bluish-green under Wood's light. No culture is necessary, so diagnosis can be made readily. If for some reason a culture is desirable or necessary, culture of the highly lipophilic *M. furfur* is carried out on a medium rich in a lipid such as vegetable oil. Treatment will vary: most treatments are with topical preparations containing selenium sulfide. As an adjunct to the topical treatment, clothing that has been in contact with the lesions should be boiled or otherwise fully disinfected as a precaution against self-reinfection.

Beyond all doubt, dermatophytosis is the most important group of fungal diseases by virtue of its high incidence of infection. The various fungi that cause dermatophytoses affect only dead layers of skin, and hair and nails, but that means they can evoke lesions literally from the top of the head to the tip of the toes and at all points in between. Thus we have specific dermatophytoses such as tinea capitis (ringworm of the scalp), tinea facialis (facial ringworm), tinea barbae (ring-

Table 16.1 A CLASSIFICATION OF HUMAN MYCOSES

I. Superficial Mycoses

A. Cutaneous Mycoses — Nondestructive, "cosmetic" diseases of the dead layers of skin and its appendages (hair and nails)

    1. Trichomycosis[a] — Soft, "greasy" growth affecting auxiliary or pubic hairs, caused by *Corynebacterium tenuis*

    2. Black Piedra — Hard, dark concretions on hair; caused by *Piedraia hortae*

    3. White Piedra — Soft, cream-colored aggregations on hair; caused by *Trichosporon beigelii*

    4. Pityriasis versicolor — Scaling lesions of skin that fluoresce golden yellow under filtered UV light (Wood's lamp); caused by *Malasezzia furfur*

    5. Erythrasma[a] — Erythematous, scaly lesions that fluoresce a pink color under Wood's lamp; caused by *Nocardia minutissima*

    6. Dermatophytosis — Discomforting but not permanent lesions of skin, hair, and nails, caused by species of *Epidermophyton, Microsporum,* and *Trichophyton* (*e.g.,* tinea capitis or ringworm of the scalp, tinea cruris or "jock itch," and tinea pedis or "athlete's foot")

    7. Tinea nigra — Superficial asymptomatic brown or black nonscaly lesions caused by *Exophiala wernickii* (appears like a silver nitrate stain on the hands)

B. Mucous Membrane Mycoses — Mucocutaneous manifestations of subcutaneous and deep mycoses (*e.g.,* mucocutaneous sporotrichosis or mucocutaneous histoplasmosis, respectively). Thrush or candidiasis of the mucous membranes is caused by *Candida albicans*

II. Subcutaneous Mycoses — Affecting primarily subcutaneous layers, often with extensive tissue damage and disfigurement; may disseminate to deep organs

A. Chromomycosis — A disease (usually) of the extremities, following a puncture wound, and culminating in conspicuous "cauliflowerlike" hyperplastic growths. Caused by several species of nonsexual fungi in the genera *Fonsecaea, Phialophora,* and *Cladosporium*

B. Sporotrichosis — A disease characterized by open, draining "boillike" lesions following a puncture wound; subcutaneous nodules develop along the superficial lymph system draining the area; caused by *Sporothrix schenckii*

C. Mycetoma — A granulomatous disease, characterized by the development of open draining lesions in which are found microcolonies (granules) of the causal agent. These granules must be viewed microscopically to make a definitive diagnosis.

    1. Eumycetoma — Granule formed of filaments 3–5 μm wide (caused by many true fungi);

Table 16.1 (*Continued*)

	or
2. Actinomycetoma[a]	Granules formed of filament 1 μm-wide (caused by several species of actinomycetes)
III. Deep Mycosis	Usually primary pulmonary diseases that may disseminate to other deep organs; or may be only an ephemeral, unapparent, self-limited disease, with little or no lasting damage or evidence of the encounter. (The following list of deep mycoses is meant to be illustrative, not exhaustive.)
A. Candidiasis	Acute or subacute infections in which the fungus causes lesions in the mouth, vagina, skin, nails, bronchi or lungs, kidney, and occasionally a septicemia, endocarditis, or meningitis. Caused mostly by *Candida albicans*, a member of the internal or external normal flora.
B. Histoplasmosis	A primary pulmonary disease; 95% of infections are inapparent, causing a self-limited disease in which the only lasting evidence of infection is a positive skin test; worldwide distribution, but with high endemicity in the Ohio and Mississippi river valleys.
C. Coccidioidomycosis	A primary pulmonary disease; 99% of patients have complete recovery; some may develop subcutaneous granulomata or may develop progressive, disseminated infection, which are usually fatal (especially in Filipino and other dark-skinned males); causal agent is *Coccidioides immitis;* geographically limited to arid southwestern United States and a few areas in Central and South America
D. Blastomycosis	A primary pulmonary disease producing in many instances a benign, self-limited infection that induces a delayed type antibody reaction, that presumably leaves the patient immune to reinfection; a progressive disease, that may disseminate to any internal organ system except the gastrointestinal tract; caused by *Blastomyces dermatitidis;* limited to North America, Africa, and a few locales in Europe
E. Cryptococcosis	An acute, subacute, or chronic pulmonary, systemic, or meningeal mycosis, with the pulmonary form usually transitory, mild and undetected; may disseminate to other deep organs, especially the central nervous system; caused by *Cryptococcus neoformans,* an encapsulated yeast; worldwide distribution, especially in conjunction with avian feces

Table 16.1 (*Continued*)

F. Paracoccidioidomycosis	A chronic granulomatous disease of the skin, mucous membranes, lymph nodes, and virtually all internal organs, although it is considered as a primary pulmonary disease; caused by *Paracoccidioides brasiliensis;* geographically it is limited to South America, with a majority of cases reported along the Amazon River
G. Nocardiosis[a]	A disease caused by an actinomycete simulating a disease caused by eumycete; acute or chronic suppurative primary pulmonary infections that may metastasize to subcutaneous tissues and internal organs; causal agents in the actinomycete genera, *Actinomyces, Nocardia* and *Streptomyces,* with *N. asteroides* the most commonly isolated organism.
H. Actinomycosis[a]	Also not a true fungal disease, it is usually a chronic suppurative and granulomatous disease, the principal causal agent is *Actinomyces israelii* in humans and *A. bovis* in cattle.

[a]Discussed in medical mycology courses because they simulate true fungal diseases and are rarely, if ever, discussed in pathogenic microbiology courses.

worm of the beard area, or "Barber's itch"), tinea corporis (ringworm of the smooth skin of the body), tinea manuum (hand), tinea unguium (nail), tinea cruris (crotch), and tinea pedis ("athlete's foot").

There is abundant evidence that infection with the dermatophytoses may be

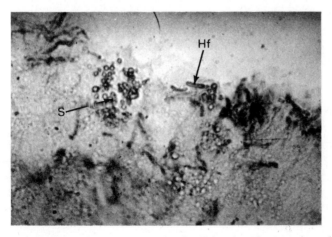

Figure 16.3 Photomicrograph of a scale of epidermis, cleared and stained by the Notchkiss-McManus procedure, revealing the hyphal fragments (Hf) and thick-walled spores (S) of *Malasezzia furfur.*

by direct person-to-person, animal-to-person, or person-to-animal transfer of fungal spores and hyphal fragments as well as by contamination from the environment. In the case of hair and skin infections, transfer from person to person or from animal to person may be mediated by combs and brushes.

There is evidence that it may take several contacts with the same dermatophyte to evoke an active lesion. The best evidence of this comes from experimental studies with mice. In gnotobiotic mice, depending on the species of fungus, it requires from four to six inoculations to produce an active lesion. This strongly suggests that the first inoculations sensitize the inoculation site to evoke a local allergic reaction. Subsequently inoculated spores or hyphal fragments then elicit typical scaly lesions. After the initial full-blown lesion has developed and subsided, it is difficult to induce further lesions on the animal, suggesting that immunity has developed.

Many of the dermatophytoses, particularly tinea manuum and some types of tinea pedis, occur unilaterally. The usual explanation for the unilateral manuum is that the pH of the skin on the two hands differs. For unilateral tinea pedis, the suggestion is often made that it is due to the unequal abrasion on the soles of the feet due to favoring one foot over another.

Often cases of dermatophytosis clear spontaneously. Tinea capitis (ringworm of the scalp) is primarily a disease of children. It varies from a benign scaly, noninflamed subclinical condition to an inflammatory disease characterized by the production of scaly erythematous lesions that may become severely inflamed. Alopecia may occur. The condition seldom persists into adulthood.

In epidemic tinea capitis, the usual picture is of a disease rampant on the scalps of children who have not yet reached puberty; after puberty, the disease clears spontaneously. The changes in the fatty acids constituting the scalp oils, from short-chain, even-numbered carbon fatty acids to long-chain, odd-numbered carbon fatty acids that occur during maturation may be a factor in these cures.

Some apparent spontaneous cures are merely a reflection of the balance between the rate of growth of the organism in the dead layers of the skin and the rate of shedding of the skin. These fungi exist in a state of *balanced saprobism*, that is, they grow inwardly at about the same rate as cells die and are sloughed off. During periods of quiescence, aggressive action in favor of enhancing sloughing affects this balance. Either chemical action by the application of keratinolytic agents or mechanical action by washing followed by vigorous abrasion with a coarse towel—or both—may help to control, if not cure, tinea pedis.

Subcutaneous Mycoses

Sporotrichosis (Figure 16.4) is an example of a subcutaneous mycoses. Sporotrichosis is a disease of worldwide distribution that is caused by the opportunistic dimorphic fungus *Sporothrix schenckii.* The natural reservoir of *S. schenckii* is the soil, so the history of a case of sporotrichosis will always include a puncture wound or skin abrasion, and contamination with soil particles.

There are several types of the mycosis, the most common of which is cutaneous lymphangitic sporotrichosis. The initial puncture wound may heal over, but after

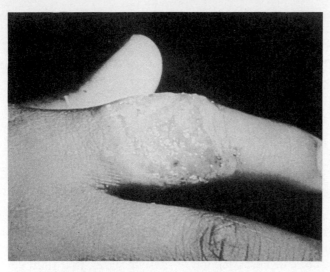

Figure 16.4 Photograph of the chancrelike primary lesion of sporotrichosis, which may develop following a puncture wound.

about 7 to 10 days a boil-like lesion usually develops, from which a sero-purulent exudate drains. This "boil" resists the usual forms of therapy. Without effective treatment, subcutaneous nodules develop along the superficial lymph ducts draining the area. If the primary lesion is curetted (a practice often used to treat recalcitrant "boils"), the subcutaneous nodules ulcerate and lesions develop further up the lymph system.

It is often difficult to detect the yeast cells in a stained smear of the exudate from the primary lesion. If the exudate is plated out on appropriate isolation media, a colony develops. If injected into an experimental animal, minute caseous lesions develop on the surfaces of organs in the peritoneal cavity. In cultures maintained at room temperature (20°–25°C) a mycelial colony develops. The colony is slow-growing and, at first, creamy, later developing brown or black sectors. The mycelial mass of the colony will ultimately produce conidia, either singly along the hypha or in a rosette arrangement on a short conidiophore. *In vivo* or *in vitro,* between 35° and 37°C *S. schenckii* grows as a single-budding yeast that is from 2 to 4 μm in length. Because the morphology of the yeast cells (Y-cells) is not unique to *S. schenckii,* the Y-phase growth must be converted to the M-phase to make an identification.

Sporotrichosis is perhaps the most readily cured of the mycoses. Although new antifungal drugs have emerged, the drug of choice for sporotrichosis remains saturated aqueous potassium iodide (KI). As with any mycosis, treatment should be continued for four weeks after the symptoms have abated.

Several immunological tests are available to help in the diagnosis of sporotrichosis. About two weeks after infection, the patient will react positively to a sporotrichin skin test. Sporotrichin is a product of the growth of the M-phase in a nonallergenic broth. It is standardized by testing in a known reactor after tests for pyrogenicity and sterility have been carried out. Caution must be exercised in interpretation of the skin test since in highly endemic areas skin test hypersensitivity develops in persons without clinical signs of an infection. Immunodiffusion and latex agglutination tests are also available. They are the easiest to perform and are the most specific serological procedures available. Cross reactions with other mycotic, bacterial, or parasitic infections do not occur. The various immunological tests are an aid in diagnosis, but for definitive diagnosis the organism must be cultured and identified.

Deep Mycoses

Among the various deep mycoses, most seem to be primary pulmonary diseases from which the organisms may disseminate hematogenously to various other organs, where metastatic lesions develop. However, there is abundant evidence, at least for several of the most common of these diseases, that from 90 to 95 percent of the infections remain subclinical, inapparent, self-limiting infections. In some respects such an encounter is desirable since it renders the patient immune to exogenous reinfection from all but massive exposures. The fungi causing these diseases are opportunistic; that is, they do not cause overt disease in a normal, healthy person, but rather in individuals whose immune systems are compromised.

Only three of the deep mycoses will be discussed in any detail: histoplasmosis, blastomycosis, and candidiasis.

Histoplasmosis

Histoplasmosis is worldwide in occurrence, although there are several areas where infection is particularly prevalent. For example, in the United States, the lower Ohio and the Mississippi river valleys have a high incidence of histoplasmosis. Any soil carrying much aged avian feces or bat guano is an ideal site for the causal agent, *H. capsulatum.* Thus caves frequented by bats, or soil under trees used as roosts by blackbirds, are ideal areas from which to recover *H. capsulatum.*

From the primary pulmonary sites the disease can spread to virtually all internal organs, although there is a predilection for infection in the cells of the reticulo-endothelial system. *In vivo* the fungus grows as a small, single-budding yeast between 2 and 4 μm in length; growth may be intra- or intercellular. The intracellular parasites are usually so abundant as to cause disruption of the host cells by their presence. The parasite is easily demonstrated in stained smears of blood, where it is usually found in the mononuclear cells.

In those instances when overt disease develops, it may be a chronic progressive lung disease, a chronic cutaneous or systemic disease, or an acute fulminating, rapidly fatal systemic disease. The latter condition is especially common in children. In addition to the signs of pulmonary infection revealed by x-rays, there is almost always hepato- and splenomegaly, an irregular fever, low red blood cell and lymphocyte counts, and emaciation.

Serologic data can be useful in the diagnosis of histoplasmosis. About the only time a delayed type hypersensitivity reaction may be of value is in a patient with disseminated histoplasmosis. Then the absence of skin-test reactivity following a prior positive skin test is an indication of anergy and is a grave sign.

Complement fixation is valuable for both diagnostic and prognostic purposes. Complement-fixing antibodies appear at two to four weeks after infection. A rising titre indicates dissemination; a titre of 1:32 or higher that remains constant or rises is indicative of active progressive disease. As antigen, either a heat-killed Y-phase or an M-phase preparation of the organism (histoplasmin) may be used; reactivity with the Y-phase preparation is retained longer than is reactivity with the M-phase preparation. Serum from people with histoplasmosis reacts with the organisms that cause cryptococcosis, blastomycosis, and coccidioidomycosis. To obtain a specific reaction, the serum must be absorbed with cells of the causal agents of the other three mycoses.

Immunodiffusion and latex agglutination tests for histoplasmosis are available. In the immunodiffusion plates, serum from patients produces two lines of significance: an *m* line is produced by serum from patients who have recovered or from patients who are in early stages of the disease; and an *h* line, closer to the serum well, is produced by serum from patients with active disease. The *h* line disappears with resolution of the disease. In the latex agglutination test, serum is mixed with latex particles coated with histoplasmin; this test becomes positive before or at the same time as the CF test becomes positive.

Data on the immunoglobulin content of the patients' serum may be helpful. In new infections, IgM specific for the parasite appears first, followed by IgG and IgA. In patients with chronic histoplasmosis, serum IgM and IgG levels remain normal, but there is an absolute increase in IgA.

Treatment of patients with disseminated histoplasmosis is difficult. In any but highly disseminated cases, bed rest and supportive therapy frequently are sufficient to effect a cure. When drug treatment is indicated, amphotericin B or amphotericin-methyl ester is used. The drawback to amphotericin B is that it is almost as toxic to host cells as to the parasite. Undesirable side effects vary from severe headaches to irreversible liver damage.

To make a definitive diagnosis, the causal agent must be isolated and identified by the micromorphology of the mycelial phase: for *H. capsulatum*, a beige colony producing tuberculate macroconidia or an albino colony producing smooth macroconidia between 8 and 14 μm in diameter is characteristic. Ideally, both phases of the organism should be examined. The M-phase should be converted to the Y-phase by transferring it to a rich medium and incubating it under 5 percent CO_2 at from 35° to 37°C. It may require several serial transfers to convert the M-phase to the Y-phase. The Y-phase cells are from 2 to 4 μm in size. When the Y-phase cultures are returned to room temperature, the M-phase will grow out. The dimorphic interconversion and examination of the two phases is necessary to differentiate *H. capsulatum* from a genus (*Sepedonium*) of soil saprobes that produces very similar macroconidia. Identification of the organism based on micromorphology of the mycelial phase must be verified by examination of the Y-phase to confirm the diagnosis of histoplasmosis.

Blastomycosis

Blastomycosis is a primary pulmonary mycosis that is usually an inapparent, subclinical, self-limiting infection. When disease develops, lesions may be cutaneous, subcutaneous, or occur in deep organs. The disease is worldwide in occurrence, with known foci of high endemicity. Until the 1950s, all reported cases had been in the United States, especially in Kentucky and Tennessee. Autochthonous cases have since been reported from 10 countries in Africa, and from Poland, England, and Switzerland.

Blastomycosis is a granulomatous and suppurative disease in its extrapulmonary forms. When dissemination occurs, other body sites become involved, especially skin and bone. The cutaneous disease is characterized by the presence of microabscesses closely spaced in a circular pattern; this causes the lesion to have an elevated border that is usually reddish-purple in color. As the lesion enlarges radially, spontaneous healing occurs in the older portions of the lesion, leaving a very transparent, "tissue paper" scar. Differential diagnosis requires differentiation from various other chronic granulomatous or suppurative pulmonary diseases such as histoplasmosis and bronchogenic carcinoma. The cutaneous form may also resemble a variety of other skin diseases.

As with all subcutaneous and deep mycoses, a diagnosis is made by demonstrating the fungus in smears of specimens of exudate or of tissue sections, and is confirmed by the positive identification of the etiologic agent by culture.

The hematoxylin-eosin (H&E) stain routinely used in pathology laboratories does not differentiate fungi at all well. It is ideal for demonstrating human tissue structure, but the H&E stain has little affinity for fungal cell walls or cytoplasm. Although hematoxylin, which is a nuclear stain, does stain the nuclei of the fungi fairly well, they are so small that even an experienced pathologist may fail to detect fungi in an H&E-stained slide. Accordingly, where a mycosis is suspected and specimens or tissue sections are to be used, special fungal stains should be employed. All fungi are Gram-positive, so the Brown and Brenn modification of the Gram stain works well. Such special stains as the periodic acid Schiff (PAS) or Gomori's methenamine silver (GMS) are especially useful for staining fungi; if cryptococcosis is suspected the mucicarmine stain is ideal since it stains the polysaccharide capsule of *Cryptococcus neoformans*. For blastomycosis, either the PAS or GMS stains are fine. The former procedure stains the yeast cell wall magenta; in the latter the fungal cell wall stains black due to the deposition of the silver nitrate and the host cells are stained a light green by the counterstain.

The causal agent of blastomycosis is *B. dermatitidis. In vivo* and *in vitro* at from 35° to 37°C, the organism develops as a single-budding yeast cell in which the bud has a broad-based attachment to the parent cell. *In vitro* at room temperature, a mycelial colony develops, but its micromorphology is not unique. Since *B. dermatitidis* is a dimorphic fungus, the *in vitro* techniques previously outlined for identification of *H. capsulatum* may be used to effect the conversion of the organisms from the M-phase to the Y-phase. This will permit identification by examination of the two phases of the organisms.

The causal agent of blastomycosis has more proteolytic enzymes in the M-phase than in the Y-phase. Yet whether the inoculum is a conidium or a mycelial fragment, the organism does not become invasive until a yeast phase forms. There are mycoses in which the invasive form is mycelial—aspergillosis and zygomycosis, for example—but no yeast phase is known for these organisms. The invasive stage in most cases of candidiasis is pseudomycelial; that is, elongate yeast cells that fail to separate.

B. dermatitidis elaborates a chemotactic factor in culture. *B. dermatitidis* filtrates have greater chemotactic activity than do *H. capsulatum* or *C. neoformans* filtrates. *B. dermatitidis,* however, is more resistant to killing by phagocytes than are the other two.

A factor in the serum of patients with untreated blastomycosis inhibits neutrophil locomotion. The factor is not present in patients with histoplasmosis, coccidioidomycosis, cryptococcosis, sporotrichosis, or treated blastomycosis. A specific lymphocyte-transforming principle also has been isolated from *B. dermatitidis.*

Blastomycosis is treated with amphotericin B. For children or patients with mild disease, dihydroxystilbamidine may be used. Several of the newer imidazoles have some activity against the fungus, but to date not enough cases have been treated with these drugs to ascertain their effectiveness.

Candidiasis

Our last example of a human mycosis will be candidiasis, which is caused primarily by *C. albicans;* a low incidence of cases is evoked by six other species of the genus. Candidiasis will be used to illustrate several aspects of the interactions of human beings and zoopathogenic fungi. Candidiasis may assume many forms; it may be superficial, as in thrush, or it may invade deeply into the body.

C. albicans is part of the normal flora of the skin and gastrointestinal tract of many humans. About 35 percent of normal, healthy people have *C. albicans* in the oral cavity; up to 85 percent of normal, healthy people have *C. albicans* in their feces; and it is common in the vagina and in the epidermal microflora. In each instance, *C. albicans* may exist in the absence of any overt signs of candidiasis. Thus, the fungus may exist as a commensal on or in the human body.

Several conditions are known to predispose to overt candidiasis. For example, extreme obesity may lead to cutaneous candidiasis; a *Candida* superinfection is not uncommon in babies with diaper rash. The avitaminosis common in the elderly, due to malnutrition, may result in perleche, a mucocutaneous form of the disease with lesions forming characteristically at the corners of the lips. There is evidence that vaginal candidiasis is exacerbated during pregnancy and by the pregnancylike changes that occur in the vaginal mucosa of women taking oral contraceptives. There are cases of congenital, generalized candidiasis in newborn infants. These usually occur following delivery by a mother with overt vaginal candidiasis who has had a prolonged labor after the fetal membranes burst. Any event that immunologically or mechanically compromises the individual may lead to overt candidiasis. For example, *C. albicans* is the bane of existence of individuals with genetically deficient immune systems. Candidiasis is common in acquired immunodeficiency syndrome (AIDS) patients, also. Severely burned children often develop generalized deep candidiasis four to six days after the burn. *C. albicans* can become an insidious pathogen when conditions allow the organism to invade.

The Candidas are dimorphic fungi. They are pseudomycelial *in vivo* and *in vitro* at 35°–37°C and are single-budding yeasts when cultured at room temperature. The mere cultural recovery of *C. albicans* does not warrant a diagnosis of candidiasis; the organism must be shown to have become invasive by demonstration of the pseudomycelial forms and the yeast cells that sometimes accompany them in stained sections of tissue from the lesion.

The Candidas are among the few zoopathogenic fungi for which the results of a battery of physiological tests are necessary to determine the species of the causal agent. Both fermentation and assimilation patterns are used, along with pellicle formation, the utilization of ethanol, and the splitting of arbutin.

Because *C. albicans* is the cause of perhaps 90 percent of all cases of candidiasis, routine identifications made in many hospital microbiology laboratories are simply reported as: *"C. albicans"* or *"Candida* not *albicans."* Treatment is usually the same regardless of which species is the causal agent, so differentiation is unimportant. Two procedures are used to distinguish *C. albicans* from other Candidas. The quickest and best is the serum filamentation test. From 1 to 2 ml of a one-in-two dilution of human serum is inoculated with the unknown Candida and incubated at 37°C for two hours. Only *C. albicans* will form a pseudomycelium (germ tubes) within two hours; this procedure distinguishes *C. albicans* from other Candidas in at least 95 percent of cases. Growth of the Candidas on corn meal/Tween 80 agar also helps identification. The site of inoculation is covered with a sterile cover slip and incubated at room temperature for 12 to 18 hours; only *C. albicans* produces a pseudomycelium with an abundance of large, thick-walled terminal chlamydospores (chlamydoconidia) under these culture conditions.

Although there is probably more literature on Candidas and the diseases they cause than on any other zoopathogenic fungus, the genus needs further taxonomic definition.

CULTURAL PROCEDURES

When clinical data lead to a presumptive diagnosis of, say, histoplasmosis, and a bronchial aspirate is sent to the laboratory with the request "Culture for fungi," the technician will routinely plate out the specimen on special culture media and incubate one plate at room temperature and the other at 37°C. Pathogenic fungi require about five days to grow out from a clinical specimen, so plates should be held at least one week before they should be considered as negative for fungi. Once the M-phase is recovered and has shown the morphology typical of one of the fungi, the M-phase growth may be transferred to a rich medium (such as chocolate agar) and incubated in a 37°C incubator in an atmosphere of between 5 and 10 percent CO_2. After one or two transfers in this new environment, mycelial growth will cease and gradual conversion to a Y-phase will occur. The conversion from Y-phase to M-phase requires simpler manipulation; it requires only that the culture vessel be removed from the incubator and that incubation be continued at room temperature. Induction of the interconversion is important, especially for fungi such as

antigens in a variety of strains of the pathogen. The cowpox virus that served as a vaccine to protect from smallpox is an example of a living agent that protects against a heterologous infection. Live vaccines that elicit humoral and cell-mediated immune responses against many different antigens and multiple epitopes are often broadly protective.

HOST RESPONSE TO VACCINATION

Antibody Responses to Vaccines

The induction of a protective immune response depends in most cases on the interaction of both B- and T-cells. This is the case with live vaccines such as those for prevention of measles. Some vaccines, however, can initiate B-cell proliferation and antibody production without inducing T-cells. This is unusual but occurs with the capsular polysaccharide vaccines against pneumococci.

The induction of lymphocytes of the various subsets results in the production of multiple types of effector systems. There may be multiplication of B-lymphocytes with production of immunoglobulins directed against the antigenic determinants in the vaccine. Memory-type B-lymphocytes may also be induced. The mechanisms of action of the antibodies induced may include direct neutralization of toxins as occurs in control of diphtheria, opsonization of pathogens as occurs in control of pneumococcal infections, complement-dependent microbial lysis as occurs in cholera, neutralization of viral infectivity as occurs in control of hepatitis B infection, and antibody-dependent cellular toxicity as occurs in the control of *Salmonella typhi* infections. If immunization induces memory cells, protection still results from the antibody the B-cells produce. The memory cells simply give the advantage of a rapid secondary response at the time of infection.

Stimulation of T-lymphocytes by the vaccine may bring about a broad range of responses that are related, in part, to the antigenic determinant's ability to induce specific T-cell subsets. Thus, the sensitized T-cells can influence B-cell activity or can act through cell-mediated immune responses. Another mechanism is to produce lymphokines that stimulate macrophage function. It is particularly important that vaccines designed for control of infections caused by intracellular microbes be capable of inducing T-cell immunity.

Artificially induced immunity may not be complete, and even with generally functional vaccines one cannot always assume that protection has developed after immunization. One way of evaluating the immune response following injection of vaccine is by measuring the quantity of circulating antibodies to the antigens in the vaccine. The process of development of antibodies is called *seroconversion.* In some instances, the presence of circulating antibodies correlates well with development of protection. This is the case with the hepatitis B and rubella vaccines. Antibody levels, however, do not tell the whole story. If there is a strong immunologic memory response, protection may exist in the absence of detectable antibody. For example, following vaccination with agents such as live attenuated measles and rubella vaccines, there will be an initial IgM antibody response, followed by a rise in IgG antibody titers. Over time, the antibody titers will fall, but even though they may fall to undetectable levels, when infection occurs there is a rapid response by the memory cells. In such situations there is both a prompt increase in IgG antibodies specific for the virus and protection from disease. The mere presence of antibody, however, may not be sufficient to assure protection from disease since a minimum level of antibody may be required. Such is the case if immunity to tetanus is to be induced by injection of tetanus toxoid.

Determinants of Response to Vaccines

Many factors determine the nature and the extent of a response to immunization. These attributes of the vaccine include the physical, chemical, and conformational state of the antigenic agent (that is, its antigenicity). Other factors include the route and timing of administration, and the condition of the host at the time of immunization.

The route of administration, which is determined in part by the nature of the vaccine, plays some role in determining the nature, extent, and duration of the immunologic response to the vaccine. The inactivated poliomyelitis vaccine (Salk vaccine), for example, is injected into the muscle, whereas the live, attenuated polio vaccine (Sabin vaccine) is administered orally. The Salk vaccine induces systemic IgG antibodies against polioviruses. In individuals given this type of vaccine, poliovirus can infect the intestines but the spread of virus to the brain and spinal cord through the bloodstream is blocked by the neutralizing IgG antibodies. On the other hand, the Sabin vaccine induces both systemic IgG and local IgA antibody production in the gastrointestinal mucosa. This type of vaccine therefore not only blocks dissemination of the virus but also prevents significant infection of the gastrointestinal tract by pathogenic polioviruses.

The timing of vaccination in relation to the anticipated exposure is important in disease control by immunization. To have optimal efficacy, vaccines must be administered far enough in advance of potential exposure to permit immunity to be induced. In general, it takes from one to three weeks for full development of the immune response following antigenic stimulation, and the induced immunity may wane with passage of time. Knowledge of epidemiologic factors is thus crucial in deciding the appropriate timing of vaccine administration. Immunization against influenza is most efficacious if the vaccine is administered in late autumn or early winter, just prior to the influenza "season." Similarly, the schedule for routine childhood immunizations against measles, mumps, rubella, diphtheria, pertussis (whooping cough), tetanus, amd polio is based on the prevalence of those diseases in childhood. Immunization is usually done before enrollment in school, where the concentration of children in classrooms favors infection. Very young infants are usually not immunized because it is generally desirable to wait for loss of maternal immunoglobulins and the maturation of the child's own immune system before immunizing them.

A factor that significantly affects the response to immunization is the overall condition of the vaccine recipient. Endogenous factors (such as age, genetic makeup, and general health status) and exogenous factors (such as infection or medication) are all important. A satisfactory response to immunization requires the recipient to be in an immunocompetent state. Those individuals with reduced immunocompetence, whether it be from an infection, hereditary defect, or treatment with immunosuppressive drugs, not only have poor immune responses but may also be at increased risk from the immunizing agent. This is especially true if live, attenuated vaccines are used. The attenuated agent may reproduce without restraint, and disease may be produced in the immunosuppressed individual. If vaccine is introduced into individuals who are incubating a disease, or if infection occurs during the period when the immune response to the vaccine is developing, severe disease may result. Living attenuated vaccines should not be given to pregnant women, for the fetus may be infected and damaged.

In summary, many factors must be taken into account when recommendations for immunoprophylaxis are developed. The recommendations must be based on the potential for exposure to particular pathogens, the probable times of exposure, and the consequences of such an exposure. The severity of the disease to be prevented must be balanced against the dangers of immunization and the discomfort and costs of immunization. The availability of a vaccine or toxoid must also be considered. The routine childhood immunizations in the United States are directed at the usual childhood diseases that occur there, such as measles, mumps, rubella, poliomyelitis, diphtheria, pertussis, tetanus, and *Haemophilus influenza* infection (Table 17.2). Immunization for various segments of the population are based on expected risk factors. Veterinarians and animal handlers receive prophylactic preexposure rabies vaccines, travelers and military personnel may be immunized against plague, yellow fever, and cholera. Elderly people may be immunized against influenza and pneumococcal pneumonia. Occupational hazards and life-style habits are thus important factors in planning immunization programs (Table 17.3).

Table 17.2 ROUTINE CHILDHOOD
IMMUNIZATIONS

Age	Immunization
2 mos.	DPT and OPV
4 mos.	DPT and OPV
6 mos.	DPT
15 mos.	DPT, OPV, MMR
24 mos.	HiB
4–6 yrs.	DPT and OPV
14–16 yrs.	
Every 10 yrs.	Td

DPT = Diphtheria and tetanus toxoids combined with pertussis vaccines; OPV = Trivalent oral polio vaccine; MMR = Measles, mumps, rubella; HiB = *Haemophilus influenza*, type B; and Td = Tetanus and diphtheria (adult type).

Table 17.3   VACCINES FOR SPECIFIC SITUATIONS OR GROUPS

Vaccine	Target group
Hepatitis B	Health care personnel
	Institutional workers
	Hemodialysis patients
	Hemophiliacs
	Homosexual males
	Illicit drug users
	Residents of correctional facilities and institutions for the mentally retarded
Influenza	Health care personnel
	Immunocompromised patients
	Patients with chronic diseases
	Elderly persons (over 65)
Pneumococcal polysaccharide	Immunocompromised persons
	Persons with splenic dysfunction/asplenia
	Chronic alcoholics
	Patients with chronic diseases
Rabies	Veterinarians, animal handlers, dogs, cats
Cholera, plague, yellow fever	Persons traveling to infected regions

PASSIVE IMMUNIZATION

Passive immunization, unlike active immunization, depends on the administration of preformed antibodies such as antitoxins to confer immediate, albeit temporary, protection. This approach is useful when exposure has already occurred (postexposure prophylaxis) or when there is either inadequate time to allow for effective active immunization before exposure or there is no active vaccine available (Table 17.4).

Table 17.4   GLOBULIN PREPARATIONS AVAILABLE FOR PASSIVE IMMUNIZATION

Product	Indications for use
Standard human immune serum globulins	
Intramuscular preparation	Prevention of Hepatitis A, measles, polio, and rubella
Intravenous preparation	Supplementation of people with immunoglobulin deficiencies and people with idiopathic thrombocytopenic purpura
Specific human immune serum globulins	
Hepatitis B	Prevention of Hepatitis B
Rabies	Prevention of Rabies
Tetanus	Prevention or treatment of tetanus
Varicella-zoster	Prevention of chickenpox

Passive immunization with antibodies occurs naturally by transplacental transmission or by passage in breast milk. It is only the very young who can assimilate antibody through the digestive tract. In older individuals administration of antibodies must be by injection. These antibodies may be in the form of antisera derived from animals who have been immunized with specific pathogens or toxins. While these heterologous sera have some use when administered prior to exposure or very early in the disease course, the hypersensitivity reactions that result from the administration of heterologous protein frequently outweigh the benefits to be derived from their administration.

In the 1940s, immune serum globulin prepared from pooled human plasma became available. It was and continues to be used in the prevention of infectious hepatitis, measles, rubella, and poliomyelitis. Immune serum globulin is often given to pregnant women who have contact with children infected with rubella as women now of childbearing age did not receive rubella vaccine as children. Immune globulin is given, for vaccine is not administed to pregnant women or women of childbearing age due to risks to the fetus. The antibodies protect the fetus from infection, which is a common cause of birth defects.

Immune serum globulin is a sterile solution containing antibodies from human blood; it is a 15–18 percent protein suspension derived by cold ethanol fractionation of pooled plasma. For years, immune serum globulin was available only as a preparation for intramuscular injection. This is because the ethanol precipitation procedure used for fractionation aggregates the immunoglobulin, yielding clumps that can activate complement and cause a shocklike condition when given intravenously. Intramuscular administration keeps the aggregates in the muscle but allows single immunoglobulin molecules to enter the circulation. The main problem with this is that only from 10 to 20 ml can be comfortably administered by the intramuscular route.

New techniques for separating gamma globulin from plasma that do not cause aggregation of antibodies have been developed. These immunoglobulin preparations can be administered intravenously so that large volumes and high levels of antibodies can be given. In fact, physiologically normal levels of immunoglobulin can now be achieved in patients who completely lack the ability to generate their own antibodies.

Human-origin immune globulins directed against specific diseases have been developed. These specific immune globulins are prepared from donors with high antibody titers against specific diseases. For example, individuals who have just recovered from varicella-zoster (shingles) will provide high titer antibody to that virus. Homologous antibody preparations are available for use in the prevention of tetanus, rabies, hepatitis B, and varicella-zoster infection of humans, for example.

Veterinarians use homologous sera to protect animals that have been exposed to various infections or that will be at immediate risk. For example, dogs taken to shows or housed in boarding kennels will be given canine-origin antidistemper serum if they have not been immunized against distemper. Any horse that is injured or that undergoes surgery receives equine-origin antitetanus serum.

COMPLICATIONS RESULTING FROM VACCINATION

Immunization is not completely free of problems. As noted previously, immunologically incompetent individuals may develop infections and disease following injection of attenuated live vaccines, and fetuses may also be adversely affected by these agents. Inactive or killed vaccines are simply ineffective in immunologically incompetent individuals.

On some occasions the vaccine may induce the disease it is designed to prevent. This occurred with some of the early Salk polio vaccines in which some virus was not inactivated during production. Other undesirable reactions may occur following immunization. Some cases of Guillain-Barre syndrome followed the swine influenza vaccination effort in 1976, for example. These undesirable or, as they are sometimes called, *idiosyncratic* reactions are particularly common with certain vaccines. The pertussis vaccine, for example, sometimes induces paralysis as a result of toxicity to the brain.

Allergic responses to vaccine components, independent of any protective responses, may result in immunologic disease in the vaccine recipient. Hypersensitivity reactions occurred following immunization with the original rabies vaccine prepared by Pasteur. This vaccine was composed of rabbit nervous tissue infected with rabies virus. After treatment to inactivate the virus, the entire preparation of nervous tissue was used to inoculate the patient. The neural tissue in the vaccine produced an immune response that cross reacted with host neural tissue and damaged the recipient's nervous system. Damage to vaccine recipients as a result of hypersensitivity to immunizing agents has also occurred following administration of killed measles vaccine. Occasionally this vaccine induced incomplete humoral immunity and, following infection by the measles virus, a cell-mediated hypersensitivity sometimes developed, causing a severe atypical measles syndrome.

VACCINE DEVELOPMENT AND PRODUCTION

Introduction

Vaccines for active immunization are of various types (Table 17.5). Vaccines may consist of suspensions of live attenuated microbes; of killed, inactivated microbes; of fractions of microbes; or of microbial products. Live vaccines generally evoke a durable immunologic response most like that resulting from natural infection. The currently available measles, mumps, and rubella vaccines are live attenuated agents. Living agents engender good immunogenicity because their growth results in continuous formation of antigen and prolonged antigenic stimulation. As infection is induced by the attenuated agents, the immunity generated resembles that resulting from natural infection. There is extensive stimulation of the immune system by the antigens produced by the infection; consequently, live vaccines usually require just one dose to induce protection.

Killed or inactivated vaccines that consist of whole organisms include cholera

Table 17.5 TYPES OF IMMUNOGENS AVAILABLE OR BEING DEVELOPED FOR ACTIVE IMMUNIZATION

Type of vaccine	Disease prevented
Live, unattenuated vaccines	Anaplasmosis, babesiosis, hog cholera
Live, attenuated vaccines	Measles, mumps, rubella, polio, yellow fever, tuberculosis
Killed or inactivated vaccines	
Whole organisms	Cholera, pertussis, plague, influenza, polio
Subunits of organisms	Influenza, hepatitis B
Soluble capsular polysaccharides	Pneumococcus, meningococcus, *Haemophilus influenza*
Recombinant DNA–type vaccines	Hepatitis B, malaria (sporozoite)
Toxoids	Diphtheria, tetanus
Synthetic polypeptide vaccines	*S. pyogenes* infection, foot-and-mouth disease, cholera, malaria (sporozoite and blood stage)

and pertussis vaccines; those that consist of components or subunits of an organism include influenza and hepatitis B vaccines. Vaccines made from soluble capsular polysaccharide material include those against pneumococcal pneumonia and meningococcal meningitis. Vaccines prepared from microbial products include the toxoids that are prepared by modifying bacterial exotoxins to make them nontoxic. Toxoids are used for prevention of diphtheria and tetanus.

As a rule, to achieve strong immunity with toxoids and killed vaccines multiple doses of vaccine must be given. To maintain adequate protective antibody levels for prolonged periods, booster injections are frequently required.

The goal of vaccine development is to obtain the purest preparation of the critical immunologically active materials with minimal contamination by nonessential materials. The objective is to assure an appropriate antigenic stimulation and to minimize the likelihood of undesirable side effects. The earliest vaccines were composed of live, wild-type organisms; most conventional modern-day vaccines, however, consist of either live, attenuated, or inactivated forms of microorganisms. Vaccines are currently being developed that take advantage of recent advances in immunology and molecular biology. Genetic engineering and chemical synthesis procedures show great promise as methods for vaccine production. The products produced by these techniques may prove to be advantageous in terms of good antigenicity, high specificity, and low ability to induce hypersensitivity.

Live Vaccines

Attenuated-type vaccines were classically produced by growing the pathogens in an "unnatural" host, by growth in culture, or by some other procedure that would select for mutant forms of the pathogen. Viruses have also been attenuated by being selected for their inability to grow well at temperatures present in the host and their ability to grow at lower temperatures, a process called *cold-adaptation*. The desired end result of these processes is the selection of a microbe that has decreased virulence and pathogenicity but is able to induce an immune response capable of protecting against the naturally occurring isolate. Until recently, the attenuation process was entirely by trial and error. An organism was repeatedly passaged in the unnatural host or other selective environment, then tested for virulence and antigenicity. As the science of molecular genetics is now providing information about the specific genes responsible for virulence and antigenicity, site-directed mutagenesis is being employed to produce microorganisms that lack only the genes responsible for virulence.

Inactivated Vaccines

Microbes to be used in inactivated vaccines may be inactivated by subjecting the pathogens to heating; by treatment with chemical agents such as formaldehyde, methanol, or beta-propiolactone; or by irradiation. As with attenuation, the goal of inactivation is to block infectivity yet preserve the major antigen determinants that induce the protective immune response.

Toxoids

Toxoids, as previously mentioned, are detoxified bacterial exotoxins. Soluble toxins, most notably from diphtheria and tetanus-causing organisms, are converted to toxoids by treatment with formalin and moderate heating. Though no longer toxic, toxoids have the ability to stimulate antitoxin formation. Immunization with toxoids protects by blocking the disease-causing process rather than by preventing infection by the microbe. To prepare toxoids for use as vaccines, they are usually precipitated by alum, which serves as an adjuvant. The primary immune response to most toxoids is generally very good, and anamnestic increases are appreciable when booster injections are given.

Subunit Vaccines

Although both attenuation and inactivation have produced many satisfactory vaccines, there are still many diseases for which vaccines do not exist, and many currently available vaccines produce undesirable side effects. In the continuing search for new vaccines and for improvement of existing vaccines, procedures for production of useful fractions of microbes are being sought. Vaccines that consist of fractions of microbes are called *subunit vaccines.* Subunit vaccines may be fractions of the infecting organism that are biochemically purified or that may be produced by genetic engineering. Since subunit vaccines do not contain actively replicating material, the risk of inducing infection is eliminated. They also lack microbial nucleic acids that may be potentially carcinogenic. One of the first successful subunit vaccines for use in humans is that for prevention of hepatitis B infection. It contains only purified hepatitis B surface antigen, the portion of the virus that elicits neutralizing antibodies. In one type of this vaccine, the antigen is derived from the plasma of chronic hepatitis B carriers; in another, it is produced by genetically modified plasmid-bearing yeasts. The efficacy of both types of this vaccine has been well-documented in controlled trials.

The polysaccharide capsules of encapsulated organisms such as pneumococcus, meningococcus, and *H. influenzae* are the virulence factors for those microbes. Vaccines were prepared from whole inactivated microbes. The soluble components of the capsules from these bacteria, however, have been shown to evoke type-specific protective responses as strong as those induced by the whole microbe. The polysaccharide capsule vaccines now in use induce antibodies that protect the recipient by enhancing phagocytosis of the organisms. These vaccines are used primarily to protect people in high-risk groups, such as the elderly and the very young. A recently developed subunit vaccine consists of a conjugate of *H. influenzae* type B polysaccharide with diphtheria toxoid. The protein toxoid serves as a carrier for the *Haemophilus* capsular polysaccharide, greatly improving its immunogenicity. This vaccine provides good protection against invasive hemophilus infection in young infants who, as a group, respond poorly to the unconjugated capsular antigen.

Recombinant DNA technology has great promise as a means of producing subunit vaccines. The process requires isolating the gene for the antigen, inserting that gene into a plasmid or other suitable carrier, introducing the complex into some host cell such as a bacterium, a yeast, or a mammalian or other animal cell that will express the gene. After the desired material is produced, it must be isolated from the culture or cell in which it was formed. Yeast and animal cells are able to add carbohydrate residues to the protein, yielding a glycoprotein that better mimics naturally occurring antigens. Bacterial host cells lack the ability to glycosylate the protein.

The recombinant hepatitis B vaccine is an example of a subunit vaccine produced by these procedures. As already noted, the plasma-derived vaccine is an effective vaccine, but high production costs and patient reservations regarding the unfounded possibility of transmission of the acquired immunodeficiency syndrome (AIDS) virus, HIV, has limited its use. The hepatitis B surface antigen has been synthesized in bacteria and in yeasts, as well as in monkey and mouse fibroblast cell lines. The yeast-derived vaccine was chosen because the surface antigen produced by the yeast is glycosylated and because there is the possibility that the animal cell lines may carry oncogenic viruses. The Food and Drug Administration licensed the recombinant hepatitis B vaccine produced in cultures of the bread yeast *Saccharomyces cerevisiae* in July 1986. The two forms of the vaccine have identical efficacy.

Another example of a currently available genetically engineered vaccine is that for immunization of piglets against enterotoxigenic strains of *Escherichia coli*. These bacteria secrete an enterotoxin that is responsible for severe diarrhea. The toxin consists of two subunits, an A subunit that is responsible for the toxic activity and a B subunit that is responsible for binding the A subunit to the intestinal epithelium. Following cloning of the toxin gene, the A subunit sequences were deleted, and the B subunit gene was transfected into *E. coli* K12. The result was that the genetically altered *E. coli* K12 produced a purified B subunit that, when collected from the culture, was an excellent toxoid.

Infectious Agents as Carriers of Genes for Antigen Production

Although recombinant DNA technology is proving to be a useful means of producing subunit vaccines such as those just described, in general these products produce immunity only equal to that of conventional inactivated vaccines. To obtain the type of immunity that results from the prolonged antigenic stimulation associated with infection, genetically modified microbes are being produced. The vaccinia virus is a popular agent for this work. Genes programming the production of the desired antigen are inserted into the virus and the modified virus is then used as the vaccine.

The concept is an attractive one. An attenuated live carrier—for example, a virus or bacterium that can infect but not harm the host—is engineered to express an added gene. When it produces infection, this recombinant microbe will then evoke long-lasting immune responses directed at both itself and the additional antigens. Vaccinia virus has been found to have a fairly broad capacity for accommodating foreign DNA without losing its infectivity. Vaccinia virus recombinants carrying genes for hepatitis B surface antigen, influenza virus hemagglutinin, herpes simplex virus glycoprotein D, and the gp120 surface antigen of HIV have been reported. In fact, because of the urgent need for development of an AIDS vaccine, the vaccinia–HIV antigen recombinant is already being tested in humans.

An avirulent *Salmonella* strain has also been tested as a carrier of genes producing antigens against infection by a variety of other microbes. This system has been used to induce immunity to infection by virulent strains of *Salmonella*. The avirulent *Salmonella* has also been used as a carrier for a plasmid-encoded gene for production of a toxin of *Shigella sonnei* and as a carrier of the gene coding for the B subunit of the toxin of enterotoxigenic *E. coli*.

Use of the heterologous recombinant carriers is still in its infancy, and field testing of these vaccines may reveal limitations that will detract from their usefulness. New virulence factors and tropisms might arise, and the antigenic nature of the carriers themselves may cause problems. For example, it has been suggested that development of antibodies to the gp120 HIV protein produced following immunization with a recombinant vaccinia virus may lead to an autoimmune-based attack on antigen-presenting cells that share some epitopes with gp120. The potential of viruses for promoting tumors is another possible problem with this type of vaccine.

Synthetic Antigens

Although it is not a new concept, the production of synthetic polypeptide vaccines has become more feasible with the advent of the techniques of molecular genetics. Anderer showed many years ago that short polypeptide fragments of the protein coat of tobacco mosaic virus could block inactivation of the virus by antiserum. This was the first demonstration that small fragments of a protein could bind antibodies. Subsequent studies showed that a hexapeptide from one fragment, when coupled to bovine serum albumin, would induce production of virus-specific neutralizing antibodies.

The first step in developing synthetic polypeptide vaccines is to identify the relevant "protection-inducing" antigen. Next, the amino acid sequence is determined, and the critical epitope is then synthesized chemically. The polypeptide, when attached to an appropriate carrier, induces production of antibody with specificity to the primary amino acid sequence. The induction of a protective immune response is not solely related to the primary amino acid sequence of an antigen, however. Antibodies to conformational determinants of the antigen expressed on the native pathogen may also be important. Although no synthetic polypeptide vaccines have been approved for use, some have been tested on humans under controlled conditions. An antimalarial vaccine is currently being tested at the vaccine center of the University of Maryland and by the United States Army (Table 17.5).

OTHER VACCINE CONSTITUENTS

In addition to the antigenic components, vaccine preparations usually contain other constituents, some active and some inert. These may be important because they may induce allergic or other undesirable reactions. These ingredients include suspending fluid that may be as simple as sterile water or saline, or may be a complex containing small amounts of protein or other constituents derived from the medium or biologic system in which the vaccine is produced. Serum proteins, egg antigens, or cell culture–derived antigens are often present in vaccines. Preservatives, stabilizers, and antibiotics are sometimes used to prevent or inhibit bacterial growth in the viral culture or the final product, and to stabilize antigens. The suspending fluid and stabilizing agents may cause allergic reactions if the recipient is sensitive to any of their components. Adjuvants are also usually added to nonliving vaccines. The only adjuvants approved for use in human medicine are aluminum compounds. They are used to enhance the immune response to vaccines that contain inactivated microorganisms or their products. Adjuvants are especially important in subunit or synthetic peptide vaccines that are often, by nature, weakly immunogenic. Alum adjuvants probably act by aggregating the antigen and causing its slow release, prolonging antigenic stimulation. It is possible that alum adjuvants also mobilize phagocytes to the site of antigen deposition.

SUMMARY

Progress in vaccine development has been characterized by simplification and purification of immunogenic agents; materials not needed for immunization are deleted from the vaccine. Attempts are being made to increase antigenicity through the use of more effective adjuvants. Attempts are also being made to develop vaccines for diseases for which none currently exist, such as malaria, herpes simplex infection, and AIDS. As our body of immunologic knowledge expands and our technologies become more sophisticated, new vaccines, based on simple synthetic peptides, for example, may become a reality. Immunization is and will remain our major tool in the prevention of disease in humans and animals.

SUGGESTIONS FOR FURTHER READING

American Academy of Pediatrics Committee on Infectious Diseases. *Report of the Committee on Infectious Diseases,* 19th edition. Evanston, Illinois, 1982.

D. C. Anderson and E. R. Stiehm. "Immunization." Journal of the American Medical Association *258*(20):3301, 1987.

K. J. Bart, W. A. Orenstein, and A. R. Hinman. "The current status of immunization principles: Recommendations for use and adverse reactions." J. Allergy Clin. Immun. *79*(2):296, 1987.

Immunization Practices Advisory Committee. "General recommendations on immunization." MMWR *32:*1, 1983.

F. Y. Liew. "New aspects of vaccine development." Clin. Exp. Immunol. *62:*225, 1985.

Chapter 18

Disease Transmission and Epidemiology

WILLIAM COLLINS

Malaria Branch
Division of Parasitic Diseases
Centers for Disease Control

INTRODUCTION

Disease transmission is the movement of diseases between individuals in populations of people or other animals. Disease can be considered to be any deviation from what is considered to be normal for the human or animal population and may include such conditions as sickle-cell disease, lead poisoning, asthma, yellow fever, acquired immunodeficiency syndrome (AIDS), cancer, heart disease, sleeping sickness, or foot-and-mouth disease.

The study of disease transmission in human populations is called *epidemiology*; in animal populations, *epizootiology*. Diseases that occur at a consistent low level in a human or animal population are called *endemic* or *enzootic* diseases, respectively. A very large-scale and devastating epidemic is called a *pandemic* or *panzootic* outbreak. Diseases that normally occur in animals rather than humans but that may infect humans are called *zoonotic diseases*. Many major diseases of humans are zoonotic. Bubonic plague, the "Black Death" of medieval Europe, is a zoonotic disease that survives in rodents between human epidemics.

The epidemiologist collects data that not only are useful for the control of epidemic diseases but are required for the practice of preventive medicine. It is the practice of preventive medicine through immunization, environmental modification, and sanitation that has made human life so much better in the advanced industrial countries in recent times. We take it for granted that most children will survive and that we will seldom have diarrhea, food poisoning, or infectious disease. When we visit the tropical world and become sick, or when we read about infant death rates of 50 percent or more in sub-Saharan Africa, we should think about the contributions that epidemiology and epidemiologists have made to our lives.

DISEASES CAUSED BY DEFECTS IN GENES

Genetically induced diseases include such afflictions as sickle-cell anemia and hemophilia. They are transmitted to offspring by parents whose germ cells contain the genes for the disease. At the present time, there is no way to prevent transmission of genetic diseases other than to provide genetic counseling to parents carrying such genes so that they may forego producing children if they so choose.

DISEASES CAUSED BY ENVIRONMENTAL CONTAMINATION

Exposure to contaminated air, water, or food is a major cause of disease in some populations. This is an area in which industrial development has actually increased problems in many cases. Manufacturing activities often produce toxic waste products that must either be detoxified or removed and isolated to prevent contact with humans. Nonetheless, many toxic substances escape into the environment, causing widespread disease in certain communities. Lead poisoning of children has been well documented. It may result from ingestion of paint used on children's playpens and furniture or from inhalation of lead in fumes from motor vehicles burning leaded gasoline.

Absorption through the skin may be the route of intoxication in some cases. The inadvertent release of toxic chemicals from manufacturing plants has been responsible for many illnesses and deaths. Extensive lung damage has occurred in people engaged in the mining and use of coal and asbestos. Diseases associated with the environment are often epidemic in nature but are usually restricted to individuals or populations doing specific work or living in specific areas. In many instances it has been difficult to identify the specific cause, and severe economic hardship often results from attempted corrective measures. Corrective measures may increase costs, and manufacturing plants may be closed.

The environmentally associated diseases are not transmissible from person to person but rather are individual responses to contamination. Unfortunately, in some cases removal of the chemical or agent from the environment may not be feasible, and only removal of the people from the contaminated area will eliminate the disease. Asthmatics who cannot tolerate the smog of major urban and industrial areas, for example, must move to cleaner areas because elimination of smog is not economically possible in most areas.

INFECTIOUS DISEASES SPREAD DIRECTLY BY PERSON-TO-PERSON CONTACT

In addition to the genetically transmitted and environmental diseases, there is the severe problem of infectious diseases caused by specific organisms such as viruses, bacteria, fungi, or protozoans that spread infection among members of the animal or human community.

Disease is spread most readily when the disease-causing agent is specific for humans or another animal species and is transmitted directly from individual to individual. Infection by inhalation is the mode of spread of many diseases, including colds, influenza, smallpox, measles, and pneumonic plague. Infection by ingestion of food and water contaminated with feces is also common (Figure 18.1). Cholera, typhoid, and giardiasis are spread by this route. Infection by injection of contaminated blood is a recently developed mode of spread. Hepatitis and AIDS are spread by this means. Transmission by sexual activity increases in importance with reduction in limits on sexual activity. Syphilis, gonorrhea, and AIDS are sexually transmitted.

Environmental and social factors greatly influence the transmission of these diseases. Since this type of transmission depends on direct contact or exchange of body fluids, many public health measures such as quarantine and isolation, treatment of sewage and water, and large campaigns of immunization and treatment with drugs and antibiotics greatly influence the maintenance and spread of these diseases. Indeed, these diseases often create serious problems in humans and animals. Theoretically, they should be the easiest to control, yet they are still common.

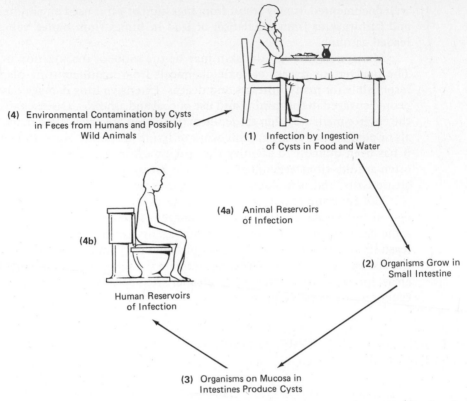

Figure 18.1 Life cycle of giardia. This organism enters its host with ingested food and water contaminated with encysted parasites (1). Parasites now in the intestine (2). Cysts produced are passed in the feces (3). Environmental contamination occurs. Food and water may be contaminated. Animal hosts as well as humans may serve as sources of infective cysts (4a&b). Control of the disease thus requires prevention of ingestion of cysts through programs of environment sanitation. Elimination of wild animal reservoirs of the parasite is not possible.

VECTOR-BORNE DISEASES

The vector-borne diseases are among the major public health problems of the world. They are particularly important in the tropics, where they have widespread distribution. Among these diseases are many caused by viral, protozoal, filarial, and rickettsial organisms. Some microbes are transmitted by bite, some by contamination with insect feces, and some by ingestion of the vector. Infection by some agents in some vectors must occur anew in each generation; in other cases infections are transmitted to the vector's offspring through the vector's ovaries.

Vector-borne Viral Diseases

Mosquitoes and ticks transmit an array of viruses such as those causing yellow fever, dengue, Japanese B encephalitis, and Congo-Crimean haemorrhagic fever. In general, the vector ingests infected blood from a person, monkey, bird, or some other host with the virus in the blood. After a period during which there is a reduction in the amount of virus in the vector, the virus begins to multiply and then becomes concentrated in various organs of the arthropod, including the salivary glands. After the virus has concentrated in the salivary glands, when the insect or other arthropod takes a blood meal the agent is transferred to the new host. If susceptible, the host may develop an infection and possibly disease.

In many cases the new host supports the agent while it awaits transmission to a new vector. Thus, in order to maintain the disease, the virus must be present in the blood of the primary host for a period long enough to infect the vector. If the viremia is of short duration or the amount of virus in the blood is low, the chances of transmission are small. Alternatively, if the viremia is maintained for many days or weeks, the likelihood of transmission is greatly increased.

Normally, a period of development of one week or more is required in the vector before the virus can be transmitted by bite. Therefore, a longer-lived vector will be more capable of transmitting the virus than a short-lived vector. As the number of hosts with immunity to the infection increases, however, the number of successful transmissions decreases. In areas where few people are capable of developing a viremia, possibly as a result of previous infection or immunization, the rate of transmission decreases (Figure 18.2).

Some individuals may actually escape infection because their contacts and the contacts of vectors are only with immune individuals. This type of protection is called *herd immunity.* The interrelationships between individuals with different levels of immunity and vectors with different thresholds of susceptibility and

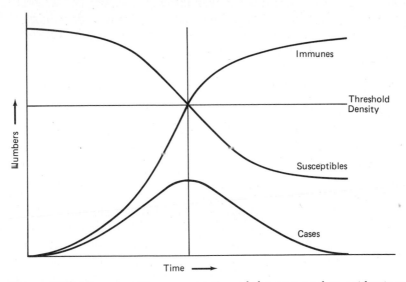

Figure 18.2 Diagrammatic representation of the course of an epidemic wave in terms of numbers of cases, numbers of susceptibles, and numbers of immunes. As the epidemic proceeds the number of susceptibles decreases and the number of immunes increases. The peak of the epidemic wave occurs at the threshold density of susceptibles.

periods of longevity are major factors determining the spread of the infection. Epidemiologists must study these factors during outbreaks and epidemics if they are to develop effective control plans. Control activities depend on identification of the vectors responsible for transmission and of the alternate hosts serving as reservoirs of infection. Efforts to interrupt transmission may be made either by vector control or through the use of vaccines. Vaccines may act by preventing humans or animals from supporting viral development, and thereby preventing infection of blood-feeding vectors.

Vector-borne Protozoal Diseases

In the world at large, the vector-borne protozoal disease of most importance to humans is malaria. This disease no longer occurs in the United States. In some areas of the United States, such as the New England coast, babesiosis of humans is a concern, but it is rare. Babesiosis of wild and domestic animals such as mice, dogs, horses, and cattle occurs in the United States and is the source of the human infection. Malaria annually infects hundreds of millions of people in Asia, Africa, and the Americas. Malaria in humans is transmitted by mosquitoes of the genus *Anopheles* and is caused by four different but related agents: *Plasmodium falciparum, Plasmodium vivax, Plasmodium malariae*, and *Plasmodium ovale.* All four of these protozoa have the same basic epidemiology. Humans are the obligate and essentially the only host for the four species that infect them. There are a large number of species of *Plasmodium* that infect birds, reptiles, and mammals other than humans, but most are highly specific in their host preference. Only a few of the Plasmodia of monkeys can infect humans.

When the mosquitoes feed on the host during certain periods of the infection, sexual stages of the parasites are taken into the mosquito gut, where the sporogenic, or sexual, cycle begins (Figure 18.3). After a period of development lasting from 7 to 15 or more days depending on the temperature, stages of the parasite infective to humans develop and migrate to the salivary glands, from which they are injected when the mosquito takes its next blood meal. Infected mosquitoes remain capable of transmitting the infection as long as they live. Like virus-infected mosquitoes, mosquitoes infected with Plasmodia vary in their ability to transmit the parasite. The ability to transmit depends on the susceptibility of the vector, the number of infective stages present in the blood of the host at the time of the initial feeding, and the longevity of the vector. If the mosquito dies before completion of the developmental cycle, the agent cannot be transmitted and no disease will be produced.

Public health measures to control or eliminate malaria depend on a thorough knowledge of the local environment, including the climatic and social conditions. In areas where environmental conditions are ideal for survival of the agent, such as West Africa, all individuals in the population may be continuously infected. Treatment with drugs, water management, widespread use of insecticides, screening of homes, and use of bed nets all contribute to making transmission difficult. In areas where the environmental and climatic conditions for malaria are less than ideal and where people have been in a position to use those means, widespread

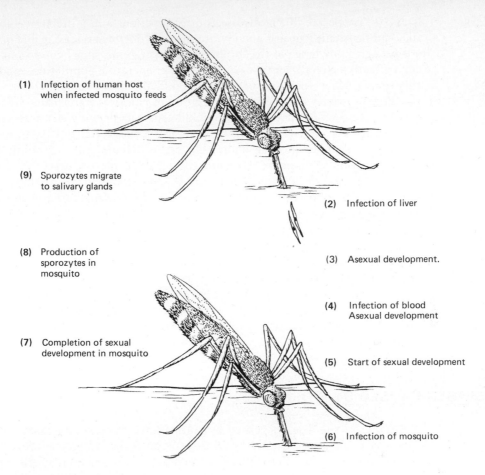

(1) Infection of human host when infected mosquito feeds

(9) Sporozytes migrate to salivary glands

(2) Infection of liver

(8) Production of sporozytes in mosquito

(3) Asexual development.

(4) Infection of blood Asexual development

(7) Completion of sexual development in mosquito

(5) Start of sexual development

(6) Infection of mosquito

Figure 18.3 The mosquito is the vector of malaria. It injects sporozoites when feeding (1). The sporozoites enter the liver (2) where they develop asexually into meronts (3). The merozoites which develop in the meront in the liver invade red blood cells (4) where they develop asexually. some of the merozoites become gametocytes (5) capable of infecting mosquitoes (6) in which sexual development is completed (7). When the sporozoites produced (8). Migrate to the salivary glands (9) the mosquito becomes infective. Infection may be controlled by reducing the mosquito population, by reducing contact between humans and mosquitoes, and by treatment of humans to prevent infection of mosquitoes. As human malaria has essentially no nonhuman reservoirs other than mosquitoes, control measures are directed to mosquitoes and humans.

reduction in mortality and morbidity has occurred. In most of Europe and North America, for example, this disease has been eliminated by the use of public health measures and environmental sanitation. However, in areas where the population will not or cannot cooperate, or where there are no good health services and no good treatment delivery systems, the disease continues to thrive.

To control any infectious disease one must have an informed population which is able to cooperate in the disease control programs and an effective government that can maintain a health and environmental control service capable of obtaining a thorough knowledge of the local environmental and social conditions. Without such effective governmental agencies and a cooperative population, eradication of this or any other vector-borne disease is difficult if not impossible.

Trypanosomes are another major group of parasites transmitted by insect vectors. Trypanosome-caused diseases include African sleeping sickness, transmitted by the tsetse fly and, in South America, Chagas' disease, transmitted by kissing bugs (Figure 18.4). Like the Plasmodia that cause malaria, the infectious organisms causing trypanosomiasis are taken into the vector as it feeds. After they are ingested there is a period of development before the vector is capable of transmitting the trypanosomes to another susceptible host. In this as with other vector-borne diseases, the vectors must take a number of blood meals over a period of time if they are to be effective in transmitting the disease agent. If the vector takes only three or four blood meals in its lifetime, it is apparent that the infective blood meal must be its first or second if more than one subsequent feeding is needed to transmit the agent. During epidemics, or in areas where there are very high infection rates, the chances of the vector being infected by the first blood meal are great. This contributes to the maintenance of the high level of endemicity. Only when natural immunity or medical intervention reduces the rate of vector infection can the level of infection decrease.

DISEASES CAUSED BY WORMS

A number of the diseases caused by worms have more complicated transmission cycles than do those caused by viruses or protozoa. Complex life cycles make epidemiologic studies more difficult and control measures more challenging. Schis-

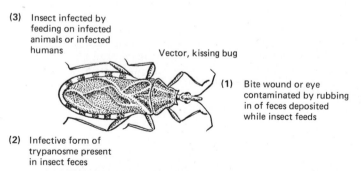

(3) Insect infected by feeding on infected animals or infected humans

Vector, kissing bug

(1) Bite wound or eye contaminated by rubbing in of feces deposited while insect feeds

(2) Infective form of trypanosme present in insect feces

Figure 18.4 Infection by Chagas' disease–causing trypanosomes occurs by contamination of a bite wound with the vector's feces or by contamination of eye with the contaminated insect feces (1). As the vector insect feeds on man or other animals control measures require prevention of human–insect contact. As a major reservoir of the parasite is present in animals other than man, treatment of human cases may have little effect on the maintenance of the infection.

tosomiasis is a major debilitating disease of the topical areas of Africa, Asia, and parts of the Americas. It is caused by a flatworm. In this case, infected humans pass the worm's eggs in their urine and feces. If these eggs enter water that contains susceptible species of snails, the snails may become infected. There then follows a cycle of development in this secondary, or alternate, host. The snail sheds infective stages that invade humans who work or bathe in the contaminated water (Figure 18.5).

Guinea worm disease also has a complicated life cycle. Infected humans shed the eggs of the parasite when they enter water. The parasites invade copepods that live in the water. After an obligate cycle in the copepod, stages infective to humans are produced and invade humans who drink the copepod-contaminated water.

To control these diseases, public health measures to eliminate the alternate hosts from the area and to prevent the introduction of the eggs into the water are required. Filtration of drinking water to remove copepods is itself an effective control measure for Guinea worm disease. Chemotherapeutic treatment to reduce the incidence of infection of people and to prevent the production of the forms infective to the alternate host supplement water sanitation efforts.

EPIDEMIOLOGY

Epidemiology is concerned with (1) how diseases are transmitted to individuals within populations and between populations, (2) when transmission is most likely to occur, and (3) where the diseases and the causative agents occur during both low and high transmission periods. Epidemiologists study the effects of partial and complete susceptibility on transmission of disease agents. They determine how epidemics spread through populations of susceptible and resistant individuals and

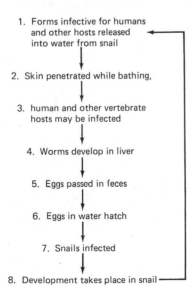

1. Forms infective for humans and other hosts released into water from snail

2. Skin penetrated while bathing,

3. human and other vertebrate hosts may be infected

4. Worms develop in liver

5. Eggs passed in feces

6. Eggs in water hatch

7. Snails infected

8. Development takes place in snail

Figure 18.5 Infective forms of the *Schistoma mansoni* that are released into water from infected snails (1) penetrate the skin (2). There may be nonhuman reservoirs of infection (3) in some regions. The worms develop in the liver (4). The eggs leave the liver by way of venules. From the venules the eggs reach the intestine. They are passed from the intestine with feces (5). In water the eggs hatch (6) releasing stages infective for snails (7). After development in the snail, stages infective for man are released (1). Those penetrate the skin of people bathing in the contaminated water. Control depends on preventing fecal contamination of water, eradication of snails, preventing bathing in contaminated water, and treatment of infected humans.

which factors govern the development and diminution of outbreaks. Epidemiologists may also study nontransmissible diseases to determine environmental and other factors responsible for their occurrence.

An environment favorable to the parasites is essential if the parasite is to multiply and spread. Many parasites survive desiccation, freezing, and, in some cases, extremes of heat. Many can survive long periods of dormancy. In order to cause disease, however, the parasite must be able to survive long enough to infect a suitable new host, must enter or attach to the host, and must there encounter an environment favorable to its growth and multiplication. Epidemiologists must determine which factors govern the survival of the parasite in the environment and determine how and when they move into and among the human or animal population. Climatic and geographic factors as well as behavior are major factors governing the spread of a parasite among individuals and populations.

Mortality and morbidity are two basic measures of the effects of disease-causing organisms on populations. Death is recorded as mortality, the most severe result of a disease. Mortality is often considered the easiest measurement to obtain in well-organized societies, and mortality rates are used to measure the impact of epidemics. However, in many instances it is very difficult to determine the specific cause of death in an individual. In urban areas of the tropics, mortality data for populations of various age groups can often be obtained. However, determination of the number of deaths due to a specific disease, such as measles, may be very difficult to determine since individuals may, in fact, also have malaria, filariasis, diarrhea, pneumonia, or other diseases. Death may thus be the result of a combination of infections, and the particular contribution of any one of them may be hard to estimate. Often mortality rates caused by a particular disease can be determined following introduction of medical programs; for example, an immunization program against a specific childhood disease or an intensive drug-treatment program with a drug specific for a particular disease. In this instance, the reduction in mortality that may result may give a true indication of the contribution of a particular disease or disease agent to the observed mortality.

Similarly, morbidity can be determined by measurement of a number of different parameters including fever, physical pain and discomfort, long-lasting physical impairment, loss of work time, incidence of abortion or sterility, and so on. Often data derived from a variety of observations must be used to determine the contribution of a disease agent to the morbidity within the population.

There are two basic measurements of the presence, severity, and impact of a given disease upon a population of people or animals. These are the *prevalence rate* and the *incidence rate.* These rates are based upon the presence of characteristic symptoms or upon the identification of the disease-causing agents themselves. The *prevalence rate* is the number of cases of a disease at a specified period of time in a particular population. It is one of the most often used statistics. It is based upon surveys or case reports of the numbers of individuals either sick or showing signs of infection, or upon the number of actual isolations and diagnoses of specific agents. This statistic is normally expressed as the number of cases per 1000 or 100,000 population. A *point prevalence rate* is the rate of infection or disease at a particular time (such as on one day or during one week) and is usually obtained from an intensive survey. A *period prevalence rate* is the rate of disease or infection over a longer time period, such as one year. By these statistics, the number of people having a particular disease during a particular time may be determined. One may find, for example, that 500 per 100,000 people in a large city or district had influenza during a particular week, or that during the year, 2500 per 100,000 people had influenza. These numbers do not indicate change from previous time periods nor do they indicate rate of change of incidence of infection within a specified time period.

Many different signs of infection may be measured to determine the prevalence rate; fever is commonly used as an indication of malaria, influenza, and various viral and bacterial infections. Actual diagnosis based on clinical signs is used to determine prevalence rates of measles, mumps, parasitic infections, and certain bacterial and mycotic infections. Clinical diagnosis may be based on physical evidence such as blindness, leprotic lesions, or elephantiasis. Serologic studies are often made on serum samples collected during point prevalence surveys and contribute data on the level of experience and degree of immunity of a population to a particular disease-causing agent.

The *incidence rate* is the number of new cases of a disease that occur in a particular population within a certain time period, divided by the number of people who may be exposed to infection during the same time period. This rate is usually expressed per 1000 or 100,000 persons or animals per year. It is possible to predict the number of expected infections with such diseases as influenza or syphilis if one has a great deal of data from previous years on the same or similar populations.

Seroepidemiology has become an important tool for the measurement of both prevalence and incidence rates within populations. A number of types of serologic tests have been developed that measure the recent or past experience of individuals with specific organisms. These tests are based on the presence of antibodies to the agents in the individual's serum. When a serological survey is to be made, the usual procedure is to collect sera from a statistically significant sample of individuals representing the different age or exposure groups in the population. The sera are examined for the presence of antibodies to the specific agent of interest and, possibly, to a number of related organisms.

Many different serological tests have been developed, including tests based on complement fixation, haemagglutination inhibition, and fluorescent-labeled antibody binding. Tests based on radiolabeled and enzyme labeled antibody binding are also widely used. With these tests, the numbers of individuals with antibodies to particular parasites can be determined. By determining the amount of antibody present, it is possible to estimate whether there has been recent exposure or repeated infection.

In areas of endemic infection there will usually be a higher number of older individuals who test positive than of younger ones. If one has test samples for the same individual taken at about one-week intervals, then the changes in titer will give much information. A higher titer in the second sample indicates current infection; a lower titer, recovery. A steady low titer indicates an old experience. The titers will usually be higher in the adults because of the effect of repeated exposure to the agent. To determine prevalence rates by serologic means, specific individuals are identified and repeatedly sampled over one or two years. The rates of infection over long periods of time can be calculated based on the assumptions that antibody responses only occur in response to infection and antibody titers are only boosted in response to reinfection or reexposure. Using this system, seasonal year-to-year rates can be determined just by examination of sera from a statistically valid sample of identified individuals in the population.

Point prevalence studies using serologic tests can determine the presence of a disease-causing agent in a population and the percentages of the various age or risk groups exposed. Incidence data may be obtained by periodic sampling. Usually, serologic studies are much easier to perform than are studies based on other diagnostic procedures.

An additional advantage of serologic studies is that centrally based laboratories can perform large numbers of tests on samples from different geographic areas using standardized reagents and procedures. This allows the epidemiologist to obtain a broad knowledge of increases or decreases in disease incidence and makes it possible for him to predict spread of disease on an almost worldwide basis. Diseases such as influenza may move around the globe within a few years and serologic studies can determine the relative risk to unexposed populations of new variants of the virus.

Serologic tests are a major tool in the planning of programs for intervention to stem the spread of many diseases. Serologic tests for antibodies to hepatitis or human immunodeficiency viruses on blood supplies, for example, provide data useful in preventing the spread of these agents through blood transfusions.

The simplest epidemiologic situation that presents itself for analysis is the introduction of a new disease-causing agent into a totally susceptible population. For example, a new strain of influenza may develop to which all people under a certain age are susceptible since they have never been exposed to this or a related variant of the virus nor have they been immunized against it. Another example of such simple epidemiologic situations occurs with cholera; there may be an interval of many years between outbreaks, thus allowing time for development of a large pool of totally susceptible individuals. Normally, however, the epidemiologic situation is complicated because many individuals within a population have some level of immunity against either infection by most agents or the development of the diseases they cause. When resistance is relatively low and there are many susceptible individuals, the disease may spread rapidly within the population. When the rate of immunity is relatively high through previous infection or immunization and there are thus few susceptible persons, transmission may be rare. Widespread usage of antibiotics and similar medications and the existence of social practices that prevent infection also reduce the likelihood of infection. Under such conditions, a disease-causing agent with a relatively complicated transmission cycle or with strict requirements for multiplication and survival will have a very difficult time causing infection when the level of immunity is only moderate. Even when major pandemics of disease occur with such agents, some individuals may escape infection merely because they are surrounded by those who had been infected previously and who are therefore now immune.

Epidemiologists must take into account many factors in planning control of disease outbreaks. Information about many of these factors is difficult to obtain or unavailable without great effort. In practice, the most easily obtained information is usually used rather than the most complete and best information.

Regardless of the agent or the transmission cycle, epidemiologists who wish to develop a disease control program for a given disease must determine what agents are involved, when they are infectious, how they are propagated within a population, and how they are maintained during periods of latency if they wish to develop a program that will work. In short, they must understand the life cycle of the parasite in order to control it. Once the life cycle is understood, then the drugs, vaccines, and vector control measures available must be assembled. To work, a program must be acceptable to the people concerned and must be within their social and economic capabilities. It is the mission of epidemiologists to determine the most logical, practical, and economical approach to reduce the mortality and morbidity of the diseases or group of diseases that plague the population with which they are working.

SUGGESTIONS FOR FURTHER READING

R. H. Fletcher, S. W. Fletcher, and E. H. Wagner. *Clinical Epidemiology: The Essentials.* Williams & Wilkins, Baltimore, 1982.

A. M. Lilienfeld and D. E. Lilienfeld. *Foundations of Epidemiology,* 2nd edition. Oxford University Press, London, 1980.

G. L. Mandell, R. G. Douglas, Jr., and J. E. Bennett. *Principles and Practice of Infectious Diseases,* 2nd edition. John Wiley, New York, 1985.

J. M. May. *The Ecology of Human Disease.* MD Publications, New York, 1958.

K. J. Rothman. *Modern Epidemiology.* Little, Brown, Boston, 1986.

Chapter 19

The Immunological System and Neoplasia

JAMES R. BLAKESLEE, JR.

Department of Veterinary Pathobiology
College of Veterinary Medicine
The Ohio State University

INTRODUCTION

Cell-mediated immunity based upon the actions of thymus-dependent lymphocytes plays a major role in defense against infection with fungi, protozoa, mycobacteria, and viruses. Thymic lymphocytes and other leukocyte populations also function in killing of tumor cells. Natural killer cells function alone, whereas K-cells function with the aid of specific antibodies directed toward surface antigens on the tumors. Non–T-, non–B-cells (Null) that are devoid of normal T- or B-cell surface antigens also lyse tumor cells directly or with the aid of antibody coating. The killing of tumor cells by antibody-dependent cellular cytotoxicity mechanisms is particularly prominent in elimination of virus-induced tumors.

The elimination of tumors by the cell-based systems of defense can be considered to be a form of rejection of foreign tissue; such rejections are a manifestation of the inducible or adaptive immune response.

Specific immunization against tumors was a popular idea at the end of the nineteenth and the beginning of the twentieth centuries. The belief was that if one could immunize an individual against parasites foreign to a host, one should also be able to immunize against a tumor, which is also foreign to the host. In 1895, two French scientists, Richet and Hericourt, inoculated a donkey and two dogs with cells from a human osteosarcoma and tested the sera from these animals in human patients with the same types of tumors. There was some evidence of improvement in some of the treated patients, but no cures occurred.

Other investigators at about the same time made the discovery that certain mammalian tumors could be transplanted from one animal to another. Some of the animals that received tumor fragments either failed to develop a tumor or showed spontaneous regression of the tumor after it had grown for a period of time. It was not until Little and Tyzzer in 1916 established the basic principles of tissue transplantation genetics that it was realized that the immunological responses reported from studies with random-bred animals were directed primarily against normal transplantation antigens present both in the tumors and in normal tissues. After this time it was realized that only studies on homozygous inbred strains of animals could distinguish between antigenic differences in tumor and normal host tissue.

EXPERIMENTAL TUMOR IMMUNOLOGY

Chemically Induced Tumors

The development of inbred mice, in which all mice of a strain are genetically identical, permitted studies of chemically induced tumors in mice. When tumor cells induced by 3-methyl-cholanthrene were injected into C3H mice, for example, the tumor cells grew and then regressed after a period of time. When these same mice were reinjected with the same tumor cells, either no growth or temporary growth followed by rapid regression of the tumors occurred; all the nonimmunized control mice behaved like the original group of mice. These findings were not fully accepted because it was believed that the induced tumor line had mutated during passage in the mice. However, it was finally accepted that the induced tumors contained antigens not present in the normal mouse and, furthermore, that each induced tumor was immunologically distinct. Other researchers showed that allogeneic inhibition, which is based on differences between donor and recipient mice, played no role in establishing immunity to tumor challenge in inbred mice injected with irradiated methyl-cholanthrene–induced autochthonous tumor cells. Thus, it was established that chemically induced tumors contained new or neoantigens on their surfaces that were responsible for immunity to the tumors. These neoantigens are called *tumor-specific antigens (TSA)*.

Oncogenic DNA Viruses

Polyoma virus (*poly,* meaning "many" and *oma,* "tumors") is capable of inducing various types of tumors when inoculated into newborn mice, hamsters, rats, or rabbits. The virus is a double-stranded DNA virus and, as with most oncogenic DNA viruses, DNA virus–induced tumors only arise in cells that are nonpermissive for virus replication and do not shed virus. This situation is distinct from that of the oncogenic RNA retroviruses that induce leukemias and sarcomas in cells that are permissive for virus replication and shed infectious virus when transformed.

Early studies with oncogenic polyoma virus–induced tumors demonstrated the existence of virally induced tumor-specific antigens and provided information on their role in tumor immunity. Adult hamsters with antibodies to polyoma virus do not develop tumors after injection of polyoma-transformed cells. The resistance to challenge with tumor cells is relative and can be overcome by injection of large numbers of the tumor cells. The immunity is specific as inoculation of inactivated virus induced immunity to challenge with isologous polyoma-induced tumor cells but not to tumors induced by other viral or chemical agents (Figure 19.1). The tumor-specific antigens in tumors induced by a given polyoma virus are identical regardless of the species of host in which they are induced and therefore are coded for by the polyoma virus. The tumor-specific antigens are different from the structural proteins of the virus, however, and thus represent virally induced proteins that play a role in the development of the virus but do not become incorporated into it.

It is clear that different mechanisms are involved in chemically induced than in virally induced cancers. In chemical induction, the cellular DNA is modified; whereas in the case of viral induction, exogenous DNA is integrated into the host cell, where it may be transcribed and translated.

Oncogenic RNA Viruses and Oncogenes

As noted in Chapter 14, the family of viruses known as the *Retroviridae* are RNA-containing viruses that are unique in that their RNA is transcribed "backward" (*retro* is the Latin word meaning "backward") into DNA through a unique enzyme, reverse transcriptase, an RNA-dependent–DNA polymerase. The retroviruses are found in individuals of a large number of vertebrate species and induce many types of tumors that can serve as models for many human cancers. Some retroviruses have a "transforming" gene and others do not. Those with a

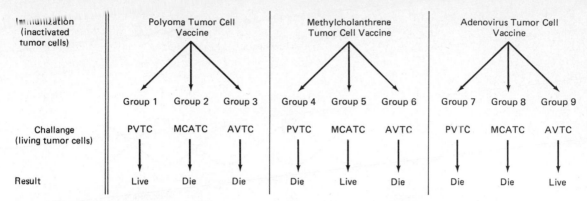

Figure 19.1 The specificity of tumor-associated antigens. Mice were immunized with inactivated polyoma virus–transformed cells, methylcholanthrene-induced tumor cells or adenovirus-induced tumor cells. The mice were challenged with living polyoma virus–transformed cells (PVTC), methylcholanthrene-induced tumor cells (MCATC), or adenovirus-transformed cells (AVTC). Only mice immunized with the tumor cells homologous to the tumor used for challenge were resistant; heterologous immunization did not protect from challenge.

transforming gene transform cells *in vitro* or induce tumors very quickly *in vivo.* These transforming genes have been given the collective name *oncogenes.* Those viruses without an oncogene do not transform cells *in vitro.* In either case, the viral genome persists in the cell after infection.

The oncogene hypothesis was proposed in the mid-1960s by Huebner and Todaro of the National Cancer Institute to explain the induction of cancers by agents such as viruses, chemicals, and radiation. They hypothesized that retroviral oncogenes were part of the genetic makeup of normal cells. They postulated that these genes had been acquired through a viral infection early in the evolution of the species. They postulated further that as long as these genes were not activated, normal growth ensued, but if stimulated, the gene products converted the cell to a transformed cell.

Oncogenes have indeed been found in many cells. It has been shown through very elegant studies, however, that cellular oncogenes are not a result of virus infection but that the viral oncogenes were obtained by the viruses from the cell. In order to distinguish viral from cell oncogene types, distinct names were required. The cellular oncogenes are therefore called *protooncogenes* (*proto* is the Greek word meaning "first") and the viral oncogenes retained the name oncogenes. The fact that the protooncogenes had survived through the cells' evolution suggested that they had something to do with the cells' normal function and well being. Thirty or more of these protooncogenes have been identified, and most are active in normal cells. Thus, the induction of neoplastic growth by protooncogenes requires something to upset the normal cells' genetic function. The cancer-gene concept and several scenarios of cancer induction are outlined in Figure 19.2. In a scenario involving mutagens or other nonretroviral agents, it is proposed that the

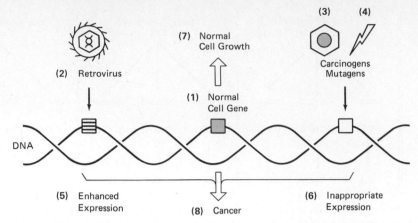

Figure 19.2 One unifying concept of the causation of cancer proposes that cancer results when a (1) normal cellular gene is modified by any one of a variety of potentially carcinogenic agents such as (2) viruses, (3) chemicals, or (4) radiation. Such agents may cause (5) enhanced or (6) inappropriate expression of the gene causing, instead of (7) normal growth, (8) a cancer.

agents mutagenize or otherwise affect the regulation of the protooncogene, permitting inappropriate expression. Retroviruses, on the other hand, may provide an oncogene that may integrate into the host cell DNA and there cause overproduction of a regulatory protein. In both scenarios, overproduction of a regulatory substance occurs, leading to cancerous growth.

IMMUNOSURVEILLANCE

Some oncologists believe that there is immune surveillance of neoplastic processes that results in natural resistance to tumor cells. The immunosurveillance hypothesis proposes that new tumor cells constantly arise but are destroyed by the immune system. When immunity fails, the normally arising tumor cells are not recognized and destroyed. If this view is correct, the problem is not just the induction of cancers, but the failure of the host to control them. The immune system can be compromised due to age, inborn genetic defects, by stress, by infection, or by drugs. An inverse relationship has been shown between the efficiency of the immune system and the development of some tumors. The immune system loses efficiency with increasing age, and with aging there is a concomitant increase in the incidence of malignant disease. Individuals with some genetic defects in the immune system, particularly defects in T-cell and thymus development and function, also have an increased incidence of some cancers, for example cancers of the type called *lymphoreticular neoplasias.* Studies have also shown that individuals treated with immunosuppressive drugs so that they will accept organ transplants have a higher than normal incidence of malignant disease.

One of the major reasons for not accepting the immune surveillance concept is the observation that athymic mice and rats, or mice and rats thymectomized at birth, do not have an increased susceptibility to chemically induced or "spontaneous" tumors. This suggests that the concept that tumor cells arise constantly may not be correct. It is more probable that neoplastic change occurs once or several times in a lifetime. It is probable that many of the tumor cells that do arise and survive to grow may be weakly immunogenic or nonimmunogenic and thus fail to elicit an effective immune response. Some lymphoid tumors even produce lymphokines that disrupt the immune response by stimulating cell sets that are inappropriate for cell killing.

In vivo passaged tumor cells of lines that have a relatively dense concentration of tumor-specific antigens, such as the RNA virus-induced tumors, elicit stronger immune responses than do tumor cells of lines with less dense tumor-antigen concentrations, such as those that are chemically induced or induced by oncogenic DNA viruses. It has been suggested that during animal passage the tumor cells with high concentrations of tumor-specific antigens are eliminated from the lines, leaving the weakly immunogenic cells. Thus selection during passage may produce tumors that are weakly immunogenic and thereby avoid immune elimination.

Some tumors may survive because they grow so rapidly that they outstrip the host's ability to mount an immunological attack. Other tumors may elicit "blocking" antibodies that prevent cytotoxic killing. Antibodies that do not fix complement may prevent binding of antibodies that do, thus preventing complement-mediated lysis of the cell. Both tumor-bearing rodents and humans are usually immunosuppressed and are thus anergic (*an,* meaning "negative," plus the Greek *ergon,* or "work"). Such hosts fail to respond to tumor antigens even if they are present in large amounts.

ACQUIRED IMMUNITY TO CANCER: FELINE LEUKEMIA

Until recently, the immunosuppressed state had been viewed in terms of its contribution to tumor cell survival rather than being considered a disease entity in itself. The recent discovery of the retroviral etiology of human acquired immunodeficiency syndrome (AIDS) has stimulated reexamination of the pathogenesis of all of the animal retroviral diseases for information that may be useful for developing programs for prevention and treatment of this devastating disease. Feline leukemia is a disease caused by a retrovirus. It, like the AIDS virus, is a horizontally transmitted exogenous retrovirus. Furthermore, feline leukemia is the first mammalian cancer for which a vaccine has been developed and is now licensed by the federal government and marketed by a commercial firm.

Feline Leukemia Virus

Feline leukemia virus (FeLV) was first described by Jarrett and his colleagues in 1964. Unfortunately it was named, as was the custom with retroviruses, after the leukemia that is only one of the diseases it causes. Leukemia is probably the least frequent result of infection with this virus. Much more prevalent are the nonneoplastic diseases caused by the virus, which include nonregenerative anemia, thymic atrophy, hemolytic anemia, glomerulonephritis, and a panleukopenialike disease.

Cats infected with feline leukemia virus may present a complex clinical picture, with one or more diseases present. Immunosuppression accompanies virtually all feline leukemia virus infections, rendering the infected cat susceptible to many opportunistic pathogenic agents. The hallmark of infection with the virus, which perhaps could more appropriately be called "feline AIDS," is the unusual number of secondary viral, bacterial, and parasitic infections that occur associated with the viremic state. Association of feline leukemia virus infection with disease caused by opportunistic pathogens is strong evidence that the virus causes immunodeficiency.

The first objective evidence that the virus causes immunosuppression was the demonstration that allograft rejection is very slow in infected cats. Infected cats lose their ability to reject skin grafts at the same time that they develop severe thymic atrophy and paracortical lymphoid depletion.

As previously mentioned, the virus is transmitted directly from cat to cat under natural conditions. Infection occurs predominantly by contact of uninfected cats with salivary and nasal secretions of cats with persistent infections. Because these viruses are readily inactivated in the environment, transfer requires direct cat-to-cat contact, contact through common feeding and watering dishes, or contact with a person who has recently handled an infected cat. Within six weeks after infection, an infected cat will either develop a persistent or a self-limiting infection. A persistent infection is characterized by a persistent viremia. Viral structural proteins can be detected in blood from infected cats by an indirect immunofluorescent antibody (IFA) test. The virus is in neutrophils and platelets. Persistently infected cats usually produce no or very little virus-neutralizing antibody. Viremia may persist for months or years, and the cat eventually dies from an intercurrent disease. The majority of cats exposed to feline leukemia virus develop a self-limiting infection. These cats develop neutralizing antibodies, do not shed virus in body fluids, and do not develop any associated disease. In some cases cats will develop a transient viremia with high antivirus antibody titers that may last from days to weeks.

Structure of Feline Leukemia Virus

All retroviruses have common features. All of them are similar in size and morphology, all have reverse transcriptase, and are released from internal and external plasma cell membranes during active infection by a process called *budding*. During infection, viral gene translation products accumulate just under the cell membrane. Through a series of biochemical steps that include cleavage of precursor molecules and reassociation, mature complete virus particles are budded through the cell membrane in association with "unused" virus components and cellular molecules. The structural proteins of FeLV and their location are summarized in Table 19.1.

Vaccination against Feline Leukemia

The early vaccines were made from "killed" virus or were attenuated virus vaccines. They were patterned after successful vaccines against diseases produced by nononcogenic viruses. In addition, vaccines that consisted of cells induced by the virus were developed.

Table 19.1 STRUCTURAL PROTEINS
OF FELINE LEUKEMIA
VIRUS AND THEIR
LOCATIONS

Location in virus	Protein component
Envelope	gp 70[a]
	p15E
	p12
	p12E
Core	p30
	p15C
RNP[b]	p10
	p85

[a]gp = glycoprotein; p = protein; molecular weight × 1000 (e.g., gp70 is a 70,000-dalton glycoprotein); E = envelope; and C = core.

[b]RNP = Ribonuclear protein.

Those naturally infected cats that develop immunity to feline leukemia virus are immune for life. The immune response is mediated by antibodies to both the virus and to virus-induced materials not incorporated into the virus particle. Most likely cell-mediated immunity also develops that is directed against virus-infected cells, but if it does, its existence has not been proven. Neutralizing antibodies for the virus are present in the colostrum of mothers of newborn kittens and protect the kittens that ingest it. Neutralizing antibodies administered passively also protect. Successful vaccines induce antibody that neutralizes the virus at the time of exposure.

As mentioned previously, the early vaccines consisted of inactivated or live attenuated virus. The inactivated virus vaccines induced sufficient neutralizing antibody in adult cats to prevent infection but failed to protect kittens and did not prevent tumor development in them. Kittens vaccinated with killed virus vaccines were actually more susceptible to infection than were nonimmunized kittens. The significance of this observation was not understood until it was shown that a component of the virus—the 15,000-dalton envelope protein (p15E)—was immunosuppressive in kittens.

As various of the early attenuated virus vaccines were shown to be effective in preventing persistent infections in adult cats but caused disease in kittens, a search for a vaccine composed of purified virus components (a subunit vaccine) was undertaken. The early subunit vaccines were not effective in inducing protective immunity; a subunit vaccine prepared from purified pg70 envelope glycoprotein, for example, failed to elicit immunity.

In an attempt to elicit immunity, four-month-old kittens were injected with cells of a virus-transformed lymphoid cell line designated FL-74. The tumor cell vaccine induced good virus-neutralizing antibody titers and antibodies that reacted with tumors; however, the vaccine was pathogenic for young kittens. A killed tumor cell vaccine elicited an antitumor response but did not inhibit the development of persistent viremia. The addition of killed virus to the tumor cell preparation did not improve it. Cats given this preparation developed tumors or other signs of infection and died.

An analysis of virus development in the FL-74 cell line revealed that the various FeLV components appeared at different times in the virus replication cycle. These antigens, which are released into the medium, were collected and tested for immunogenicity. They were found to elicit a good immune response against both the tumor cell antigens and virus structural proteins. More than 80 percent of the cats vaccinated with these preparations were protected against challenge. They developed neither persistent viremia nor tumors when challenged with virulent virus.

Vaccine made from the virus material secreted by the FL-74 cell line is safe and effective in protecting cats against feline leukemia virus–induced disease.

Nature of the Vaccine Yielding Protection against Feline Leukemia

The immunogenic components of the vaccine that were shed from the FL-74 cell line were shed as individual components and not as a part of the intact virus particle. These components of the vaccine were conformationally different from similar proteins incorporated into the virus itself. Vaccinated cats responded to the material in the culture fluid sooner and developed higher antibody titers than did cats given equivalent amounts of whole virus. The protein in the culture fluid was different from that in the virus particles as it was not immunosuppressive. The difference in immunogenicity between the intact virus and the secreted components that are not incorporated into the virion is probably related to the conformational and other changes that viral proteins undergo during incorporation into the virus.

MAREK'S DISEASE

Marek's disease is a leukemia of chickens induced by a herpesvirus. The infection is characterized by loss of nerve insulation (demyelination) and the development of tumors in visceral organs, muscles, and skin. It is an extremely common neoplastic condition that probably occurs in all poultry-producing countries. In 1970 the first vaccine for Marek's disease was introduced, and the monetary effects four years later were striking: The estimated benefits from reduced bird and egg losses in the United States alone were $168.5 million. A conservative estimate of the total cost of Marek's disease worldwide before introduction of the vaccine was $943 million.

Types of Marek's Disease

There are two major recognized forms of Marek's disease: acute and classical. The acute form affects young birds from one to two months of age, whereas in the classical form, birds are usually from three to five months of age when they develop disease. In the acute form, one finds high tumor incidence along with atrophy of the thymus and the Bursa of Fabricius. There is also liver and spleen involvement and high mortality. Birds may have respiratory problems due to tumor infiltration of the lungs. The classical form has low mortality, with the major symptoms being paralysis of the wings and legs. The paralysis is caused by infiltration of the nerves with neoplastic and inflammatory cells. As a result of the infiltration, there is enlargement of peripheral nerves. In both forms, the tumors are lymphomas that are found in most organs. In addition, lymphomas are sometimes found in the skin around the feather follicles.

Marek's Disease Virus

Marek's disease virus is a typical herpesvirus. It has icosahedral symmetry and is enveloped. The envelope is loose and contains spikes. The herpesviruses contain double-stranded DNA. There are at least three envelope glycoproteins of molecular weights from 50,000 daltons to 115,000 daltons and at least four major capsid proteins of from 30,000 daltons to 140,000 daltons in Marek's disease virus. These proteins are produced by host cells undergoing lytic infections. In some cases the virus does not lyse the cell but rather induces a latent infection in which a few copies of viral DNA are produced, but no virus proteins. If latently infected cells are removed from the host and cultured *in vitro*, synthesis of viral antigens and DNA occur. It is probable that expression of virus antigens and DNA *in vitro* is a result of the removal of the suppressive effect of the host's immune system. In addition to lytic and latent infection, a third type of infection called *transformation* may occur. Transformation may be a preneoplastic process. The tumor that may be produced is a lymphoma. It has been shown that part of the DNA from transformed cells is similar to DNA isolated from the virus. This suggests that the viral DNA in transformed cells is virtually intact and is either integrated into the host cell DNA or is carried within the cell cytoplasma as an episome. When lymphoma results from infection, Marek's disease virus components may be produced, as well as viral genome–programmed materials that are not incorporated into the virus. One of these materials is a tumor-associated surface antigen called *MATSA*. MATSA is also expressed on transformed cell lines that are not fully developed lymphomas. All strains of Marek's disease virus induce MATSA production in infected cells, including the nononcogenic strains.

After Marek's disease virus was isolated, an antigenically related herpesvirus was isolated from healthy turkeys (herpesvirus of turkeys). Strains of Marek's disease virus that did not produce disease were also found in chickens. Strains isolated from chickens can be divided into two distinct serological groups, with the turkey virus comprising a third group. Viruses of serotype 1 are all oncogenic, those of serotype 2 from chickens are nononcogenic, and the viruses from turkeys fall into serotype 3 and are also nononcogenic.

Resistance to Marek's Disease

The outcome of infection of chickens is dependent upon a number of factors including age, sex, passive immunity received from maternal sources through the yolk sac, the genetic makeup of the chicken, environmental factors, and virus strain. Young chickens are more susceptible than older birds, and females are more susceptible than are males. Passive immunity mediated by maternal antibody causes a delay in onset of disease, a reduction in death rates, and low levels of tumor formation. Environmental factors such as stresses brought on by manipulations that are a part of normal management, such as debeaking, vaccination for other diseases, and handling of birds, increase a chicken's susceptibility to Marek's disease.

Humoral Immunity to Marek's Disease

Following infection, antibodies of the IgG and IgM classes specific for the virus develop. The IgM antibodies develop before the IgG. Virus-neutralizing antibodies are present. The antibodies are specific for the free virus and have little effect on virus-infected cells.

Cell-mediated Immunity to Marek's Disease

Natural killer cells are active in effecting immunity to Marek's disease. Transfer of natural killer cells to chickens confers on them the ability to destroy tumor cells. Macrophages also have a role in immunity to Marek's disease. Macrophages from infected chickens restrict Marek's disease virus replication in cells *in vitro* and inhibit DNA synthesis and proliferation of lymphoma cells in the spleens of infected chickens. Growth of virus-infected cells is also inhibited by antibody-dependent cell-mediated cytotoxicity. Normal lymphocytes kill virus-infected cells in the presence of serum from Marek's disease virus–infected chickens under natural conditions of infection, but lymphocytes and serum are not active *in vitro* against cultured tumor cells.

Vaccination against Marek's Disease

Vaccines are prepared from attenuated oncogenic and nononcogenic strains of the virus. Vaccines have also been prepared from both living and killed tumor cells, from membranes of infected cells, and from extracts of various infected cell components. The most successful and widely used vaccine is simply a preparation containing the live herpesvirus of turkeys. The turkey virus is antigenically similar to Marek's disease virus but is not identical to it. Herpesvirus of turkeys spreads easily from turkey to turkey, its natural hosts, but it spreads poorly among chickens. As a result of poor spreading, every chicken in a flock must be vaccinated.

The turkey virus vaccine does not protect the birds against infection. One usually thinks of a vaccine as protecting against infection, but in this case, chickens vaccinated with turkey virus, if they come into contact with Marek's disease virus, become infected for life. They shed the virus and can be a source of infection to susceptible chickens. The value of the vaccine lies in its ability to prevent the diseases caused by infection with Marek's disease virus and, in particular, to prevent tumorigenesis. The vaccine induces immunity to tumor formation in bursectomized chickens but not in those that have been thymectomized. The antitumor immunity established by the turkey virus vaccine is thus probably T-lymphocyte mediated.

CONCLUSIONS

The control of cancer by establishment of immunity through vaccination has long been a goal of scientists working in cancer research. Feline leukemia in cats and Marek's disease in chickens are the first neoplastic diseases to be controlled through vaccines. A vaccine that protects squirrel monkeys against virus-induced lymphoma has also been developed. These vaccines are preventive, however, not curative. There is presently no vaccine effective in preventing neoplastic disease in humans. Success with these two vaccines holds out hope that immunological means of tumor control may be possible with at least some neoplastic diseases.

SUGGESTIONS FOR FURTHER READING

J. A. Bellanti. *Immunology, Vol. 3 .* W. B. Saunders, Philadelphia, 1985.

J. M. Bishop. "Cellular oncogenes and retroviruses." Ann. Rev. Biochem. *52:* 301, 1983.

W. Okazaki, H. Purchase, and B. Burmester. "Protection against Marek's disease by vaccination with a herpesvirus of turkeys." Avian Dis. *14:* 113, 1970.

R. G. Olsen, M. Lewis, J. Mastro, R. Sharpee, M. Tarr, and L. Mathes. Feline Retrovirus Vaccine. In *Leukemia: Recent Advances in Biology and Treatment, Vol. 28,* R. Gale and D. W. Golde, *eds.* Alan R. Liss, New York, 1985.

R. G. Olsen, *ed. Feline Leukemia.* CRC Press, Boca Raton, Florida, 1981.

L. M. Payne, *ed. Marek's Disease: Scientific Basis and Methods of Control.* Martinus Nijhoff, Boston, 1985.

H. G. Purchase. Clinical Disease and Its Economic Impact. In *Marek's Disease: Scientific Basis and Methods of Control,* L. M. Payne, *ed.* Martinus Nijhoff, Boston, 1985.

C. G. Wormser, R. E. Stahl, and E. J. Bottone, *eds. AIDS, Acquired Immune Deficiency Syndrome and Other Manifestations of HIV Infection: Epidemiology, Etiology, Immunology, Clinical Manifestations, Pathology, Control, and Prevention.* Noyes Publication, Park Ridge, New Jersey, 1987.

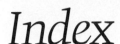

Index

Page numbers in italic type indicate references to illustrations. A *t* following a page number indicates a reference to a table.